OXFORD MEDICAL PUBLICATIONS

Neurodisability and Community Child Health

T0202124

Oxford Specialist Handbooks published and forthcoming

**Oxford Specialist Handbooks
in Paediatrics**

Neurodisability
and Community
Child Health

SECOND EDITION

EDITED BY

Srinivas Gada

Consultant Paediatrician in Neurodevelopment and
Neurodisability, Nuffield Health Oxford and HCA
Healthcare London
Honorary Senior Clinical Lecturer, University of Oxford
Honorary Consultant, Oxford University Hospitals NHS
Foundation Trust, Oxford, UK

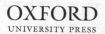

OXFORD
UNIVERSITY PRESS

OXFORD
UNIVERSITY PRESS

Great Clarendon Street, Oxford, OX2 6DP,
United Kingdom

Oxford University Press is a department of the University of Oxford.
It furthers the University's objective of excellence in research, scholarship,
and education by publishing worldwide. Oxford is a registered trade mark of
Oxford University Press in the UK and in certain other countries

First Edition published in 2012
Second Edition published in 2022

Impression: 1

Published in the United States of America by Oxford University Press
198 Madison Avenue, New York, NY 10016, United States of America

British Library Cataloguing in Publication Data
Data available

Library of Congress Control Number: 2021945282

ISBN 978–0–19–885191–2

DOI: 10.1093/med/9780198851912.001.0001

Printed in Great Britain by
Ashford Colour Press Ltd, Gosport, Hampshire

Dedication

I dedicate this book to my parents, Sulochana and Shankerappa, for their countless sacrifices for my education, and without whom I would not be here.

Foreword

It is a privilege to offer a foreword to this new Handbook for the ever-expanding field of neurodisability—what I like to call the field of 'Applied Child Development'.

As Dr. Gada rightly notes in his Preface, child-onset neurodisability and community child health has seen remarkable change and development in the past decade. Fundamental shifts—more accurately characterized as expansions in our thinking—have made the field almost unrecognizably richer than was ever imagined possible by those of us trained in twentieth-century thinking! Among the contributing forces in these developments one can cite, in no implied order of priority, the WHO's 2001 International Classification of Functioning, Health, and Disability (ICF) framework for health; the recognition that parents must be equal partners with professionals, and the importance of our engagement with them at every step of the journey; seeking and heeding the voices of children; seeing 'childhood' issues in a life-course perspective; and promoting the functioning and participation of young people with impairments who were traditionally assumed to be sentenced to lives of limited possibility.

This Handbook provides readers with accessible notes and guides to a myriad of topics, with detailed cross-linking of each section to many others. In this respect, the Handbook is a refreshing complement to the traditional textbook, with discursive writing on background, placing ideas in context with the history of the topic, detailed explanations, justifications, interpretations of the arguments, and so on. (Full disclosure, I have experience with such textbooks and believe they also have a place!)

What makes this current volume so useful is the immediacy of access to whatever the user seeks to know right now. As a Handbook, the focus is on the practical application of the available knowledge and ideas it offers. As noted, there are always links to other parts of the text where the reader can recognize the ways that concepts discussed in relation to a particular impairment or diagnosis almost always have wide-ranging 'non-categorical' relevance across the field.

Finally, I believe it is essential to celebrate, with this Handbook, the accumulation of what Dr. Gada notes as the 'insights, experience, and knowledge'—indeed, it is fair to call this 'clinical wisdom'—of colleagues across a wide range of disciplines and from many countries. Their rich contributions blend together the modern scientific developments of our ever-expanding field with the humanism and art of caring for children with complicated lives and their families. This is a much-appreciated achievement.

Peter Rosenbaum, MD, FRCP(C), DSc (HC)
Professor of Paediatrics, McMaster University
Canada Research Chair in Childhood Disability 2001–2014
Co-Founder, CanChild Centre for Childhood Disability Research
Editorial Board, Mac Keith Press

Preface

A lack of a concise, easy-to-use, and updated resource on child neurodisability and community child health motivated me to write this book. This book is a sequel to the *Oxford Specialist Handbook of Community Paediatrics*, published in 2012, but this edition focuses more on neurodevelopmental disorders. Thus, this book contains hundreds of topics on neuroplasticity, child development, neurobehavioural disorders, sensory impairments, neuro-orthopaedics, neuro-genetics, neurorehabilitation, mental health and allied therapies.

This book is a culmination of my twenty plus years of clinical experience in child neurodisability and community child health at Oxford University Hospitals NHS Foundation Trust, Oxford and previously at Royal Free Hospital and Royal London Hospital in London. During the past two decades, I have had the privilege to work with my colleagues in Oxford and learn in my various professional capacities, such as consultant community paediatrician, child development team lead, course director, hon senior clinical lecturer, educational supervisor, clinical governance lead, editor, reviewer and a team member. This book contains all my clinical experience enriched with informative, up-to-date and concise summaries on hundreds of topics written by experts across the globe. I have been honored to work with this team of specialists from the USA, Canada, Australia, India, and the UK who have decades of medical experience and abundant clinical wisdom. Therefore, this book will serve as an essential companion and first point of reference to both established practitioners and trainees in neurodisability, community child health, paediatrics, general practice and professionals from multidisciplinary and multiagency teams.

Changes in the field of neurodisability and community child health can seem slow, feel imperceptible and even go unnoticed. Yet, so much has changed since this book's predecessor in 2012. There has been the launch of the DSM-5, ICD-11 and numerous new guidelines from authoritative sources such as NICE, AAP, RCPCH, and EACD. This book has been completely revamped to reflect this updated guidance. In addition, this book has been presented in an intuitive, easily readable format, with extensive use of bullet points, tables, boxes, flow charts, sample reports, clinical tips, and signposting to valuable resources.

This book is a portable guide focusing on practical advice that is clinically effective, helping you know what to do and how to do it. Furthermore, this book contains the insights, experience, and knowledge of experts from various disciplines such as neurodevelopmental paediatricians, neurology, psychiatry, orthopaedics, genetics, rehabilitation specialists, child protection, safeguarding, adoption and fostering, special educational needs, and therapists from multidisciplinary teams. Consequently, this book supports you in working collaboratively with other professionals, thus enabling you to deliver holistic care and make a positive difference in the lives of children and the families you serve.

Dr Srinivas Gada
Oxford
November 2021

Acknowledgements

After serving at Oxford University Hospitals NHS Foundation Trust from 2005, I stopped working at this prestigious institute in 2019 to focus on completing this handbook and be more available to my ageing parents. I want to offer my special thanks of gratitude to my parents, both of whom passed away during the writing of this book and couldn't be around to see this book in print. Like many around the globe, the COVID-19 pandemic was brutal, and it affected the production of this book in many ways. Nevertheless, reminding myself of the patience and perseverance of my parents helped me to conclude this book.

This book would not have come into being without the expertise and assistance of the editorial team at OUP, namely Nicola Wilson, Nic Williams (freelance copyeditor), Clement Raj (Newgen Knowledge Works), and especially Sylvia Warren. Sylvia's patience and support were crucial for this project.

As a practising neurodevelopmental paediatrician, much of the information in this handbook was drawn from my two decades in clinical practice. Therefore, my utmost thanks go to all the children and their families who shared their challenges with me.

I would like to extend my sincere gratitude to all the contributors for their hard work and for offering their valuable time and expertise, despite challenging work conditions at their institutes due to the pandemic. Their commitment was crucial for the conclusion of this project.

My special thanks go to Professor Georg Hollander, Dr Ivor Byren, Dr Martin Smith, and Nicki Sullivan for offering me professional support. My thanks also go to all my ex-colleagues at Oxford University Hospitals NHS Foundation Trust.

I am indebted to my wife, Vaishali, and my daughters, Ritu and Pooja, for their numerous sacrifices, encouragement, and practical help while I spent countless evenings and weekends working on this book.

Dr Srinivas Gada
Oxford
October 2021

Acknowledgements

Contents

Contents

Contributors

William J. Barbaresi

Professor of Pediatrics, Wade
Family Chair in Developmental
Medicine
Department of Pediatrics, Division
of Developmental Medicine
Harvard Medical School, Boston
Children's Hospital
Boston, MA, USA

Mohan V. Belthur

Associate Professor and Director,
Neuroorthopaedic Unit/Bubba
Watson and Ping Motion Analysis
Laboratory
Department of Orthopedics
Phoenix Children's Hospital and
University of Arizona College of
Medicine—Phoenix
Phoenix, AZ, USA

Elaine Burfitt

Consultant Community Paediatrician
& Named Doctor for Safeguarding
Children
Department of Community
Paediatrics
Salford Care Organisation
Northern Care Alliance NHS
Foundation Trust
Salford, UK

Robert Chapman

Consultant Child and Adolescent
Psychiatrist
Oxfordshire CAMHS NDC Pathway
Oxford Health NHS
Foundation Trust
Oxford, UK

Srinivas Gada

Consultant Paediatrician
in Neurodevelopment and
Neurodisability

Nuffield Health Oxford and HCA
Healthcare London
Honorary Senior Clinical Lecturer
University of Oxford
Honorary Consultant
Oxford University Hospitals NHS
Foundation Trust
Oxford, UK

Suneel Godbole

Developmental Pediatrician
Head of the Department,
Small Steps Morris Autism &
Child Development Centre,
Deenanath Mangeshkar Hospital &
Research Centre
Pune, India

Praveen K. Goyal

Consultant Paediatrician
Department of Community
Paediatrics
Oxford Children's Hospital
Oxford, UK

Emily Harrop

Consultant in Paediatric Palliative
Care & Medical Director
Helen & Douglas House
Honorary Consultant Oxford
University Hospitals NHS Trust
Oxford, UK

Usha Kini

Associate Professor
University of Oxford
Consultant Clinical Geneticist
Oxford Centre for Genomic
Medicine
Oxford University Hospitals NHS
Foundation Trust
Oxford, UK

Olaf Kraus de Carmargo

Associate Professor
Department of Paediatrics
McMaster University
Hamilton, ON, Canada

Mike Merzenich

Professor Emeritus
University of California
San Francisco
Chief Scientific Officer
Posit Science Founder & President
Brain Plasticity Institute
University of California
San Francisco

Waheeda Pagarkar

Consultant in Audiovestibular
Medicine
Department of Audiology
University College London
Hospitals and Great Ormond Street
Hospital
London, UK

Vijay Palanivel

Consultant in Paediatric
Neurodisability
The Children's Trust
Tadworth, UK

Jeremy Parr

Professor in Paediatric
Neurodisability, Neurodevelopment
and Disability Team
Sir James Spence Institute, Royal
Victoria Infirmary and Newcastle
University
England, UK

Sithara Ramdas

Consultant Paediatric Neurologist
and Honorary Senior Lecturer
Department of Paediatric
Neurology
John Radcliffe Hospital
Oxford, UK

Ashish S. Ranade

Consultant Orthopaedic Surgeon
Blooming Buds Centre for Pediatric
Orthopaedics
Deenanath Mangeshkar Hospital
Maharashtra, India

Marie Reilly

Instructor and Attending
Developmental-Behavioral
Pediatrician
Department of Pediatrics, Division
of Developmental Medicine
Harvard Medical School, Boston
Children's Hospital
Boston, MA, USA

Jenefer Sargent

Consultant Paediatrician and
Speciality Lead, Neurodisability
Neurodisability Service, Department
of Neurosciences
Great Ormond St Hospital for
Children
London, UK

Doug E. Simkiss

Medical Director and Deputy Chief
Executive
Birmingham Community Healthcare
NHS Foundation Trust
Birmingham, UK

Martin Smith

Consultant Paediatric Neurologist
Department of Paediatric
Neurology
John Radcliffe Hospital
Oxford, UK

Neil Wimalasundera

Consultant in Paediatric
Neurodisability and Rehabilitation
Victorian Paediatric Rehabilitation
Service
Royal Children's Hospital
Melbourne, Australia

Symbols and abbreviations

⊃	cross-reference
▶	important
❶	warning
℘	website
♀	female
♂	male
AABR	automated auditory brainstem response
AAC	augmentative and alternative communication
ABR	auditory brainstem response
AC	air conduction
ACE	adverse childhood experience
ACP	advance care plan
AD	autosomal dominant
ADD	attention deficit disorder
ADHD	attention deficit hyperactivity disorder
ADOS	Autism Diagnostic Observation Schedule
AFO	ankle–foot orthosis
AHT	abusive head trauma
ANSD	auditory neuropathy spectrum disorder
AOAE	automated otoacoustic emissions
AR	autosomal recessive
ASD	autistic spectrum disorder
BC	bone conduction
BCG	bacillus Calmette–Guérin
BMD	Becker muscular dystrophy or bone mineral density
BMI	body mass index
C&YP	children and young people
CAMHS	child and adolescent mental health services
CBT	cognitive behaviour therapy
CCE	child criminal exploitation
CCG	clinical commissioning group
cCMV	congenital cytomegalovirus
CCN	children's community nurse
CD	conduct disorder
CDC	child development centre
CDOP	Child Death Overview Panel

CDR	Child Death Review
CDRM	Child Death Review Meeting
CDT	child development team
CGH	comparative genomic hybridization
CHARGE	choanae, heart, anal, growth, and ear anomalies
CIN	child in need
CMA	chromosomal microarray
CMAP	compound motor action potential
CMV	cytomegalovirus
CNS	central nervous system
CP	cerebral palsy
CSA	child sexual abuse
CSC	children's social care
CSE	child sexual exploitation
CT	computer tomography
CVI	cerebral visual impairment
DA	domestic abuse
DCD	developmental coordination disorder
DLD	developmental learning disorder
DGE	delayed gastric emptying
DLA	disability living allowance
DMD	Duchenne muscular dystrophy
DS	Down syndrome
DSH	deliberate self-harm
DSM-5	*Diagnostic and Statistical Manual of Mental Disorders*, fifth edition
DXA	dual-energy X-ray absorptiometry
ECG	electrocardiogram
ED	eating disorder
EEG	electroencephalogram/ electroencephalography
EHC	Education, Health and Care
EMG	electromyogram/ electromyography
EPO	Emergency Protection Order
EYSENIT	Early Years special educational needs inclusion team
FBC	full blood count

FGM	female genital mutilation
FII	fabricated or induced illness
FISH	fluorescent *in situ* hybridization
FMS	Functional Mobility Scale
GDD	global developmental delay
GI	gastrointestinal
GMDS-ER	Griffiths Mental Developmental Scales–Extended Revised
GMFCS-E&R	Gross Motor Function Classification System—Expanded and Revised
GMFM	Gross Motor Function Measure
GOR	gastro-oesophageal reflux
GP	general practitioner
H2RA	histamine type 2 receptor antagonist
HINE	Hammersmith Infant Neurological Examination
HKAFO	hip–knee–ankle–foot orthosis
HL	hearing loss
HV	health visitor
ICC	initial case conference
ICD-11	*International Classification of Disease,* eleventh revision
ICF	International Classification of Functioning, Disability and Health
ID	intellectual disability
IEM	inborn error of metabolism
Ig	immunoglobulin
IQ	intelligence quotient
KAFO	knee–ankle–foot orthosis
LD	learning disability
LRTI	lower respiratory tract infection
MASH	Multiagency Safeguarding Hub
MCAD	medium-chain acyl dehydrogenase deficiency
MDT	multidisciplinary team
MELAS	myopathy, encephalopathy, lactic acidosis, and stroke
MERRF	myoclonic epilepsy with ragged red fibres
MPS	mucopolysaccharidosis
MRC	Medical Research Council
MRI	magnetic resonance imaging
nAHT	non-abusive head trauma
NF1	neurofibromatosis type 1

NF2	neurofibromatosis type 2
NHSP	newborn hearing screening programme
NICE	National Institute for Health and Care Excellence
NICU	neonatal intensive care unit
NSPCC	National Society for the Prevention of Cruelty to Children
OCD	obsessive–compulsive disorder
ODD	oppositional defiant disorder
OFC	occipitofrontal circumference
OME	otitis media with effusion
OSA	obstructive sleep apnoea
OT	occupational therapist
PCHI	permanent childhood hearing impairment
PCR	polymerase chain reaction
PICU	paediatric intensive care unit
PKAN	pantothenate kinase-associated neurodegeneration
PKU	phenylketonuria
PPO	Police Protection Order
PSG	polysomnography
PT	physiotherapist
RCPCH	Royal College of Paediatrics and Child Health
SD	standard deviation
SEGA	subependymal giant cell astrocytoma
SEN	special educational needs
SEND	special educational needs and disabilities
SHUEE	Shiners Hospital Upper Extremity Evaluation
SIDS	sudden infant death syndrome
SIGN	Scottish Intercollegiate Guidelines Network
SLT	speech and language therapist
SMA	spinal muscular atrophy
SMART	Specific, Measurable, Achievable, Relevant, and Time specific
SNHL	sensorineural hearing loss
SPD	sensory processing disorder
SPECT	single-photon emission computed tomography
SSRI	selective serotonin reuptake inhibitor

SUDC	sudden unexpected death in childhood		TORCH	toxoplasmosis, other (syphilis, varicella zoster, parvovirus B19), rubella, cytomegalovirus, and herpes simplex virus
SUDI	sudden unexpected death in infancy		TS	tuberous sclerosis
T&A	tonsillectomy and adenoidectomy		UN	United Nations
TBI	traumatic brain injury		VI	visual impairment
TLSO	thoracolumbar sacral orthosis		XLR	X-linked recessive

Working with child and family

Do what you can, with what you have, where you are.
Theodore Roosevelt, 1858–1919

Communication with children

Fundamental principles for communicating with young people

- Awareness of the cultural and social background of children and their families.
- Being non-judgemental, respectful, and fair.
- Acknowledging their rights to equality and diversity.
- Understanding that communication is a two-way process.
- Patient listening to encourage their feeling of participation, empowerment, and respect.
- Using clear common language without technical words or jargons.
- Realization of the importance (and effect) of non-verbal communication (facial expression, tone of voice, body language, etc.) on children.
- Offering information to children and young people (C&YP) in a way to match their level of understanding.
- Use of real-life situations to put information in the right perspective.
- Frequently checking their understanding through discussion, and summarizing key points at the end of the meeting.
- Offer to talk to young people, especially teenagers, separately from their parents and deciding together how to involve parents or carers in decision-making process.
- Asking open questions to widen the topic of discussion and encouraging expression of their feelings.
- Use of multisensory methods of communication such as drawing and models to get important and complicated information across.
- Presenting genuine choices and options in decision-making process.

Techniques of communicating with children

Verbal

- Use of 'I'/'me' instead of 'you'.
- Third-person technique, e.g. 'Sometimes when someone is hurt, they are angry or sad. Do you sometimes feel like that?'
- By being non-judgemental and legitimizing their feelings, e.g. 'It is sometimes OK to feel hurt'.
- Story telling—telling two stories with different outcomes.
- 'What if' question—by encouraging the child to use alternative options to deal with a different situation.
- 'What would you ask if you have three wishes?' may help in exteriorizing a child's feelings and help in establishing rapport.
- Using a rating scale, e.g. 'How will you rate tummy ache on a scale of 1 to 10?'

Non-verbal

- Writing—feelings or thoughts, keeping a diary.
- Drawing.
- Play—spontaneous play with ordinary toys or directed play, e.g. to involve them in imaginative play.
- Use of models to explain complicated topics.

Communicating with children at different ages

Infants
- Mainly non-verbal, vocalization, cuddle, and careful handling.
- Beware of stranger anxiety.

Early childhood
- Focus on individual child.
- Personalize experience to them.
- May prefer to touch and feel examination equipment.
- Concrete thinking—avoid abstract concepts or language.

School-age children
- Want straight explanations and reasons for everything, but would be happy to accept if given in simple language.

Adolescents
- Respecting their views.
- Respect privacy and right to confidentiality (except if safeguarding or other serious issues involved).
- Undivided attention and good listening.
- Keeping an open mind and staying calm.
- Avoid judging.

Barriers to effective communication
- Defending a situation or opinion.
- Stereotyped comments and clichés.
- Direct/close-ended questions from the start.
- Interfering and finishing other's sentences.
- Talking more than listening.
- Frequent change of topic/focus.

Clues/signs of poor communication
- Long periods of silence.
- Constant fidgeting.
- Tapping, playing with hair.
- Looking around, yawning.

Difficult communication
See ➔ pp. 212–14 and pp. 216.

Child- and family-centred care

- During the latter half of the twentieth century, there has been a growing understanding of the family's role in a child's life. It is recognized that *each family is unique and family members are the experts and best advocate of a child's needs*.
- Family-centred care puts children and their families at the heart of care provisions and is a significant shift from the traditional *biomedical model* of care which focuses on biological rather than social and emotional aspects to deal with the disease process.

Why is child- and family-centred care important?

- To empower family to become the experts for their child.
- To manage child's condition on day-to-day basis.
- To meet child's developmental needs.
- To meet sibling's developmental needs.
- To feel comfortable in sharing ongoing stress and periodic crises.
- To assist family members in managing their feelings.
- To educate and inform others about the child's condition.
- To establish a support system.

Key principles of child- and family-centred care

- Recognition that family occupies a central and constant position in a child's life.
- Acknowledging that family members are the experts about a child's condition and that they are the best advocates of a child's needs.
- Family–professional collaboration at all levels of healthcare, professional education, policymaking, and programme development to optimize care.
- Effective communication and negotiation of care.
- Recognizing and building on the strengths of each child and family, even in difficult and challenging situations.
- Empowering each child and family by free exchange of information backed by professional support to ensure their involvement in decision-making process.
- Recognition and respect for cultural, racial, and social diversity.
- To fit various support services around the child's and family's needs rather than to suit care provider's convenience.
- Encouraging networking and family-to-family support to facilitate learning from each other's experience.

Advantages of child-centred and family-focused care

- Greater patient, family, and professional satisfaction.
- Improved patient and family outcome.
- Decreased healthcare costs.
- More effective use of healthcare resources.

Example of child- and family-centred care

Harry is a 2-year-old boy seen in clinic for developmental delay. On assessment it became clear that he has autism with general delay in cognitive development. His parents are distraught with this news and would like to know about the best way forward.

They would also like to know:
• What they can do as a family to optimize his development?
• What and how to tell their family and friends?
• How can professionals help?

A family-centred approach will involve:
• Discussion with parents (and with extended family if needed) reflecting respect, involvement, and empowerment.
• Explaining autism with details on how it is affecting Harry rather than discussing about a 'typical case of autism'.
• Highlighting Harry's unique strengths and difficulties.
• Providing the best available information (autistic spectrum disorder (ASD) support groups, benefits, etc.) for the family to go through at their own pace.
• Honest opinion about prognosis, leaving room for hope in view of Harry's young age.
• Arranging appropriate referrals to a speech and language therapist (SLT), occupational therapist (OT), Early Years special educational needs inclusion team (EYSENIT), and social services with clear information about who is going to be offering what.
• Clear overview of coordination and delivery of services.
• Discussions followed by written report/letter to the referring provider and the family containing the details of the assessment and plan.
• Clear plan for follow-up and information about contact prior to next meeting if needed.
• Making yourself available for follow-up questions that might arise shortly after disclosure of diagnosis.

Child development teams

In 1976, Donald Court's report, commissioned by the British government, drew particular attention to service provisions for children with disabilities and recommended creation of a district team which should include a number of professionals providing multidisciplinary support.

Child development team (CDT)

- A secondary level service provision for children with neurodevelopmental disability, providing interdisciplinary assessment and support in a local health district.
- Provides a cohesive service ideally from a common location.
- Makes sure that service provisions are responsive to the individual needs of families and children.
- Usually serves preschool children.

Functions of a CDT

- Specific assessment and therapy.
- Information about specific conditions and about disabilities in general.
- Emotional support.
- Link with other families with similar conditions.
- Easy access to other agencies such as education.
- Prompt, efficient supply and repair of equipment.

Structure and composition of a CDT

- Can vary but usually include staff from healthcare, education, and social care (Fig. 1.1).
- It usually includes the following:
  - Community paediatrician/developmental paediatrician.
  - Clinical (or educational) psychologist.
  - SLT.
  - OT.
  - Physiotherapist (PT).
  - Preschool teacher/Portage worker/EYSENIT.
  - Social worker.
  - Specialist health visitor (HV)/key worker.
  - Audiologist.
  - Allied disciplines, e.g. orthoptist, child psychiatrist, dietician, dentist, play specialist, etc.

Assessment by a CDT

- Assessment may take place jointly at a central facility (child development centre (CDC)) but is more commonly performed at different times by individual team members (aka a 'virtual team').
- Some teams may also assess children at a variety of sites outside the CDC including local nurseries, educational units, and at home.
- Team meetings and discussions form the core of the CDT to facilitate:
  - Coordination of appropriate service provisions and to avoid duplication (case management).
  - Discussing new referrals to plan and coordinate future assessments.
  - Reviewing policy and team organizations.

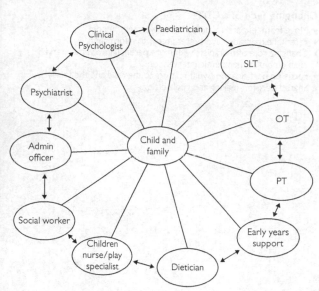

Fig. 1.1 Child development team.

- In-service training, audit, etc.
- Combined health, educational, and care needs of children attending special schools can be discussed in interdisciplinary school meetings.
- Information obtained during the assessment process is shared with the parents and (other) professionals working with the child.
- A detailed written report is provided to parents at the end of assessment and shared with partner agencies with parental consent.

Advantages of a CDT

- Detailed interdisciplinary assessments identify needs enabling appropriate service provisions.
- Seamless communication between various professionals/disciplines.
- Avoidance of duplication of assessment with improved coordination.
- Team members learning from each other (transdisciplinarity).

Disadvantages of a CDT

- Risk losing an overview of the child if not coordinated well.
- Lack of accountability and responsibility.
- Dual accountability of practitioners to the team and their line manager with potential for conflict.
- Excluding older children and those without multiple needs who may still benefit from CDT input.
- Risk of becoming CDT centred rather than family centred.

Changing face of a CDT

- Move from 'expert' model to 'empowerment' model.
- Parental expectation and better access to information.
- Changing role of therapists with more parental involvement and enablement in therapeutic interventions.
- Focus on participation (what matters to the child and the family?).
- Shared decision-making and goal-setting.

Child development centres

Some CDTs operate from a base while others gather at different locations to meet.

Advantages of a CDC

- Better communication and coordination of services.
- Purpose-built facilities and co-location of various support services.
- Recognizable point of contact for families and other professionals.
- Can be used for health promotion activities.
- Can be used as a base to provide various resources by other professionals and local community, e.g. Down syndrome (DS) support group meetings, parenting programmes, early bird courses for ASD, etc.

Disadvantages of a CDC

- Risk of isolation from families and local services.
- Increasing wait times due to bottlenecks.

Children likely to benefit from CDT/CDC input

Those with:

- Cognitive disorders (see ➔ p. 420).
- Learning disabilities/intellectual disabilities (see ➔ pp. 136–41).
- Gross motor impairment:
  - Cerebral palsy (CP) (see ➔ pp. 92–101).
  - Neuromuscular disorders (see ➔ pp. 272–6).
  - Chronic neurological conditions, e.g. post meningitis, brain malformations, survivors of severe head injury (see ➔ pp. 108–9).
- Fine motor difficulties:
  - Developmental coordination disorder (DCD)/dyspraxia (see ➔ pp. 146–9).
- Speech, language, and communication disorders:
  - Severe language disorder (see ➔ pp. 402–3).
  - ASD (see ➔ pp. 114–25).
- Paediatric feeding disorder.
- Visual impairment (see ➔ pp. 202–8).
- Hearing impairment (see ➔ pp. 170).
- Any of the above-listed conditions with associated behavioural disorders.

Interdisciplinary working

- Children with complex needs and their families require support from multiple agencies. Families can sometime get overwhelmed with multiplicity and duplication of input if these agencies work in isolation.
- Various professionals involved may represent public, private, or voluntary organizations. It is crucially important for various professionals, often working across different agencies, to work together in order to meet the family's needs in an effective and efficient manner (see ➔ p. 675).
- Multiagency support can be provided in the form of team around a child model or by assembling multiagency teams or panels.

Advantages of interdisciplinary working

- Effective and efficient provision of services with improved quality of care.
- Better coordination with minimization of duplication of assessments and support, therefore increasing cost effectiveness.
- Beneficial for families by reducing the number of different agencies they have to deal with.
- Key worker or coordinator can provide easy point of access.
- Improving skills of professionals by working together and learning from each other, e.g. joint home visit by preschool teacher and various therapists (transdisciplinarity).
- Increases patient's and family's satisfaction.

Skills required for interdisciplinary team working

- Good communication skills.
- Willingness to work with others along with commitment to team process to help children and families.
- Ability to listen and see other's perspective.
- Have mutual respect and trust other team members.
- Understanding of partner agencies' working.

Key principles which underline successful interdisciplinary working
- General knowledge and understanding of the range of organizations and individuals working with C&YP.
- Knowledge and appreciation of common principles and procedures of joint working including those for consent, assessment, confidentiality, and information sharing.
- Clarity about individual roles along with respect and value for other's contribution.
- Effective communication with appropriate information sharing, avoiding jargon and abbreviations.
- Being proactive and assertive to be able to make significant contributions.
- Confidence to challenge situations by asking considered questions.
- Putting children and their families at the centre of decision-making process.
- Common language of terminology (e.g. use of International Classification of Functioning, Disability and Health (ICF) terminology).
- Awareness of the partner agencies' policies and working practices.

- Co-location of services.
- Joint budgetary control if possible.

Potential disadvantages of multiagency working
- Lack of responsibility and accountability. This can be overcome by appointing a coordinator or key professional who can liaise with other professionals.
- Potential to confuse families and young people about whom to contact during times of specific needs. This can be overcome by appointing one team member as a key person for the family to connect.
- Time and resource intensive.

Barriers to effective multiagency working
- Poor communication and information sharing.
- Differences in organizational aims.
- Lack of support and commitment from senior management.
- Constant reorganization.
- Frequent staff turnover.
- Financial uncertainty.
- Different professional ideologies and agency cultures.

Example of an interdisciplinary team
See Fig. 1.2.

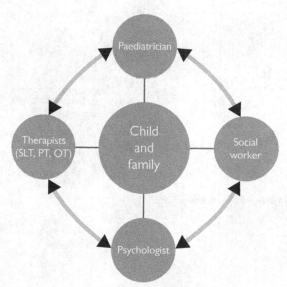

Fig. 1.2 Example of an interdisciplinary team.

Interdisciplinary team process
- Rather than working as a single discipline or as different multiple disciplines, the biopsychosocial approach in developmental care requires interdisciplinary collaboration, prioritization, and person-centred goal setting and outcomes.
- Professionals need to understand the child's and family's activity limitations, participation restrictions, as well as the barriers and facilitators of environmental factors to gain a broader understanding of the child's health in context.
- Interdisciplinary process emphasizes the team's responsibility to move beyond siloed professional paradigms and highlights the need for a diverse team of healthcare, education, and social care professionals. See Fig. 1.3.

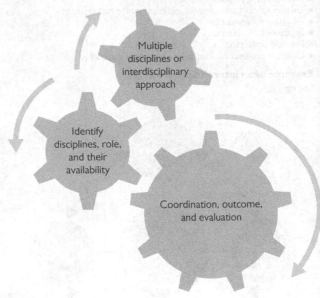

Fig. 1.3 Interdisciplinary team process.

Difficult conversations

You will often come across the term 'breaking bad news'. Consider that 'bad' is a judgement and some conditions or diagnoses that you might feel are not so bad from a clinician's perspective, actually might be devastating for parents. It can also happen that a topic you expected to be devastating might provide a long-sought clarification and closure to parents. Always be prepared that conversations might become difficult—for both family and health professionals. The following are some suggestions to consider.

Briefing
- Gather all medical information available and the timeline related to it.
- Gather information about the child and family from all team members.
- Discuss with the team why you think this conversation might be difficult—what are the expectations of the family?
- Prepare for different scenarios after the conversation—which supports might be required and how can it be ensured that they are available?

Setting the scene
- The most senior person who knows the family best should give the news.
- Collect appropriate information, anticipate likely questions, and prepare answers.
- Make sure there is no interruption during the consultation.
- Keep a box of tissues, drinking water, etc. in the room.
- This should be a sitting down, face-to-face conversation.
- Preferably both parents should be present. Suggest inviting a relative or friend especially for single parents for support.

Consultation
- Introduce yourself if you are not already known, and address the child by name.
- Establish what is already known to the family.
- Gently build up before delivering the bad news, e.g. 'As you are aware, Jack had an MRI scan of his brain. I am afraid it is not normal'.
- Avoid jargon and speak at a pace the family can understand.
- Be honest and straight to the point.
- Reassure them that everything that needs to be done is being done.
- Don't promise anything you are not sure you can deliver.
- Be sensitive to a parent's reaction.
- Provide plenty of time and opportunities for asking questions.
- Be willing to repeat information if necessary.
- Give a clear plan of action and follow-up.
- Provide contact details to the family for further questions if necessary.
- Offer to share information with the child or others involved in the child's care.
- During an interdisciplinary assessment/briefing, offer to speak to the parents privately prior to a joint meeting with other team members.

Follow-up

- Write to the family to supplement verbal discussion.
- Offer a follow-up appointment to meet the family.

Debriefing with team

- What have we learned that we did not know before?
- What needs to be documented in the chart so everyone is on the same page and re-traumatizing the family can be avoided?
- How is everyone doing? Are there any needs for support within the team?

Common scenarios—includes giving diagnosis of

- CP (see ➜ pp. 92–101).
- Autism (see ➜ pp. 114–25).
- Developmental testing revealing global developmental delay (GDD) (see ➜ p. 30).
- Genetic investigations, e.g. *MECP2* mutation detection confirming Rett syndrome (see ➜ pp. 518–19).
- Lab confirmation of an Inborn Error of Metabolism (IEM) (see ➜ pp. 150–1) etc.

Effects of illness and disability on family

- The life of families with members affected by chronic illness or disability is often perceived as extremely burdened and suffering.
- Health economists have even come up with the term 'burden of disease' and try to calculate it. This position is easily perceived as ableist.
- As clinicians, we need to realize that the chronic condition or disability is part of the life of our patients and their families.
- We cannot assume, but we need them to feel comfortable to let us know if they feel burdened.
- Consider what can be done to alleviate this burden, if that is the case.

Causes of increased number of families impacted by chronic illness and disability

- Better survival of extremely premature neonates and those born with birth defects.
- Early intervention with longer life span for some of the babies with treatments previously not offered, e.g. cardiac surgery for children with DS (see ➜ pp. 499–500).
- Better awareness and early identification of conditions such as autism (see ➜ p. 114).
- More children with disabilities are now living at home and attending mainstream schools.

Potential risks of disability for the family

A child's impairment can affect the entire family's well-being by:
- Feelings of guilt, blame, and reduced self-esteem which may either lead to rejection or overprotection of the affected child.
- Limiting and interrupting family activities.
- Feeling of helplessness due to lack of information and awareness of service provisions.
- Consuming large majority of parental time, energy, and attention.
- Relative neglect of siblings and other family member's needs (see ➜ pp. 26–7).
- Poor peer activities and cognitive development in siblings.
- Affecting family income due to parents taking time off or leaving jobs.
- It can be a source of parental emotional distress and mental health problems affecting relations and living arrangements (see ➜ p. 365).
- Social isolation from peers and neighbours due to perceived stigma attached to disability.

Potential positive effects of disability

Having a disabled child can be a unique family experience which may also have the following positive effects:
- Enhance family cohesion and encourage links with community groups.
- Increase awareness of inner strength.
- Reframe values and priorities.
- Acquire new perspectives on society and its diversity.
- Become an expert and advocate for other children and families.

Minimizing the negative effects of disability

To achieve this, health professionals need to adopt a *family-centred approach* (see ➲ p. 4). Families caring for children with disabilities can be helped by:

- Addressing their (child and family's) complex medical, developmental, educational, social, emotional, recreational, and care needs.
- Informing families about the range of services required for a particular child (see ➲ p. 68).
- Arranging required services locally as much as possible.
- By understanding and supporting families through the grieving process (see ➲ p. 481).

Sources of support

- Acute and primary healthcare services to manage long-term conditions, e.g. children's community nurse (CCN) (see ➲ p. 681), therapy services (see ➲ Chapter 7), etc.
- Social services for financial support, respite, and home adaptations (see ➲ pp. 682–3), etc.
- Education services for providing special educational needs (SEN) provisions (see ➲ pp. 656–8).
- Voluntary organizations (see ➲ p. 684).
- Parent support groups.

Further resources

Carers Trust: ℐ℃ http://www.carers.org
Sibs: ☎ 01535 645453; ℐ℃ http://www.sibs.org.uk

Using the ICF as a framework for family-centred collaboration

- The ICF can serve as a way to remind us of all the components that contribute to a healthy participation of an individual.
- The ICF allows us to capture the classic biomedical findings that interact with the usual domains of the life of our patients and the relevant environmental factors that can be acting as barriers or facilitators to such a participation.
- An easy way to introduce this framework is using the 'F-words' (Fun, Family, Function, Friends, Fitness, and Future) approach developed at CanChild (🔗 https://canchild.ca/en/research-in-practice/f-words-in-childhood-disability).

Even in a fast-paced clinic, it might be helpful to have a 'snapshot' of each patient with the main relevant aspects to their functioning:
- *Personal factors ('Fun')*: who are you? What kind of personality do you have (timid, shy, gregarious, risk-taking, etc.)? What makes you experience fun?
- *Environmental factors ('Family')*: with whom do you live? Where do you go to school? What is helpful in your life and what not so much? Do you receive any therapies/treatments? Are you on waiting lists?
- *Activities ('Function')*: what activities are you able to do, and which ones are restricted?
- *Participation ('Friends')*: what do you like to do with friends? Do you prefer to be inside or outside? What are your favourite pastimes? Do you experience any limitations?
- *Body functions and structures ('Fitness')*: what can you do to keep yourself fit? What body impairments do we need to be aware of?
- And *'Future'*: what are your next steps and goals?

This framework is also being used to discuss and make decisions about relevant therapy goals using the *F-words goal sheet* (🔗 https://canchild.ca/system/tenon/assets/attachments/000/003/061/original/FWordsGoalSheet_May1_2020.pdf).

Providing information, support, and advice

> *There was no substitute for real people, written information is nice to have as a comfort factor, but you really get your information from people, talking face to face with them.*
>
> Parent with a child with learning disabilities

> *You could talk to her about anything, and she was really good. She knew people who could help you if you were stuck, or would say 'well, you could try this, or that, or something else'.*
>
> Parent of a child with learning disabilities

Living with a disabled child presents a number of challenges even for more resourceful and well-informed parents. It is a juggling act, balancing routine parenting tasks with treatment programmes and additional physical and emotional demands (see pp. 364–5).

Adequate information is crucial:
• To understand the impact of disability on family life.
• To facilitate adjustment to disability.
• To empower parents—helps in coping and transitions.
• Non-directive information can be valuable during periods of crises.

Settings

Exchange of information can take place:
• In a multidisciplinary case conference.
• During a home visit.
• At an outpatient/school clinic.
• During a hospital admission on the ward.
• Over the telephone or by email.
• In the form of a clinic letter.

Types of information

• New diagnosis: provide information about the condition, its complications, long-term outcome, etc.
• Information regarding various management options.
• About engaging other professionals for further assessment/support (see p. 675).
• About local and national support agencies, e.g. voluntary organizations and charities such as Scope for CP (see p. 684).
• For support from statutory agencies (e.g. statutory assessment for SEN (see pp. 656–8) and Disability Living Allowance (DLA)).
• To inform about local support groups for parents, e.g. local DS groups for a child newly diagnosed with DS (see p. 23).
• Internet-based resources, e.g. ERIC (The Children's Bowel & Bladder Charity) for incontinence (see p. 311).

Ways in which families receive information

• Personal communication with professionals:
  • Most frequent and highly valued mode of information.

- Verbal information supported by written/printed material helps to reinforce the message delivered during consultations.
- Direct contact with other parents and voluntary organizations.
- Locally produced booklets (rather than general publications) are more relevant and better appreciated by families.

Advantages of appropriate and timely information

This enables parents to:
- Access suitable services and benefits.
- Enhance management of their child's condition and behaviour.
- Plan, prepare, and hence feel more in control.
- Link with support agencies to adjust emotionally to their child's disabilities and reduce the feeling of isolation.

Type of support needed by families with children with complex needs

Information
- About long-term outcome, treatment options, prognosis, and its impact on family life (see ⭢ p. 22).
- About condition-specific support groups via Contact (previously Contact a Family) directory.
- Benefits, allowances, equipment, and details of local agencies (see ⭢ p. 675).

Education
- Acknowledgement and understanding of child's difficulties in educational setting while promoting inclusion. Children's community nurses (CCNs) (see ⭢ p. 681) and school nurses (see ⭢ p. 679) play a valuable role in support.
- Good ongoing liaison between parents, school, and health services.
- Identification and provision for SEN— equipment and medications.
- Home teacher or home-school link worker for prolonged periods of absence secondary to illness (see ⭢ pp. 668–9).
- Special school provisions and support from specialist advisory teachers if necessary, e.g. autism advisory teacher or specialist teacher for visual (see ⭢ p. 207) or hearing impaired (see ⭢ p. 196).
- By providing transition programmes and specialized job training during teenage years (see ⭢ p. 471).

Financial support
- Allowances and benefits (see ⭢ p. 675).
- Home adaptation (see ⭢ pp. 392–3).

Social and emotional support
- Directing parents and siblings to local support agencies and advocacy groups (see ⭢ p. 19) to share information and meet other families affected with similar condition (e.g. autism family support).
- Respite care including support for siblings and parents (see ⭢ p. 675).
- Support from extended family and friends.
- Psychological support from counsellors and family therapy (see ⭢ p. 367).
- Spiritual support from faith leaders.

Support for practical issues
- Good liaison between hospital and community teams for issues such as home oxygen, suction, specialized bed, mobilization devices, feeding pumps, etc.
- Training of parents and other carers for managing specialized procedures such as gastrostomy feeding (see ➔ p. 442), administering rescue medications such as buccal midazolam, managing a Hickman line etc.
- Details of continuing supplies such as oxygen, medications, and other consumables.
- Contact details of key worker, link professional, and members of interdisciplinary/multiagency teams (see ➔ p. 14); arrangement of open access at local paediatric unit etc.

Further resources

Contact (Previously Contact-a-Family): ✎ https://contact.org.uk/
Council for Disabled Children: ✎ https://councilfordisabledchildren.org.uk/members/meet-our-members/parents-inclusion
Parent Champions: ✎ http://www.parentchampions.org.uk/resources/
Scope: ✎ http://www.scope.org.uk

Care of siblings

- Siblings share their culture, heritage, parents, and a whole host of environmental factors throughout their lives.
- Disability or a chronic illness in a child therefore is bound to have a significant and long-lasting impact on siblings.
- Siblings of children with disability react in different ways according to their age and understanding about their sibling's disability. Their resilience and adjustment to sibling disability is also influenced by factors affecting the family and the social environment.

Factors contributing to sibling adaptation to chronic illness or disability

- Socioeconomic status.
- Parental stress (see ➋ pp. 205–7).
- Family cohesion (see ➋ p. 18).
- Consistent routines.

Emotions in siblings of disabled children

- Worry, fear, and anxiety.
- Embarrassment and shame.
- Jealousy, anger, resentment, and a sense of injustice.
- Isolation and loneliness, especially if sibling requires/receives a significant amount of parental attention.
- A sense of loss and sadness.
- Increased levels of anxiety (see ➋ pp. 306–8), depression (see ➋ pp. 330–2), peer problems, and behavioural difficulties (see ➋ pp. 362–3).

Positive attributes seen in siblings of a disabled child

- Often more caring, empathetic, and sensitive to others' needs.
- More responsible and tolerant behaviour with maturity and independence.

Signs of difficulty in coping with the situation

- Help should be sought if a sibling is:
  - Having difficulty with sleep (see ➋ pp. 466–8) or appetite.
  - Avoiding the disabled child.
  - Apathetic with low self-esteem.
  - Has behavioural difficulties (see ➋ pp. 362–3).
- Siblings have specific needs that require attention at different stages of their lives.

Strategies which can help children cope with their sibling's disability

These include:
- Clear and factual information about the child's disability to siblings (see ➋ p. 22).
- To acknowledge and appreciate sibling's emotions and feelings.
- Parents spending some quality time with siblings especially sharing activities which mean a lot to them.

- Appreciating and encouraging good qualities and behaviours in siblings.
- Providing siblings with their own personal space.
- Ask siblings if they would like to be involved in care-giving responsibilities appropriate to their abilities and respecting their wishes if they don't want to.
- Individual sibling support or combined family intervention programmes can be helpful in protecting their physical and emotional well-being (see ➲ p. 367).

Further resources

Carers Trust: ☎ 0844 800 4361; ∿ http://www.carers.org
Sibs: ☎ 01535 645453; ∿ http://www.sibs.org.uk

Shared decision-making and goal setting

- Focus on the needs of the child and the family—'optimizing' instead of 'fixing'
- Assess for facilitators and barriers in the main life domains of the child.
- Define 'SMART' (Specific, Measurable, Achievable, Relevant, and Time specific) goals based on the needs identified.
- Establish baseline and timeframe for reassessment.
- Importance of good 'fit' between family and therapists.
- Content of intervention needs to be meaningful for child.

Tips for families when choosing therapies and providers

🔗 https://link.medium.com/cMDu77Zzu8

Child development and neuroplasticity

A stitch in time saves nine.

English proverb

Developmental delay

What is developmental delay?

- Developmental delay is a term used for a child <5 years of age who has failed to meet the expected developmental milestones. In other words, the child has not yet acquired the developmental skills as would be expected of him or her, when compared with their age-appropriate peers.
- The term developmental delay is replaced by the term 'learning disability' (LD) in a child >5 years of age. It is worth noting that not all children with developmental delay go on to have a LD.
- Developmental delays could be in a child's motor, language, communication, cognition, or social skill domains.
- Moreover, development delay can be 'isolated developmental delay', i.e. delay in a single domain, or the delay could be 'global developmental delay' (GDD), i.e. when there is a significant delay in two or more developmental domains.

How common is developmental delay?

- Developmental delay is common in children. The prevalence of developmental delay varies from 6% to 15%, in different surveys.
- The 2018 Annual Report from the US Centers for Disease Control and Prevention estimated that ~16% of children had a developmental disability or a developmental delay.

What are the risk factors for developmental delay?

The risk factors for developmental delay can be categorized into:
- *Prenatal*, e.g. exposure to alcohol, smoking, drugs, or infections in pregnancy.
- *Perinatal*, e.g. infection, low birth weight, prematurity, or lack of oxygen.
- *Postnatal*, e.g. maternal depression, substance abuse, neglect, abuse, trauma, or infections such as meningitis or encephalitis.
- *Genetic conditions*, e.g. DS, Turner syndrome, Fragile X, and many others.
- *Environmental factors*, e.g. poverty, deprivation, poor housing, lack of social support, lack of sanitation, and the state of the health service.
- *Medical conditions*, e.g. hypothyroidism, or heart, chest, or gut problems.
- *Adverse experiences*, e.g. war, food insecurity, racism, parental unemployment, illiteracy, parental mental illness, and displacement because of political or climate events.

What could be the protective factors for developmental delay?

The following factors have been shown to prevent or minimize developmental delays:
- A stable and supportive family.
- Active engagement of parents with their child's school, and learning.
- Regular household schedule for mealtimes and bedtimes.
- Regular reading of stories or visits to the local library.
- Opportunities to play with other children, participation in playgroups, visits to the local park, and outdoor activities.

How do you identify developmental delay?

Developmental delay can be identified in two ways:
- Developmental screening.
- Developmental assessment.

Identifying developmental delay

A hundred years from now it will not matter what my bank account was, the sort of house I lived in or the kind of car I drove. . . but the world may be different because I was important in the life of a child.

Forest E. Witcraft

Developmental screening

- Screening tests are used to identify children whose development is unknown or when there is a suspicion of developmental delay. Screening tests ask the question 'Is this normal? Yes/no'.
- Screening tests produce two outcomes:
  - 'Pass' (development is within normal limits).
  - 'Fail' (there is likely to be developmental delay).
- Screening tests carry a risk of false positives/negatives, either over- or under-identifying children with developmental delay.
- Screening tests can take the form of either:
  - A questionnaire handed out to the parent/carer, or
  - A checklist, i.e. ticking the milestones achieved by the child.
- Screening tests are carried out by HVs (see ➔ pp. 676–7), general practitioners (GPs), EYSENITs (see ➔ p. 5), and professionals in primary care.
- The following tests are widely used:
  - The 'Ten Questions' test (widely used in developing countries).
  - 'Schedule of Growing Skills' (widely used in the UK).
  - 'Denver Developmental Screening Test' (widely used outside the UK).

Developmental assessment

- Developmental assessments are used to answer the question 'At what level (i.e. mental age/developmental age) is this child functioning and why?'
- Assessment is an in-depth evaluation of a child's abilities and is carried out by trained professionals such as developmental paediatricians, educational psychologists (see ➔ pp. 666–7), neuropsychologists (see ➔ p. 414), neurologists, etc.
- Developmental assessment is usually part of a process of establishing developmental diagnosis.
- Developmental assessment gives a detailed understanding of a child's strengths, weaknesses, and attainment levels by providing developmental results in the following forms:
  - Percentiles.
  - Quotients.
  - Standard deviation (SD) or 'z' scores.
  - Age equivalent scores etc.
- The following tests are more widely used for developmental assessment by paediatricians, psychologists, and therapists:
  - Griffiths Mental Developmental Scales–Extended Revised (GMDS-ER).
  - Bayley Scales of Infant and Toddler Development-III.

Establishing developmental diagnosis

- **❶** In developmental assessment, there is no place for 'spot' diagnoses.
- Diagnosis consists of not only observing what a child does but how he/she does it, and the degree of maturity he/she shows.
- Developmental diagnosis should never be made on clinical impression alone, but should be based on:
  - History.
  - Examination.
  - Developmental assessment.
  - Clinical observations.
  - Special investigations, where relevant.
  - 'Interpretation' of all of the above points.

How does developmental assessment help us?

- Certain developmental profiles (see following section) are suggestive of specific developmental disorders/diagnoses and hence help in formulating a diagnosis of developmental disorder/disability.
- Developmental profiles help our understanding of the child by providing the developmental age/mental age, strengths, and weaknesses.
- Guides our decision to undertake further investigations for delay/disorder, e.g. if the results show a severe delay/deviation, you are more likely to consider investigations (see ➜ p. 32) versus if the results were to reveal mild delay.
- Results of assessments help in making appropriate referrals for therapeutic interventions, e.g. PT (see ➜ pp. 374–6), OT (see ➜ pp. 390–1), SLT (see ➜ pp. 402–3), audiologists, psychologists, etc.
- Leads us in our referrals to educational/early intervention programmes (see ➜ p. 68).
- Helps in assessing the impact of the interventions, programmes, and therapies offered to the child.
- Directs our decisions about educational placement/options (see ➜ p. 23 and pp. 656–8) to be offered to the child.

Developmental profiles

Relative discrepancies in the percentile score from a mean of the 50th percentile by more than 2 SD or by comparison between the domains or over several assessments give valuable indications of the child's strengths, weaknesses, and rate of progress.

The following *developmental disorders* are more likely to produce *typical developmental profiles* on developmental testing, if there are no added comorbidities:

- Autism/ASD (see ➜ pp. 114–25): very low scores in language (Lang) and social (PS) scales. Low scores in eye–hand coordination (EHC) and patchy abilities in practical reasoning (PR).
- ASD (High functioning) (see ➜ pp. 300–3): low in PS, average in Lang. Low in performance (Perf), EHC, and locomotion (Loco) if they are also dyspraxic.
- General LD (see ➜ pp. 136–41): low scores (the degree depends on the severity of LD) across all skill areas, i.e. locomotor (Loco), PS, Lang, EHC, Perf, PR.

- Hearing impairment (see ➜ pp. 168–9): low scores on Lang, PR, and PS subscales in items which are language dependent.
- Vision impairment (see ➜ pp. 202–8): very low scores in EHC and Perf which are more vision dependent. Low scores in PS, Lang, and even PR, if autistic features.
- Developmental coordination disorder (see ➜ pp. 146–9): low scores (depends on the severity of the disorder) in EHC, Perf, and Loco.
- Specific LD (see ➜ p. 142), e.g. dyspraxia: Lang good, low on EHC, Perf, and PR.
- Physical disability (see ➜ pp. 92–101) e.g. CP, hypotonia: low in Loco, EHC, and Perf. Lang, PS, and PR are not affected to similar extent.

Cautions when using developmental tests

- Compare one's findings with the history given before reporting the results of developmental assessments.
- Shyness and failure to cooperate should not lead to hasty conclusions. In doubtful cases with unusual features, it is better to repeat the test after an interval.
- Important aspects such as the alertness, the rapidity with which tests are performed, the degree of the understanding displayed by the child, the interest shown in their surroundings, and his/her personality are usually not recorded quantitatively by many developmental tests.
- Don't make 'predictions'! Mental subnormality can never be diagnosed on account of delay in any one skill such as sphincter control, locomotion, or speech. It can largely be eliminated by the normal or early development of speech. There are many variables, hence one cannot predict the effect that opportunity, education, personality, motivation, illness, injury, and care received will have on the development of the child.
- 'Milestones' are just milestones! It is wrong to say that a child should pass a certain milestone at a certain age. All one can say is that the further away from average the child is in anything, the less likely they are to develop normally.
- The maturity and quality of speech has the highest correlation of all aspects of behaviour with the child's later intelligence. Gross motor development with the age of sitting and walking has the lowest correlation with subsequent intelligence.

! Failure to present the tests correctly can affect the performance of the child and lead to fallacious results.

Principles of neurodevelopmental testing

Aims

- Ask yourself what are you really testing and why? Is the testing to screen the child's development so far or is it to assess and quantify the exact degree of developmental delay?
- This will help you to choose an appropriate developmental test, i.e. a screening test or a detailed/diagnostic test to address the given question.

General advice on testing

- Speak slowly and clearly.
- Engage the child's cooperation.
- Do the test only. Do not engage in prolonged general discussion or chatting during the test.
- Attract the child's attention before asking a question.
- The test items are not toys. Put away each piece of equipment after testing, having only one item before the child at a time. Put the equipment, e.g. picture cards, in the correct order after finishing. (If you lose one test item, e.g. a piece of a form board, then a whole sequence of test items across a wide range of ages may be inaccessible!)
- Hygiene: clean the soiled test items with warm water and soap/ antiseptic solution. Follow local infection control guidance.
- Safety: watch children so that they do not put small beads in their mouth etc. Be careful on stairs. Children need to be supervised at all times.

Testing environment

- Most developmental tests can be administered in a variety of settings, e.g. clinic, home, school, nursery, etc.
- The testing room/adjoining corridor should be large enough to administer locomotor scales.
- The room should have adequate lighting, heating, and ventilation.
- There should not be any distractions, e.g. posters, on the walls or non-test items within view of the child during the test itself.
- Seating: there should be a table and chair of suitable height, i.e. the child's feet should be on the floor and the child should be able to place elbows at right-angles and hands on the table surface.
- Additional equipment: paper, pencils, crayons, story books for different ages, and access to stairs may be needed in addition to the test items/ equipment.

Method of administration

Success comes when preparation meets opportunity.

Henry Hartman

- Follow the standardized procedure as mentioned in the administration manual/section.
- Practise the presentation of items in the way that was used to standardize the test. If the instructions are not followed exactly then the results of the developmental assessment would be unreliable and not comparable to the standardization norms in norm-referenced tests.

- Save time by administering all tests using the same equipment consecutively.
- Test sequence: generally use non-verbal items, e.g. form boards, before verbal items, e.g. comprehension questions. Also leave the locomotor scales to last as the child may not re-engage easily once he/she gets off the chair.
- Time taken to administer the test varies according to the skill of the examiner in selecting correct age range of items, ability to move efficiently between different scales to reach a basal/ceiling score, the child's concentration, cooperation, and ability.
- Do not hurry the test.

  ▶ Refer to 'administration' instructions on a regular basis.

Scoring

Score each item marking '√' for 'pass' and more discrete '–' for 'fail'.

- Know the principles of scoring. Get the baseline and 'ceiling' for each scale before moving to the next scale/domain wherever possible.
- Be careful in transferring and calculating the scores. Inaccuracy unsurprisingly leads to false interpretation and a wasted opportunity to help the child.
- ❶ Re-check if scores are contradictory to the clinical picture.
- Add the scores correctly for the test used to get 'RAW scores' for each scale.
- Obtain relevant standard scores, e.g. 'percentiles', 'z-scores', 'age equivalent/mental/developmental age', etc.
- The same record book may be used for reassessment of the same child at a later date, using a different coloured pen, to demonstrate new skills or regression.

Interpretation

> All human knowledge takes the form of interpretation. All meanings, we
> know, depend on the key of interpretation.

George Eliot

- ❶ Do not interpret the results in isolation.
- Take all the history, parental/school concerns, your general observations, and the child's interaction and behaviour into consideration before you draw conclusions. There is more to developmental testing than meets the eye. You could gain a great deal of information from testing situation from:
  - A: Attention, alertness.
  - B: Behaviours and mannerisms.
  - C: Cooperation/refusal, Concentration.
  - D: Dysmorphism, Disabilities.
  - E: Eye contact, Exploratory behaviour.
  - F: Family interaction with primary carer.
  - G: General aspects, e.g. spontaneous speech, articulation, etc.

- Relative discrepancies in the percentile score from a mean of the 50th percentile by >1 SD or by comparison between the subscales gives an indication of the *child's strengths, weaknesses, and profile.*
- Interpret the results obtained using item analysis of each scale—the *'construct model'* of the test, e.g. in GMDS-ER test:
  - *Practical reasoning* subscale would give information about moral/ social/everyday reasoning, sequential reasoning, analogical reasoning, concept formation, and general cognitive functioning (memory, attention, learned knowledge).
  - *Locomotor subscale* would give information on power, strength, agility, depth perception, gross visuomotor coordination, balance, etc.
- Each developmental disorder can create a specific profile or signature on developmental assessment (see ➜ p. 32–pp. 40–1).

Conclusions

In addition to the uses of developmental screening (see ➜ p. 32), detailed neurodevelopmental assessments help us by:

- Providing corroborative evidence for 'developmental diagnosis'.
- Identifying comorbidities/hidden disabilities, e.g. a child assessed for language delay could also show moderate/severe coordination difficulties.
- Giving an opportunity to identify additional features, e.g. sensory processing disorder, hypermobility, neurocutaneous markers, asymmetric weakness, hemihypertrophy, dysmorphic features, involuntary movements, etc.
- Alerting us to the need for further investigation of the child's circumstances when results are 'odd' or inconsistent, i.e. when profile/ scores contradict the history or clinical picture.

Tips for real-world developmental assessments

Starting points

Involving the child

Tips for 'real-world' developmental assessments

Starting points

- Having some information/knowledge about age-appropriate and current TV programmes, fads, toys, computer games, music, books, etc. will help you engage the child and provide conversational content.
- Be prepared to talk about school likes/dislikes, friendships, 'sleep overs', whether they are invited to play or parties, etc.
- Humour can be helpful.
- Consider having age-appropriate toy selection, drawing materials, puzzles, blocks, toy animals, etc. available to occupy the child while consulting the parent/carer so as only to use test equipment for assessment.
- Personally collect the child and parent from the waiting area. Watch the gait, disposition, parent–child interaction, etc.
- Warm up! Begin by introducing yourself to parent/carer, listen to their concerns/questions, while the child warms up to the new environment.
- Sighting shot! Place a box of ten bricks on the table. While introductions are going on, the child might start exploring, manipulating, and building with the bricks. You'll get an idea of where the child's development is and this may help you decide which test items you need to administer further.

Involving the child

- Introduce yourself to the child: say 'We are going to play some games, which you will enjoy. You will find some games easy and some difficult. Just do your best'.
- Establish rapport and maintain a play-like rapport. Smile. Compliment the child. Be opportunistic.
- Mind your language! Don't give a choice to the child by saying 'Would you like to . . .' or 'Can you do this for me?' Instead say 'Now it's your turn to do this and this'.
- Encourage. Praise the efforts of the child by saying 'keep going', 'good try', 'great effort', etc. But do not say whether their answer is right or wrong, as this could influence their score on a subsequent item.
- Sustain the child's attention by knowing your presentation well. Direct them to the equipment or test items you want them to play with. An appropriate testing environment (see ➔ p. 36) will help.
- If the child loses concentration or appears tired then move on to different scales or test items or give them a short break/food/drink accordingly. Do not show your dissatisfaction with the child's response.
- Administer tests or items that utilize his/her curiosity or interest of the moment.
- Observe, observe, observe! OWL approach = Observe, Wait, Listen. Observe for any unusual behaviours, mannerisms, carer–child interaction, engaged–withdrawn, impulsivity, overactivity, social interaction/disinhibition, etc. Listen for any spontaneous speech.

❶ Beware of the parent talking 'over' or for the child.

Involving parents/carers

- Always begin by asking parents what their 'concerns' are (see → p. 364).
- Parents should then sit out of the child's view.
- Involve them only where necessary, i.e. on the staircase/steps etc.
- If the child refuses to attempt a number of items repeatedly, then ask the parent/carer to administer those items according to your instructions.

Simple tests

- Goodenough–Harris 'Draw a man test' (general mental level 3–15 years, standardized in the 1980s).
- Verbal fluency, e.g. test by number of different types of 'food' child could say in 60 seconds; mean:
  - 6 years = 10 (SD 3).
  - 8 years = 11 (SD 3).
  - 10 years = 14 (SD 2).
  - 12 years+ (approximate adult levels) = 18 (SD 4).
- Describe a picture (note: naming, narrative, perception, articulation).
- Three-part instruction (most can manage by 4 years).
- Literacy/numeracy: check reading, reading comprehension, spelling, times tables, addition/subtraction, and writing. Levels of expected attainment strongly dependent upon age and quality of education.
- Copying shapes, e.g. Aston Index Test.
- Read analogue clock face, left–right, and other person left–right orientation.
- General screening questionnaires, e.g. 'Strengths and Difficulties'.
- Develop selection of simple tests that can be applied across age bands (i.e. describe a picture), and stick with it; if given to enough children in a consistent fashion you will in time develop a sense of what a broadly 'average' performance is for a given age.

Useful general questions for parents/carers

- How much do you think the child is behind other children in development?
- What do you think is the child's biggest problem?
- Have I seen a fair picture of what the child can do?
- How does he/she spend her time/interests/concentration?
- Does the child pretend or show imagination/humour? Could you give an example?

Gross motor milestones

- Gross motor skills involve the ability of humans to sit, stand, walk, run, jump, kick, climb, throw, catch, ride, swim, and undertake exercise, among others.
- Gross motor skills involve the use of large muscles in our core, arms, and legs.
- Gross motor skills are essential for mobility, independent living, self-care, undertaking exercise, participation in sports, and to maintain fitness.
- Assessment of a child's gross motor skills gives us information about his/her postural control, muscle tone, strength, agility, flexibility, balance, and visual–motor coordination.
- There is a wide variation in the acquisition of gross motor skills (Table 2.1).
- Delay in acquiring these milestones can occur in various neurodevelopmental disorders such as GDD/ID(see ➡ pp. 136–41), CP (see ➡ pp. 92–101), DCD (see ➡ pp. 146–9), myopathies (see ➡ p. 274), neuropathies, muscular dystrophies (see ➡ pp. 272–5), various genetic disorders/syndromes (see ➡ pp. 516–19), and following insult or trauma to the developing brain, among others.
- Identifying and addressing gross motor delays is important as delays can have an impact on child's development of fine motor skills, self-care skills, peer-relationships, ability to participate in exercise/sports, maintain fitness, engagement in learning, inclusion, and psychosocial well-being, among others.

Table 2.1 Gross motor milestones. These milestones should only be used as a guide to average development. There can be variation within normal development. These milestones do not replace the role of detailed 'neurodevelopmental assessment', which should be undertaken if there are concerns regarding a child's development or behaviour

0–3 months	• Supine: turns head side to side
	• Brings hands to midline
	• Prone: lift chin. Lifts head up momentarily
	• Prone: props on forearm, lifts head and face vertical
	• Pulled to sit: minimal head lag
	• Pushes with feet against hands
	• Kicks actively in baths
	• Rolls from side to back
	• Holds head steady briefly when held
3–6 months	• No head lag when pulled to sit
	• Rolls prone to supine or front to back
	• Followed by ability to roll back to front
	• Prone: pushes up on extended arms
	• Sitting: sits with trunk support
	• Sitting: sits with pelvic support
	• Later sits alone for a short time, can prop arms in front for support
	• Turns around when left on floor, i.e. pivots in prone/on front

Table 2.1 (Contd.)

6–9 months	• Can get into sitting position • Sits steady without support • Can put arms out to sides for balance • Crawls: tries vigorously to crawl • Crawls: then make progress moving forward or back • Commando crawls on hands and knees • Followed by crawl on all four limbs straightened, i.e. bear walks • Bounces when held • Stand: when held up • Pulls self to stand up • Can stand holding on to furniture
9–12 months	• Can pivot in sitting • Can climb on a low ledge or a step • Followed by ability to crawl up some stairs • Can side-step inside of cot or holding rails • Cruise around furniture holding both hands • Stand: with one hand led • Stand: for a few seconds on own • Walk: with two hands held • Walk: with one handheld
12–18 months	• Can climb into a low seat • Can climb some stairs, both up and down on all fours • Can stand up without support • Walk: arms high and out • Walk: able to walk independently • Walk: carrying a toy • Walk: backwards pulling a toy on a string • Can stoop to pick up a toy or object • Can run stiff-legged
18–24 months	• Can seat self in small chair • Run: start, stop • Followed by ability to run well • Kick: walks into ball • Kick: a small ball with demonstration • Kick: a ball on own • Stairs: can walk up and down, two feet to a step • Stairs: walk up one foot to each step with one handheld • Can jump off a step • Throw: a ball over arm • Can squat in play

(Continued)

Table 2.1 (*Contd.*)

2–3 years	• Kick: with force
	• Run: turn around obstacles
	• Can pedal a tricycle
	• Stairs: walks up with alternating feet, down 2 feet to a step
	• Can balance on one leg: momentarily
	• Stand and walk on tiptoe
	• Catch: large ball on extended arms
	• Can jump off the bottom step
	• Can jump in place
	• Can throw overhand
	• Can walk upstairs, holding rails with alternating feet
	• Stands with both feet on balance beam
3–4 years	• Stairs: walk or run up and down with alternating feet
	• Can balance on one leg for 3–5 seconds
	• Can hop
	• Can throw and catch: large ball, bounced ball to/from another person
	• Start using a bat
	• Can sit cross-legged on floor
	• Can walk on a straight line for 4–6 steps
	• Can run and kick a medium size ball
	• Can jump off 2 steps
4–5 years	• Can balance on one leg for 8–10 seconds
	• Can walk downstairs one foot to each step
	• Can walk heel-to-toe along a straight line
	• Large ball: can throw, catch, and bounce to self
	• Can hop on each foot for 3+ hops
	• Can broad jump 1–2 feet wide
	• Can bend and touch toes with knees straight
	• Can run fast outdoors
5–6 years	• Can run upstairs
	• Can jump off 3 steps
	• Can balance on each leg for 15–20 seconds
	• Can ride a bicycle
	• Tennis ball: can throw, catch, and bounce to self
	• Can jog at a steady pace in a playground
	• Can hop and skip
	• Can walk in a march, swinging arms with opposite legs
	• Can hop on one foot for 12–15 feet
	• Can skip using rope

(Continued)

Table 2.1 (*Contd.*)

6–8 years	• Can run downstairs
	• Can walk backward heel-to-toe
	• Can jump backwards
	• Can balance on one leg for 20+ seconds
	• Can throw a tennis ball up and catch it
	• Can hop and skip in an open area
	• Can jump off 4 steps
	• Tandem walks
	• Can skip with a rope 3+ skips
	• Can do somersaults

Fine motor milestones

- The ability of humans to write, draw, paint, feed, dress, compose music, use a keyboard, or write a code for artificial intelligence requires the use of hands that differentiate them from their closest evolutionary cousins, the chimpanzees.
- Fine motor skills involve the use of small muscles in our fingers, hands, and wrists.
- Fine motor skills are patterns which include reach, grasp, carry, and voluntary release, as well as more complex skills of in-hand manipulation, form perception, and bilateral coordination.
- The development of fine motor skills depends on adequate postural functions and sufficient visual-perceptual and cognitive development.
- There is a wide variation in the acquisition of fine motor skills (Table 2.2).
- Fine motor skills are essential for independent living, self-care, learning, and academic achievement.
- Delay in acquiring these milestones can occur in various neurodevelopmental disorders such as DCD (see ➜ pp. 146–9), ASD (see ➜ pp. 114–25), ADHD (see ➜ pp. 126–34), and ID (see ➜ pp. 136–41).
- Identifying and addressing these delays can prevent the development of secondary consequences for the child, such as disengagement from learning, low self-esteem, anxiety, and poor psychological health.

Table 2.2 Fine motor milestones. These milestones should only be used as a guide to average development. These milestones do not replace the role of detailed 'neurodevelopmental testing' which should be undertaken if there are concerns regarding a child's development or behaviour

0–3 months	• Infant can reflexively grasp things placed in their hands
	• He/she can focus eyes on parent/mother's face
	• They are beginning to open hands occasionally
	• They can have voluntarily grasp at 3 months
	• Extensor movements of limbs cause fingers and toes to fan out
3–6 months	• Infants are visually more alert
	• He/she can regard and look at their own hands when lying supine
	• They can bring hands into midline over their chest or chin
	• He/she can clasp and unclasp hands and press palms together
	• They can hold a rattle for a few moments
	• An infant can visually regard a rattle at the same time as holding or moving it
6–9 months	• An infant's eyes move in unison to follow activities across the room
	• Can be alert for a purpose and have developed controlled reach
	• Can grasp toys or objects within 15–30 cm using a palmar grasp
	• They can put objects in their mouth
	• He/she can pass a toy from one hand to another

Table 2.2 (*Contd.*)

9–12 months	• They can manipulate a toy by passing it from one hand to another
	• They can explore a toy by turning it over
	• Start pointing with the index finger at distant objects
	• Can pick small objects up between index and thumb (inferior pincer grasp)
	• Can release a toy by dropping but are not yet able to place a toy down voluntarily
12–18 months	• He/she can now pick-up small objects, e.g. a raisin, between the tip of their index finger and thumb (pincer grasp)
	• Can play pushing little cars along
	• Can play at rolling a ball
	• They are developing a right- or left-hand preference
	• Can hold one cube in each hand using three fingers (tripod grasp)
	• Can bang cubes together
	• Can build a tower of 2–3 cubes after a demonstration
	• Can scribble more freely
	• Can throw a ball towards a person
18–24 months	• Can use a spoon well
	• Can hold a cup and drink
	• Can do spontaneous to-and-fro scribble with either hand holding crayon/pencil in a fisted grasp
	• Can build a tower of 5–6 bricks
	• Can place pegs in a pegboard
	• Can turn several pages of a book at a time
	• Hand preference is becoming established
	• Can turn a doorknob
	• Can point with the index finger to demonstrate interest or demand objects out of reach
	• Can help actively to dress and undress
24–36 months	• Can build a tower of 6–10 bricks
	• Can imitate a vertical and horizontal line, copy a circle
	• Can do circular scribbles, holding pencil proximally with all fingers and thumb pointing downwards towards the tip of a pencil
	• Can pick up tiny objects accurately and quickly and place them down neatly
	• Can turn pages of a book one at a time
	• Can thread large wooden beads on a shoelace
	• Can cut with toy scissors
	• Beginning use of one hand consistently in most activities
	• Can roll, squeeze, or pull playdough
	• Can eat without assistance if food is chopped into manageable chunks

(Continued)

Table 2.2 (Contd.)

3–4 years	• Can build a tower of 8–10 bricks • Can build a bridge of three cubes from a model using two hands • Can manipulate clay material to make balls or cookies • Can hold a pencil in their preferred hand • Can copy a cross (+) • Can draw a person with a head and 3–4 body parts • Can handle scissors to snip paper • Can thread 6+ beads • Can undress without assistance
4–5 years	• Can build three steps with six cubes from a model • Can hold pencil distally between first two fingers and thumb with precise opposition of pads of thumb, index, and middle fingers • Can draw a person with head, trunk, legs, arms, and usually fingers • Can imitate their thumb touching each finger with either hand • Can copy a ladder • Can copy a square • Can wash their own hands and face with some assistance • Can do up their buttons • Can put their socks and shoes on • Can dress and undress with minimal or no assistance
5–6 years	• Can now copy a triangle • Can draw a picture of a house • Can copy several letters and even write a few letters spontaneously • Can write their first name • Can draw a person with a head, trunk, legs, arms, and features • Can cut a thin strip edge of the paper • Can brush their teeth without assistance • Can get a drink of water from the tap without help • Can wear a cardigan or topcoat unaided • Are able to pick up and replace tiny objects carefully • Are able to colour within the lines
6–8 years	• Can draw a person with features • Can draw a house with features • Can copy a window and a diamond • Could draw more complex and unfamiliar shapes • Can write their full name • Can use their dominant hand while stabilizing paper with their non-dominant hand • Can tie their shoelaces and can tie a double bowknot • Can bath or shower and dry themselves without assistance • Posts coins into a slot quickly and accurately • Thread beads onto a string quickly and accurately using in-hand manipulation to turn beads in fingertips

Development of vision/visual milestones

- The first few years of life are crucial for visual development (see ➔ pp. 202–8).
- Adequate stimulation of both eyes in the first 6–8 years of life is essential to achieve normal visual acuity as adults.
- Visual deprivation of one or both eyes from any reversible cause can result in amblyopia (lazy eye).

The various stages of visual development are listed in Table 2.3

Table 2.3 Stages of visual development

0–3 months	• Briefly holds gaze • Takes interest (stares) in surroundings • Blinks at bright lights • Tracks vertically and horizontally • Makes eye contact at 6–8 weeks • Fixes on mother's face
3–6 months	• Follows adults or moving objects with eyes across midline • Observes own hands • Displays interest in human faces • Briefly fixes and reaches for small objects
7–12 months	• Recognizes objects at home • Tracks vision across the room • Interested in pictures, and inspects toys • Enjoys hide-and-seek (recognizes partially hidden objects) • Responds to smiles and voices • Develops stranger anxiety
1–1½ years	• Enjoys picture books and points to pictures • Holds objects close to eyes to inspect
2–3 years	• Recognizes faces in photographs • Begins to inspect objects without touching them • Likes to watch moving objects, such as wheels on toy vehicle • Watches and imitates other children • 'Reads' pictures in books
3–4 years	• Copies patterns • Recognition of colours • Can close eyes on request and may be able to wink
4–5 years	• Draws recognizable person and house and names pictures • Uses eyes and hands together with increasing skill • Moves and rolls eyes expressively • Can place small objects into small openings • Demonstrates visual interest in new objects

Social–emotional and self-care milestones

- A child learns to communicate with their parent/caregiver socially and emotionally, well before they learn to communicate using speech and language.
- Social–emotional and self-care skills can give us an insight into a child's communicative intent, temperament, interpersonal skills, concept of self, self-care skills, and domestic skills (Table 2.4).
- As these milestones develop on a well-established trajectory, a good knowledge of 'social-emotional' milestones can help in identifying neurodevelopmental conditions such as ASD (see ➜ pp. 114–25) much earlier.
- Assessing children using these milestones as a guide forms an essential part of preventative health and development supervision visits by HVs.
- A delay or lack of development of several of these milestones in a child should guide the HV (see ➜ p. 32) or GP to refer for a neurodevelopmental assessment by a community/neurodevelopmental paediatrician.

Table 2.4 Personal–social milestones. These milestones should only be used as a guide to average development. These milestones do not replace the role of detailed 'neurodevelopmental assessment' which should be undertaken if there are concerns regarding a child's development or behaviour

0–3 months	• Can recognize their mother/parent • Develop their first observable social milestone, i.e. develop the ability to offer social smile in response to their parent's smile • Can follow a moving person at close distance with their eye gaze • Can bring their hand to their mouth
3–6 months	• Can now spontaneously smile at their parent • Can enjoy 'to and from' communication with sounds • Begin turn-taking with their parent using vocalizations • Can recognize primary caregivers by their smell and sight • Can greet their parent with squeals and vocalizations • Can hold their bottle briefly • Can respond to gentle calming when distressed. They learn to regulate their emotional stress with a sensitive and firm response from parent/caregiver
6–9 months	• Joint attention develops, i.e. can follow parent's gaze in the same direction as the object and then look back at parent/caregiver to share or acknowledge their experience • Gaze monitoring develops, i.e. they can follow an adult's gaze with their own • Effective attachment is beginning to be established with a responsive parent/caregiver. Hence, separation anxiety starts emerging with strangers or unfamiliar faces • Begin vocalizing to seek attention from their caregiver • Can hold their own drink bottle • Begin to finger-feed themselves • Can pull off their hat

Table 2.4 (Contd.)

9–12 months	• 'Proto-imperative pointing' is beginning to be formed. Can now request by pointing to ask for an item of interest and integrate their pointing with eye contact between the object and the parent
	• Secure attachment is formed with a primary caregiver. Hence, separation anxiety is established
	• Can put their arms up to be picked up
	• Can recognize and consequently respond to their own name being called
	• Can recognize self in a mirror, smile, and reach out to their image in the mirror
	• Can engage in interactive play with games such as 'peek-a-boo' and copies 'pat-a-cake' with a parent
	• Can give affection to their parent with a kiss, a cuddle, or snuggle up to them
	• Can use gestures such as waving 'bye-bye' to communicate needs and interests
	• Become interested in watching other children
	• Can drink from an open cup if held to lips
12–18 months	• Can engage in a 'solitary play' and can play away from a caregiver for a short while
	• 'Functional play' becomes well established, i.e. a child's manipulations become object specific rather than indiscriminate banging
	• 'Proto-declarative pointing' emerges at this stage when a child points with eye gaze coordination to show an object of interest to others
	• Enjoy sharing a book with parent/caregiver
	• Can respond to simple commands, e.g. 'Give me the spoon' and brings objects to show or give to their caregiver
	• Can use a spoon with some spilling. Can pick up and drink from a lidded cup
	• Can now remove sock/shoe or a garment
	• Can explore his/her surroundings independently and help with household chores or simple tasks
	• They become more aware of their own emotions and develop empathy for others. Can become upset if others cry or feel proud when applauded for helping with tasks
18–24 months	• They learn to partake in 'pretend play', e.g. talking on a toy phone or 'pat-a-cake'
	• 'Symbolic play', e.g. feeding a doll, is emerging
	• Can demonstrate the development of self-identity with concepts such as 'I' or 'Mine'. Hence, they become possessive of their own toys. Cannot share or play cooperatively or imaginatively with peers yet. Play is more alongside a parent or a peer, i.e. 'parallel play'
	• Can help put toys away on request. Imitate household chores
	• Can indicate toilet needs by pointing or gestures
	• Can help with dressing by putting their arms and legs through
	• Can use a spoon nicely. Can drink from an open cup
	• Can suck drinks through a straw

(Continued)

Table 2.4 (Contd.)

24–30 months	• Begin to share and join others briefly in a cooperative or imaginative play
	• 'Symbolic play' is now well established, e.g. ride a broomstick for a horse
	• Understanding of social etiquette is emerging, e.g. saying 'thank you'. They are now beginning to regulate their emotions by minimizing or exaggerating these according to the social setting
	• Know their gender and gender awareness is emerging
	• Can participate in simple group activities
	• Can use a fork and a spoon well
	• Can wash their hands and dry them
	• Can pull-off a tee shirt
30–36 months	• Cooperative play is emerging. Beginning to take turns in play
	• Can share their toys or an item with siblings/peers. Impulse control is emerging
	• Sensitive and thoughtful caregiving helps a child learn self-control, autonomy, initiative, and a sense of control
	• Can know their age
	• Many become toilet trained by this age
	• Can wear a dress, but they need help with buttons and zips
	• Can finish a meal unaided if food is cut into 'bite-sizes'
	• Can brush teeth with assistance
3–4 years	• 'Imaginative play', i.e. child's imagination, is doing the work versus design and function of the toy by playing with dolls. Their play can have a theme or a storyline
	• Learning to manage their aggression. Can share and cooperate without prompts
	• Become independent with their toileting needs. Can take themselves to the toilet in a setting familiar to them
	• Can wash their hands and face on their own
	• Can unbutton. Learning to button up
	• Can put their shoes on without laces
4–5 years	• Can play in small groups or with 1–2 peers, with turn-taking and joint goals. Can join in play with other children. Hence, time when peer relationship issues emerge
	• Can distinguish between imaginary and real games. Imaginary play is becoming more complex
	• Can give their family name or last name
	• Can brush their teeth without assistance
	• Can put on an overcoat or cardigan
	• Can fasten buckle of a shoe

(Continued)

Table 2.4 *(Contd.)*

5–6 years	• Can play with 3–4 peers. Have a special playmate. Can choose their friends and spend more time in their peer groups
	• Beginning to learn adult social skills such as praising others for their excellent work or apologizing for their unintended mistakes
	• Have developed an understanding to choose their clothes according to the weather, i.e. for summer/winter
	• Can follow simple rules and instructions. Hence, can now take part in competitive games
	• Demonstrate increasing social awareness, and most know their address by this age
	• Can spread with a knife
	• Can wash hands and face and dry them with no help
6–7 years	• Can relate more to a group of friends and, consequently, prefer to spend more time with them. There is an increasing understanding of relationships and disagreements
	• Can play board games with rules
	• Can distinguish between fantasy from reality
	• Develop an increased sense of their social self. Most should know their birthday date, month, and year
	• Can know their full address, and many know their postcodes too
	• Have become adept at dressing and undressing completely, without help
	• Can lay the table for dinner with some supervision
7–8 years	• Can understand rules and regulations. Learn from their mistakes. Moral understanding of right or wrong is becoming established
	• Show a deeper understanding of responsibilities. Can do homework on their own
	• Have developed a better understanding of relationships. Can now help others/younger children
	• Prefer to spend more time with children of same gender. Many have found a best friend. Spending time with peers and friends becomes more important than spending time with family
	• Can delay their gratification. Can wait for their turn
	• Can shampoo hair, and have a bath or shower on own
	• Can lay the table completely without supervision. Can tie shoelaces

Speech and language milestones

- *Homo sapiens* have evolved and emerged as the most dominant species of all on this planet, because of their critical ability to communicate, cooperate, and coordinate with each other using speech and language.
- 'Speech' is our ability to produce recognizable sounds using coordinated actions of muscles present in our vocal cords, palate, tongue, lips, and jaw.
- 'Language' is a communication system or a set of shared rules by which people express and share their ideas meaningfully. A delay or disorder could be due to difficulty in understanding what others are saying (receptive language) or problems sharing one's intention and thoughts using the spoken form (expressive language).
- Delay in speech and language can impact a child's ability to share and express ideas, socially interact with peers, participate in play, and learn.
- Language delay during preschool years has been shown to affect confidence, self-esteem, engagement in learning, and could have a long-term impact on a child's learning.
- Assessment of speech and language skills (see ➲ pp. 404–6) gives information about a child's receptive language, expressive language, linguistic and applied knowledge, verbal reasoning, auditory memory, and conceptualization (Table 2.5).
- Speech and language delay can occur in several neurodevelopmental disorders such as GDD (see ➲ p. 30), isolated speech/language delay, intellectual disability (ID)/LD (see ➲ pp. 136–41), ASD (see ➲ pp. 114–25), ex-prematurity, hearing impairment (see ➲ pp. 168–9), speech dyspraxia (see ➲ pp. 402–3), DCD (see ➲ pp. 146–9), and CP (see ➲ pp. 92–101).

Table 2.5 Speech and language milestones. These milestones should only be used as a guide. These milestones do not replace the role of detailed 'neurodevelopmental testing' which should be undertaken if there are concerns regarding a child's development or behaviour

0–3 months	• Cry for food, comfort, and company
	• Can listen to a bell
	• One-syllable cooing
	• Search for sound with head movements
	• Can make two different kinds of sounds
3–6 months	• Cooing and gurgling
	• Can make four different kinds of sounds
	• Developing two-syllable babble
	• Can shout for attention
	• Can listen to conversations
6–9 months	• Can have singing tones
	• Like jingles and rhymes
	• May have developed one word that is meaningful, e.g. dada, mama
	• Can have 4+-syllable babbled phrases
	• Know own name and respond on calling
	• Can shake head for a 'no'

Table 2.5 (Contd.)

9–12 months	<ul><li>Can have a babbled monologue when on their own</li><li>Most of them can now use 2–3 words meaningfully</li><li>Can have babbled conversations</li><li>Can respond to 'no'</li><li>Many develop a context-dependent understanding of language</li><li>Comprehension of everyday words is increasing</li></ul>
12–18 months	<ul><li>Can have babbled sentences with some clear words</li><li>Can use up to 12 words in context with meaning</li><li>Can identify 4–6 objects and name a couple of them</li><li>Can obey simple requests, e.g. 'Give me the spoon'</li><li>Can understand simple questions, e.g. 'Where is your cup?'</li><li>Can know 3–6 body parts and can point to them</li><li>Enjoy picture book with simple stories, rhymes, and songs</li></ul>
18–24 months	<ul><li>Can point to pictures in a book when named</li><li>Can understand many single words, nouns, and verbs</li><li>Learning new words regularly and can have up to 50 words</li><li>Can put two-words together, e.g. daddy come, more drink</li><li>Can listen to stories</li><li>Can identify several objects and name some of them</li></ul>
2 years	<ul><li>Can use 2–3-word phrase to talk or ask for things</li><li>Can use words that contain k, g, m, p, b, t, d, and n, sounds</li><li>Often word endings are omitted</li><li>But family and friends can understand their speech</li><li>Can name several objects and can ask for them by name</li><li>Can define a couple of objects by use, e.g. 'What is a cup for?' They could say 'drink'</li></ul>
2.6 years	<ul><li>Speech has many sound simplifications</li><li>Hence, speech is understood by familiar adults</li><li>Can use words with 'f', 's', 'sh', and 'ch' sounds</li><li>Can use sentences of 5–6 words</li><li>Can use some pronouns (me, he, she)</li><li>Can understand basic concepts such as big/little, on/under</li></ul>
3 years	<ul><li>Increasing clarity in speech and language</li><li>Hence, they can be understood most of the time by strangers</li><li>They begin to ask 'why' questions</li><li>Can tell a story</li><li>Can have a vocabulary of 500+ words</li><li>They have a word for most things</li><li>Beginning to understand 'yesterday/tomorrow'</li></ul>

(Continued)

Table 2.5 (Contd.)

4 years	• Can speak in fluent sentences
	• Can converse and explain at a simple level
	• Can talk about things they have done and will do
	• Can tell stories in their play
	• Can answer simple questions, e.g. who, what, and where
	• Can still make errors, especially with the past tense, e.g. falled
	• Can understand more 'time' words (morning, evening)
	• Their speech is intelligible but may have errors with blending consonants (sp, bl, gr) and sh/ch
5 years	• Can pay close attention to a story and answer questions relating to it
	• Can understand most of what is said at school and at home
	• Can communicate readily with peers and adults
	• Many have full adult grammar
	• Can have a good reciprocal conversation
	• Most speech is correct, with only some minor errors that do not affect intelligibility
	• Can still have difficulties with speech sounds 'th', 'r', 's', or 'z'
6 years	• Can answer comprehension questions such as 'What should you do if ...?'
	• Can know 8–10 colours
	• Know 20+ capital letters
	• Can use the preposition 'above'
	• Begin to master exceptions to grammatical rules
	• Can understand passive tense
	• Can give directions
	• Can ask/answer factual and inferential questions
	• Can answer complex how, who, why, when questions
	• Can take turns in conversations
	• Can listen for sustained period of time
7 years	• Can follow a series of instructions without the need for repetition
	• Can use language to problem solve and talk about their feelings
	• Can rephrase a statement if not understood
	• Can ask for clarification if they do not understand
	• Know their full address
	• Can know their birthday
	• Most have one special school friend
8 years	• Begin to understand and use idioms
	• Can use clear and subject-related vocabulary
	• Can explain what has been learned
	• Can repeat a 16-syllable sentence
	• Can describe a picture with many descriptive words
	• Can give synonyms and categories in word definitions
	• Begin to understand jokes and riddles

Cognition milestones

Cognition milestones

- Assessment of a child's 'cognition' involves looking into the child's listening, thinking, understanding, problem-solving, reasoning (moral/everyday/social), learning, and remembering (memory and learnt knowledge) skills.
- It is important to assess a child's cognition and identify any delays, as cognitive delays can affect all other areas of development and learning. A knowledge of cognitive milestones (Table 2.6) helps in identifying the presence and degree of delay.
- Cognitive delay is central to the neurodevelopmental disorders such as GDD (see ⮕ p. 30) and LD/ID (see ⮕ pp. 136–41), however, cognitive delay can also be an important comorbidity in disorders such as CP, ASD (see ⮕ pp. 114–25), ADHD (see ⮕ pp. 126–34), DCD (see ⮕ pp. 146–9), and developmental learning disorder (DLD) (see ⮕ pp. 142–5), among others.
- The way the child thinks in each stage is different. The process of development is marked by a gradual decrease in egocentrism (being able to see only one aspect of a situation). The child constructs knowledge through actions then later mental actions (operations).
- Biological adaptation: cognition is a form of adaptation to the environment through two complementary processes:
  - Assimilation (incorporating new knowledge into existing).
  - Accommodation (changing cognitive structures).
- Broadly, stages of cognitive development are as follows:
  - Object permanence.
  - Capacity for representation.
  - Symbolic language (signs/numbers/letters).
  - Decrease in egocentricity.
  - Formal operations (12 years onwards): ability to think about thinking—metacognitive activity/abstract thinking.

Table 2.6 Cognition milestones. These milestones should only be used as a guide to average development. These milestones do not replace the role of detailed 'neurodevelopmental assessment' which should be undertaken if there are concerns regarding a child's development or behaviour

0–3 months	• Recognizes mother
	• Can follow face
	• Grasps rattle when given
	• Gazes at black and white objects
	• Can look at a toy on the table
	• Visually explores environment
	• Can follow large highly contrasting objects
	• Reaches for parent's face
	• Follows objects moved in circle while lying on back

Table 2.6 (Contd.)

3–6 months	• Shows interest in toy • Reaches for a ring or a rattle • Grasps a rattle or a toy • Can shake a rattle • Passes toy/rattle from hand to hand • Can mouth objects • Can regard and look at mirror image • Stares longer at stranger faces than familiar ones • Turns head to look for dropped cube or a toy • Removes cloth on face • Can bang toys
6–9 months	• Finds a toy hidden under a cup • Observe cubes in each hand • Manipulates 2 objects or bricks at once • Tears/crumples a tissue paper • Interested in a toy car • Can explore different aspects of a toy • Casting, i.e. throws objects to the floor • Can ring a bell • Looks for object after it falls silently to the floor • Can pull a string to obtain an attached ring or a toy that is out of reach
9–12 months	• Holds pencil and can make random marks on paper • Plays with a brick box, takes lid off/bricks out • Unwraps toy under a cloth • Interested in pictures in a book • Can complete single-piece form board • Responds to simple commands, e.g. 'Give me the fork' • Tries to put cube in a cup or box • Rattles spoon in cup • Can lift the lid off box and remove bricks inside • Can play pushing toy cars along
12–18 months	• Identifies 4–5 objects • Knows function of objects, e.g. comb for hair, spoon to eat, etc. • Can obey simple requests, e.g. 'Give me the car' • Can replace bricks back into the box and put lid on • Can complete two-circle form board • Enjoys looking through a book with an adult • Can turn several pages of a book • Can dangle a ring by string • Rattles spoon in cup • Lifts box lid to find toy • Can find a hidden toy under covers

(Continued)

Table 2.6 (Contd.)

18–24 months	• Can complete a three-shape form board
	• Can complete a shape form board rotated
	• Can copy horizontal and vertical stroke with pencil
	• Can open a screw toy
	• Can make a tower of 5–7 bricks
	• Can match pairs of objects
	• Can match an object to a picture
	• Show use of familiar objects
	• Can listen to stories
	• Begin to cooperate in play
24–30 months	• Matches objects to appropriate pictures
	• Matches colours
	• Can match shapes
	• Can repeat single digits on request
	• Can repeat two digits on request, e.g. 2–5, 8–6
	• Can count to 3
	• Can compare sizes, i.e. big and small
	• Can point to pictures in a book
30–36 months	• Can count up to 4 correctly
	• Can talk about what he/she did
	• Knows gender
	• Can play well with other children
	• Assists with small household tasks on request
	• Can notice and point to small details in pictures
	• Can point to self in photos
	• Can point to body parts according to function, e.g. 'What do you see with …?'
	• Can define 1–2 objects by use, e.g. what is a cup for?
36–48 months	• Can compare two lines for length
	• Can compare two brick towers for height
	• Can draw a 3–4-part person
	• Can follow a three-step command
	• Can count up to 10 correctly
	• Moral reasoning, e.g. 'Is it right or wrong to hit someone?'—answers correctly
	• Uses 'why' and 'how' questions
	• Can draw a 2–3-part person
	• Understands big and little, long and short, more and less
	• Knows own age
	• Answers some comprehension questions, e.g. 'What should you do if you feel cold?'

(Continued)

Table 2.6 (Contd.)

4–5 years	• Can draw a 7–8-part person
	• Can count correctly up to 15
	• Social reasoning emerging, e.g. 'Which costs more money, a watch or a drink?'—answers correctly
	• Knows 6+ colours
	• Knows one or two parts of his/her address
	• Understands functional concepts, e.g. use of appliances
	• Understands concept of time, i.e. past/present
	• Can answer question regarding materials, e.g. 'What is a house made of?'
	• Answers some opposites correctly, e.g. 'A boy is big, a baby is ...?'
	• Points to letters and numbers when named
5–6 years	• Can draw a 10–12-part person
	• Knows number of fingers on both hands put together
	• Can count backwards from 10
	• Counts up to 30
	• Knows ten colours
	• Can identify ten colours
	• Knows most sounds/letters
	• Knows morning and afternoon
	• Can write first name
	• Can explain about an incident at school
	• Can name many days of the week
	• Can understand seasons
	• Knows many parts of address
	• Can identify coins/money
	• Knows which costs more, e.g. a bicycle or a ball?
6–7 years	• Can do single-digit addition and subtraction
	• Begins to spell out words/read few sentences
	• Begins to read words
	• Can count backwards from 15
	• Can name all the days of the week in correct order
	• Knows 'directions' and 'sides of a body', e.g. left hand/right leg
	• Can draws 12–14-part person
	• Count up to 30
	• Can do simple addition and subtraction
	• Can write full name
	• Can sound out regularly spelled words
	• Knows some similarities and differences, e.g. 'How are a fish and a dog different?'

(Continued)

Table 2.6 (*Contd.*)

7–8 years	• Can count backwards from 30
	• Can read sentences (without unusual words) more fluently
	• Can repeat 5 digits, e.g. 4–7–1–9–6 forward on request
	• Can repeat 3 digits backwards, e.g. 5–2–9, answer 9–2–5
	• Can arrange 4–5 pictures in correct sequence and tell a story
	• Can draw a person or house with use of creativity and imagination
	• Starts 'reading to learn' rather than just 'learning to read'
	• Can now do two-place addition and subtraction
	• Can answer many comprehension questions, e.g. 'What should you do if you were lost?'
	• Enjoys reading independently
	• Knows full address
	• Knows birthday

Warning signs: 'red flags' in child development

- Just like in many other aspects of life, there are 'red flags' in the field of child development too. Hence, it is essential to know these red flags, as being forewarned is forearmed.
- A lack of awareness of these warning signs/red flags in children's development, is hampering early identification of neurodevelopmental disorders such as ASD (see ➲ pp. 114–25), ADHD (see ➲ pp. 126–34), dyspraxia (see ➲ pp. 402–3), and many others.
- Each red flag listed in Table 2.7 would be of some concern. In the absence of anything else, they may just need continued observation or a discussion with the HV (see ➲ pp. 676–7) or GP. However, the presence of more than one red flag in an individual domain, or many red flags across more than one aspect, deserves prompt attention and an assessment.
- Early identification is crucial in optimizing outcome. Early identification helps in accessing appropriate educational interventions, family support, medical treatment of associated conditions such as sleep difficulties, inattention, and anxiety.

Table 2.7 'Red flags' in child development

Gross motor development	• Has a floppy or limp body posture compared to other children of the same age
	• Has stiffness in arms and or legs
	• Reduced movements of arms or legs
	• Uses one side of the body in preference to the other, especially <18 months
	• Is very clumsy or poorly coordinated when compared with peers of the same age, e.g. gait is wide or dyskinetic
	• Difficulties in keeping balance while sitting, walking, and playing or frequent falling
	• Involuntary or abnormal movements
Fine motor and vision development	• Turns tilts or holds head in an unusual position when trying to look at or follow an object
	• Seems to have difficulty finding or picking up small objects dropped on the floor
	• Lacks pincer grasp even after 10–12 months of age
	• Has tremor in limbs
	• Rubs eyes frequently
	• Eyes appear to be crossed or turned in or out
	• Closes one eye when trying to look at distant objects
	• Brings objects too close to eyes to see
	• One or both eyes appear abnormal in size
	• Difficulty in manipulating small objects after 3 years of age

Table 2.7 (Contd.)

Hearing and language development	• Cannot chew or choke on food or drink • Dribbles excessively • Does not startle to loud noises • Resists loud sounds, e.g. hand dryers, by covering hands over ears • Ears appear small or deformed • Talks in a very loud or incredibly soft voice • Seems to have difficulty responding when called from across the room • Does not make sounds in response to others after 12 months • Turns body so that the same ear is always turned towards the sound • Has difficulty understanding simple sentences after 3 years of age • Fails to develop sounds or words that would be appropriate at his/her age • Little variation in tone, intonation, pitch, or rhythm of speech
Social interaction and communication development	• Avoids eye contact with others • Lack of reciprocal social smile • Inability to communicate using pointing, facial expressions, and gestures, • Poor attention or inability to stay focused on an activity • Focuses on unusual objects for extended periods or observes them from unique angles • Enjoys these distinct activities more than interacting with other children or parents • Does not seek love and approval from a caregiver or parent • Lack of sharing interest or enjoyment with others • Preference to play alone • Withdraws or spends time 'in a world of their own' • Does not respond to his/her name being called • Lack of social anticipation • Gets unusually frustrated when trying to do simple tasks • Difficulty in seeing a coherent whole, instead focus on small features in a picture • Dislikes hugs, kisses, cuddles, and close physical contact • Mis-judges personal space • Frequently interrupts or intrudes on others
Behaviour/ personality development	• Unusual motor mannerisms, e.g. hand flapping, spinning, staring into space, rocking, or tiptoeing • Restricted range of interests and activities, e.g. playing with a single toy or minimal range of toys • Difficulty in coping with change or abnormal reaction to a change in routine • Displays aggressive or uncooperative behaviours • Is significantly overactive or oppositional for their age • Displays temper tantrums or violent behaviours daily • Shows unusual attachments to toys, objects, or parts of objects • Does not play with the toys in a way they are designed for • Spends a lot of time lining things up or putting things in a particular order

Early intervention

Early intervention maximizes the opportunity for the child to achieve his/her potential. Subsequent to the developmental diagnosis, a paediatrician can refer a child to a variety of different resources with the following aims:
- Involve appropriate therapy services specifically tailored to meet the needs of the child.
- Provide information, support, and advice to families to enhance the child's development.

The early intervention resources/services can include any number of the following:
- Physiotherapy (see ➋ pp. 374–6).
- Postural management services (see ➋ pp. 392–3).
- Occupational therapy (see ➋ pp. 390–1).
- Speech and language therapy (see ➋ pp. 402–3).
- Psychology (see ➋ pp. 412–13).
- Counselling services (see ➋ p. 366).
- SEN services (see ➋ p. 656).
- Audiology (see ➋ p. 178).
- Ophthalmology and orthoptics (see ➋ p. 204).
- Assistive technology (see ➋ pp. 388–9 and pp. 392–3) (wheelchair, keyboard, etc.).
- Community nursing (see ➋ p. 681).
- Dietician and nutritionists (see ➋ pp. 436–7).
- Respite services (see ➋ p. 476).
- Social services for benefits, allowances, and housing adaptations (see ➋ pp. 682–3).
- Orthopaedic services (gait analysis, spasticity/dystonia treatment/botulinum toxin, etc. (see ➋ pp. 526–8)).
- Dentist (see ➋ pp. 464–5).

Why is an early intervention programme important?

Early intervention is important for various reasons:
- Early enablement has better results/outcomes when compared to later intervention.
- A delay in one area (e.g. vision) can affect other developmental areas (e.g. gross and fine motor coordination, social interactions, etc.).
- Late/inadequate intervention can result in poor self-esteem, educational difficulties, disengagement from learning, difficulties with inclusion/integration into mainstream school/society, poor psychosocial health, and poor life outcomes. Early intervention would improve outcomes for child, family, and society.

Further resources

Department of Education. Special educational needs and disability (SEND): detailed information: ℘ https://www.gov.uk/topic/schools-colleges-childrens-services/special-educational-needs-disabilitiesDisability Matters: ℘ https://councilfordisabledchildren.org.uk/resources-and-help Get Your Rights: ℘ http://www.getyourrights.org/GOV.UK. Help if you have a disabled child: ℘ https://www.gov.uk/help-for-disabled-childNHS Choices: ℘ http://www.nhs.uk

Brain plasticity and organic brain health in the growing child

By all elementary appearances, the brain appears to be substantially physically 'adult' in most respects within 1–3 years after birth. The notion that the 'development' of brain wiring is substantially completed over the first 15–30 months of life has been a predominating view in paediatric medicine for more than half a century. By that perspective, the capacity to modify the wiring of brain circuits was believed to be primarily limited to a 'critical period' during the late fetal/infant/toddler period.

In actuality, *no human organ undergoes a more important or more dramatic progression of physical and functional change across the span of childhood than the brain*. That change progression, largely occurring on an almost invisible and unreconstructible microscale, differs from that expressed in every other human organ because it effectively defines the operational powers of the organ (and its possessor), and because its functional evolution has large-scale implications for the organic health of the brain and body.

In actuality:

- Modification by use is the brain's 'big trick'. Its emergent, refined powers are a direct product of that use.
- Every brain is a continuous work in progress, subject to large-scale plastic revision at any age, by use.
- There is great variability in the quality of young-life experiences impacting that neurological progression—which translates to substantially unrecognized large-scale variability in organic brain health and in neurobehavioral performance.
- *Brain plasticity is bidirectional.* Following the rules that govern plasticity, and with an understanding of the positive factors or unfortunate factors that impact the course of plasticity-driven neurological change, *a child's experiences can just as easily enable and empower—or disable and degrade—their neurological progression.* A large proportion of modern children have the experiential scales tilted in their young lives in a neurologically disabling and degrading direction.
- The neurological struggles of those unfortunate children (which, untreated, can last a lifetime) are not their fault.
- *Brain plasticity is bidirectional.* Remember? That means that the limitations and distortions in the brains of most struggling children can be substantially overcome by re-engaging their brain with appropriate forms of remedial neurologically targeted exercise.

Here, we'll consider some of the practical implications of the brain's native capacity to physically and functionally revise itself by use, described from the perspective of a translational neuroscientist whose attention has been focused on harnessing brain plasticity to improve, sustain, and secure organic brain health and to grow the operational capabilities of every child.

When does brain plasticity begin?

Studies in animal models born at a relatively young gestational age and studies in human fetuses and newborns have shown that the brain begins to progressively revise itself *in utero* on the basis of its experiences and primitively generated actions at about the beginning of the third trimester *in utero*. The demonstration that the child selectively responds at birth to the modulation of their mother's voice is one (of several) demonstrated consequence(s) of that prenatal plasticity.

We exposed animal infants to intense sounds whose gestational age matched a human infant 1–2 months prior to normal delivery, simulating the application of a modulated-low frequency ultrasound procedure used to gain a refined image of the head and brain *in utero*. Without damaging hearing, that intense speech-frequency range sound exposure had a dramatically negative impact on the development of the processing machinery of the young postnatal hearing brain—a clear example of the brain's capacity for expressing 'negative' as well as 'positive' prenatal brain plasticity. Without later experiential correction, that limited very early intense-sound exposure resulted in a large-scale degradation of sound processing that endured into the animal's adulthood.

Scientists who have tracked the progressions of the pseudo-random movements of the fetus *in utero* have shown that they progress in movement elaboration and fluidity as a function of gestational age. The brain is almost certainly associating and 'mapping' sensory feedback in relation to limb and body position and motion and elaborating movement control itself in this developmental epoch, as an important prerequisite for all later organized involuntary and voluntary motor behaviours.

From the perspective of the progressive development of the powers of the brain, birth is, of course, an environmental shock for that newborn baby. The eyes open to light and visual motion. A world of slowly modulated sounds is replaced by a cacophony, now including highly dynamic acoustic signals expressed by the airborne sounds of the child's native language. All of those advances in movement organization achieved in the weight-supported fluidic environment of the uterus now have to be recalibrated to deal with the forces of gravity in a new world without the same movement resistances or restraints.

Early postnatal plasticity: a rapid progression to 'adult' (outcomes-controlled) plasticity

With their 'arrival' at birth, enabled by the greater possibilities represented by the 'real world', brain remodelling advanced by the behavioural experiences of the infant takes off—if all is well—'like a rocket'.

In an initial postnatal epoch, the 'plasticity switch' is continuously *on*. Change-enabling 'neuromodulators' are being continuously produced and released, and *any* input drives connectional modifications in competitive brain networks. The rapid competitive establishment of brain circuits that selectively represent different frequently occurring sound elements—the 'phonemes'—of the infant's native language resulting from their mere exposure to several hundred thousand words, is a beautiful case in point. Note that this elegant competitively generated 'sorting' occurs well before the infant neurologically associates any specific meaning with those word-sounds. Note that in about 85% of all children born on the planet, the analytic machinery in the hearing brain selectively evolves to now accurately and highly selectively represent the modulatory and phonemic and sound-progression structures of that infant's native language in high fidelity, be it English, Hebrew, Tagalog, Urdu, or any one of the other 7000 world languages.

Under a burden of inherited gene expression limitations, impoverished language exposure, abuse/stress, and/or genetics, the remaining 15% of children acquire native language skills 'the hard way', i.e. syllable by syllable and word by word, without accurate intra-syllabic phonemic resolution. Because translation by letter in written languages is largely phoneme based, without correction these children shall later struggle to learn to read and (again, without correction) shall likely be limited for life in speech reception and production accuracy and fluency.

Across this epoch, the machinery that controls and enables plasticity (which is also plastic) advances, to progressively establish *control* over neurological remodelling processes. By the age of 2 or 3 years, the plasticity in most (not all) forebrain areas is (are) enabled by state-dependent neuromodulator release. The 'plasticity switch' was always 'on' at an earlier age. Indeed, it was even 'on' when the baby slept. Now, it is usually 'off', turned 'on' *only* when specific neurological contingencies are met.

You can think of the transition from that early postnatal period to this second epoch as an advance from 'anything goes' competitive brain remodelling, to an older-age, life-long epoch of regulated, purpose-driven, brain-controlled functional remodelling.

In effect, the older child's brain only permits change when it interprets a just-happened event to be 'good for itself'. It records, immediately after the fact, surprising, unexpected events that it is alerted (by 'surprise'-generated noradrenaline release, broadly amplifying neural excitability) to assign a valence to:

- Specifically attended inputs and actions.
- Inputs and actions adjudged to be important, or successful (and therefore self-rewarded by the brain).
- Inputs or actions followed by hedonic 'rewards', or by 'punishments'.

These enabling conditions for change all express the release of modulatory neurotransmitters (primarily acetylcholine, dopamine, and noradrenaline) that collectively 'throw that plasticity switch' to 'on'.

Plasticity 101

As noted earlier, *all* postnatal neurological progressions are shaped by our behavioural experiences. Across most of the latter half of the last century, most scientists and medical authorities viewed the first year or two of life to be a final epoch of neurological (brain) 'development'. That view primarily stemmed from three classes of studies:

- Studies of the primary visual cortex (V1) documented a rapid developmental progression that resulted in a stable pattern of representation of the inputs from the two retinae in the binocular-vision area of the occipital neocortex, and in the advance of neuronal connections and neurons themselves to an apparently 'mature' status. This basic machinery was believed to be unalterable beyond that narrow 'maturational' window (a 'critical period') by even exaggerated variations in experiential histories.
- 'Synaptic plasticity', documented in detail in the 1970s and 1980s in *in vitro* brain slices, or by time-controlled manipulations of associated inputs *in vivo*, was shown to be strongly expressed in very young postnatal brain tissue of intact brains, but only weakly expressed in older animals.
- The major white matter tracks distributing information in the brain could be rerouted by a variety of manipulations in very young animals, but that rerouting was very limited in scale in older postnatal brains.

This 'perfect storm' of misleading observations led to the conclusion that that brain was 'hard-wired' (mature; aplastic) after the first year (or two, or three) of postnatal life. Subsequent studies have shown that:

- Visual input 'sorting' to generate a balanced, overlapping representation of the two eyes—crucially supporting binocular vision—is anomalous, in the cerebral cortex. Everywhere else (and in the visual cortex, if you examine the potential to change in other ways) local-scale older age plasticity abounds.
- The brain rapidly matures to take control of its plasticity as a function of the status of attentional processes, and of the novelty of and the outcomes of its experiences. Those requisite conditions for enabling that we noted earlier—e.g. attention to the task, behavioural outcomes success, hedonic rewards, and 'punishments'—were not met in those *in vitro* or isolated *in vivo* preparations.
- While changes in the wiring of the young brain evolve from a macro to a micro scale, they continue apace, throughout life.
- Quadrillions of moments of change expressed by synaptic strengthening or weakening or by synaptogenesis give rise to our evolving and continuously changing operational personhoods, generate the 'self', and support and elaborate its executive actions.
- Every acquired or refined skill and ability is a direct product of neurological remodelling. Our operational personhoods are the grand result of this connectional revision.
- Neurological remodelling all across the span of childhood (and beyond) is a *primary* determinant of both organic brain and general health.

Because the progression of neuroplastic remodelling largely accounts for the development of the operational child under your care, and because their history of neurological remodelling largely accounts for the organic health of their brain and body, it is important that you understand how these last three decades of brain science have revised our informed perspective about the origins of neurobehavioral capabilities, about a child's personhood, and about brain-to-body impacts on general health. Let's consider those issues in a little more detail.

Creating a person

Consider what the normal brain achieves, across the first several years of life.

First, it creates a model of that specific world that the child just happens to have been born into. That world is chock full of tools and challenges that no child had to master or learn about just a few decades (much less a few centuries) ago.

Note that generally acquired abilities in this twenty-first century—like facile reading, mathematics, electric or electronic tool usage, bicycle riding, automobile driving, or keyboard usage—were a rarity or non-existent a few centuries ago. Universal reading acquisition in child populations—initiated in the eighteenth century—was an especially important advance because it added to humans' neurological advantages attributable to language that distinguish us from our advanced primate cousins. Aural language had enabled a second way (beyond sensory recognition) to identify, label, and manipulate the neurological representations of the things and actions of our world. Writing, and pictorial representation in electronic devices, added a third, then a fourth way. As deeply engrained skills, they collectively advanced the power and reliability of our neurological operations, contributing substantially to our species' rapid, collective neurological evolution.

Second, it has to advance its 'machinery' to refine and to control all of its operations and actions in that world, achieved via the acquisition and progressive mastery of the innumerable skills and abilities that define every individual's operational personhood.

Third, it has to create a 'captain'—a 'self'—and establish its agency—its executive powers—to establish control of the wilful operations of the brain. It accomplishes that through billions of moments of what become wired associations of our sensations, feelings, thoughts, and actions to their source—*our self*.

Fourth, it creates the attachments that tie us to our clan, stabilizing the lines of social and educational inculcation and support that are so crucial for the child's individual thriving and survival. This association to other heavily rewarding experiential sources is a natural extension of the child's 'self-creation'. From, those changes, the brain is set up to establish a rich source of experiential change in the social and emotion cognition and control domains.

The brain has to accomplish all of these things by physically revising the strengths and numbers of its synaptic connections, and by engendering other changes (e.g. selective myelination, changes in synaptic receptor subunits, elaboration of local circuit processes, etc.) that impact our neurological powers and efficiencies.

The fundamental strategy that it uses to accomplish all of these incredible things is to encode—and organize its coded representations of—the million-and-one things and actions it encounters in its world by:
- Selectively amplifying (or reducing) the strengths and by elaborating (or simplifying) the richness and extents of synaptic connections.
- Growing the cooperativity of neuronal populations in the elementary processing units in the cerebral cortex (its >350 million 'mini-columns'), a crucial step for increasing the brain's representational encoding accuracy, reliability, 'sampling rate', and operational speed.
- Further increasing that representational accuracy and reliability by coupling myelination and other time-dependent processes to that growing micro-circuit coordination and cooperativity. Myelinated circuit connections are faster. Faster connections are a key to reliable, high-accuracy signal transmission. They are a crucial asset for supporting 'working memory', which is requisite for generating associative and executive powers in the brain. As a rule, faster brains operating in 'high fidelity' are 'smarter'.

This remodelling is all engendered in competitive networks that are progressively refining their processing of information in the domains of place and time and intensity. The fundamental 'Hebbian' rule that applies[1]: 'What fires together, wires together.' The brain is evolving its powers by co-strengthening any synaptic action, moment by moment in time, that has contributed to performance success, or that has been otherwise adjudged to be important enough to be recorded for posterity. Plasticity is a time-coincidence-based and brain importance-based 'sorter'. By induced changes, all of those 'important' co-concurring things that define a specific thing or an action in our world are integrated to represent the whole. Because the world is structured, as we move across it our brain translates and records that structure in the domain of time. Put another way, it creates a structural landscape in which things that 'belong' (are predicted to be) in adjacency in time, in place, and in intensity are connectional 'neighbours' in place, in time, and in intensity in your rewired brain.

The neuromodulators that control plasticity in the older brain act together to enable change:
- *Noradrenaline* release, triggered by novelty and elevating arousal ('attentiveness'), broadly amplifies cortical excitability, which increases brain-change (learning) rates.
- *Acetylcholine* release more selectively amplifies the responses of all inputs in a network zone that is engaged in a behaviour, establishing the possibility of remodelling for any of the mostly silent inputs in that zone that turn out to contribute to performance success (and reward) at the new task at hand.
- *Dopamine* is the primary agent controlling permanent change, inducing moment-by-moment strengthening of all momentarily nearly synchronous inputs in a 'save it' operation immediately following the behavioural act—then in the next moment, weakening all *other* inputs

---

1 Postulated by the Canadian physiological psychologist Donald Hebb, in 1947.

in that territory that 'chattered' out of sync with those coordinated behaviourally associated moments.

It is important to understand that the processing capacities of the brain actually evolve through use. The brain could be analogized to be like a 50-year-old computer in those first days after a child's birth. *But* it has a remarkable capacity to evolve its 'information processor' *by use*, and by age 20, its owner has the equivalent of something closer to a state-of-the-art computer. I have likened[2] the brain to a factory that has the rather miraculous capacity to upgrade the machinery manufacturing its products as a direct function of the reliability, productivity, and quality of its manufacturing—with its progressively advancing machinery capable every month and year of producing more and more sophisticated and elaborated and useful products—*all achieved by physically changing itself*.

It is also important to understand that the connectional remodelling in the brain is a *selective process*. At any brain level subject to change, there must be at least weak pre-existing inputs that can be strengthened in a 'plastic' moment of change. The richer the extent of those reconnectional possibilities, the greater the potential for multiple forms of fast, experience-based remodelling. Many studies, conducted over a 60-year period, have shown that connectional enrichment is a product of experiential enrichment, and that we have life-long powers of connectional elaboration. That connectional elaboration powerfully amplifies the *possibilities* for experientially driven remodelling.

As the cerebral cortex advances in its powers at 'lower' system levels, its progressively more temporally and spatially resolved actions and the growing coordination powers of its 'mini-columns' critically enable 'higher-level' plasticity. That coordination also triggers changes in myelination that more accurately transmit those coordinated activities and thereby further amplify the plasticity-generating powers of fed-forward inputs.

Higher-level abilities—e.g. executive control—can never fully develop in a brain that is not generating salient representations of perceptual inputs. The most effective strategies for improving higher-level abilities must address limitations in lower-level forebrain system functionality.

What a gift these remarkable self-organizing brain processes are, for every child entrusted to your care.

2 *Soft-Wired*. M. Merzenich. Parnassus Publ., Amazon.

Reversible plasticity

The demonstration that brain plasticity processes are, by their fundamental nature, reversible is one of the most important practical discoveries in this research domain. There are three basic ways by which this reversibility is expressed:

1. *Neurological processes are competitive.* While synapses that contribute to 'getting the answer right' are strengthened, non-contributing synapses (now, a source of 'chatter' that impacts neurological reliability) in the same neighbourhood but 'out of sync', and 'losing in the competition' are weakened. There are 'winners' and 'losers' in every one of those trillions or quadrillions of moments of change.

2. *By following that 'what fires together wires together' Hebbian rule, within its limits, neurological operations can be refined or degraded at will.* To cite one of a thousand examples, by broadly simultaneously engaging the surfaces of the hand in a demanding, closely attended behavioural task, with not too many hours of practice, we experimentally demonstrated that it will destroy the ability to resolve the details of what is held or effectively manipulated by that hand, shrink its representation in to the brain to about half of its normal size, and utterly destroy a monkey's (or human's) ability to control that hand.[3] Or, by engaging those surfaces in a task that requires that a trainee progressively distinguish progressively finer spatial details, we showed that you can substantially enlarge that original hand-surface representation, substantially improve its representation of felt-surface details, and substantially improve the ability to recognize what is held in the hand, with improved manual dexterity. Again, following that 'Hebbian rule', within its limits, we can advance *or* degrade neurological performance abilities *at will*.

   • The 'negative' side of these two aspects of bidirectional plasticity are dramatically recorded in the emergence of the distorted movement control recorded in a child that progressively develops a CP. For a variety of neurological reasons, the fetus or infant initiates a schedule of co-contraction of the flexor and extensor muscles in the leg. By the Hebbian rule, all of the sources of feedback from the limb are strengthened (wired) together, to increasingly more strongly support that otherwise rare movement. Because that movement dominates the baby's limb-movement experiences, the neurological representation of this abnormal movement competitively grows in power, ultimately subsuming the weaker representations of differential movements around other degrees of freedom of the joints of the leg, ankle, and foot.

   • We reproduced this scenario by splinting the hind legs of a normal infant rat for 12 hours a day over a brief postnatal period. With just this limited exposure, the plastically coupled neuronal assemblies representing undifferentiated all-leg movements were competitively dominant, and after the splints were removed in the now 3-week-old infant rat, *these empowered neuronal assemblies continued to grow* at the expense of the differentiated sensory and motor cortical representations of all other leg movements. As the rat progressed

---

3 This is also the true origin of a 'focal dystonia' of the hand.

to young adulthood, its hindlimbs were like extended sticks, in continuous co-contraction all up and down the leg. By that age, no other movement around the ankle or knee could be voluntarily generated from the level of the motor cortex, and the growing neurological distortion was beginning to competitively encroach on the movement control of the trunk and forelimbs.

- By following the rules that governed plasticity, a 'CP' had been induced in this completely normal animal.

Extended histories of high-stress and fear, all too common in child populations, put the brain and body on 'high alert', engender distortions in hormonal and neuromodulator expression that 'hi-jack' neurological progressions, and degrade the machinery that supports positive brain change. *In that state, neurological progression can be dramatically slower and grossly distorted in a brain that can be radically 'specialized' for 'personal defence'.*

Again, all of these negative hormonal- and neuromodulator-driven processes appear to be *reversible*.

When I drive a brain in a 'negative' (functionally degrading) or a 'positive' (functionally empowering) direction, what, *exactly*, is reversible? We first asked this question in animal models and have been progressively extending that inquiry to humans.

The short answer: *everything*. We initially looked at 17 different physical or functional indices of neurological status, later extending that list (now including non-brain performance functions like reactive hyperaemia, blood–brain barrier integrity, brain-based immune response, etc.) to >30 indices of brain health. In a positive plasticity mode, *everything* measured was stronger, more reliable, faster, more coordinated, and more functional. In a negative plasticity mode, *everything* measured was weaker, less reliable, slower, less coordinated, and less functionally competent. It appears that we humans (mammals) have a kind of 'master switch' that throws gene regulation for the brain in a broadly positive (growth) or broadly negative (reduction) mode. We have argued that the probable survival value of this bidirectionality is the assured retention of the ability to 'get the answer right' in ways that support that survival. If the brain is usually successful in advancing its performance abilities, everything is set up to positively advance. When it begins to make many errors, it relaxes its operational characteristics, slowing down, taking longer to 'decide', adopting a more provisional and cautionary approach. In a sense, it adjusts back to an operational status that it successfully applied in its recent past. In any event, we appear to be endowed with a brain that is literally designed 'to do the best it can'.

In an analogy to physical exercise in the body, a regular regimen of physical exercise has been repeatedly and elaborately shown to have broad impacts on general somatic (and neurological) health. Almost every other somatic process and organ is positively impacted because of that physical exercise. In a life with little physical exercise, almost every organ 'takes a hit'.

So, too, for your brain. Brain exercise, in the right forms, strengthens *every* aspect of organic brain health. *An un-exercised brain is an unhealthy brain.*

In general, you want that master switch in the children that you are responsible for thrown in the 'on' position for as much of their young lives as is possible.

Plasticity in the older child

As noted earlier, beyond the age of 2 or 3 years, in most children, neuroplasticity processes in most of the forebrain are controlled by behavioural contingencies and outcomes. At the same time, as the child matures, those contingent factors play an increasingly greater role in learning and in skill development. As the child advances to more complex behaviours:

- *Prior brain-change histories have a major impact on the successful advance to a 'higher' performance level.* The child has to progress from strengthening the body core to crawling, to standing, to 'cruising', to walking, to running over hill and dale. Almost all complex skills are similarly dependent on prerequisite skill development. Year 5/ fourth-grade mathematics (multiplication/division/fractionation), for example, is built on a platform of distinguishing magnitude and number differences, number assignment, and facile, simpler arithmetic operations. Reading proficiency (as noted earlier) is dependent upon phonemic reception accuracy, and on elementary practised oculomotor scanning and visual focus and resolution abilities.

- *The power of 'rewards' or 'punishments' guiding behaviours are subject to a natural (and often-unnatural) evolution.* Enduring brain change is modulated as a function of the *strengths* of rewards. The nature, specific identities, and values of 'rewards' change as a child grows older and vary substantially in different older children.

- *The child increasingly bears the 'costs' of the weight of their historic neurological experiences.* A slowly growing increase in the difficulty in acquiring a second language represents one of many cases in point. The first language, subject to a massive schedule of brain-changing usage, is competitively dominant. An older brain has to establish phonemic sorting and the other dimensions of language-specific sequencing and voice modulation in a brain that has been long generating a progressively stronger prediction of sound and word associations in the first language. As a result, the brain of a teenager or young adult has to create a substantially non-overlapping parallel ('second') processor representing the features of that second language.
  - An important early study conducted in immigrant children in Sweden identified a second reason why acquisition of a second language can be slower in a teenager or adult than in an elementary school-age child. The younger child willingly accepts language immersion. The far more socially conscious teenager seeks companionship with children who understand them.
  - When actual times of immersion in Swedish were taken as a measure of second language acquisition time, it took only modestly longer for that older child to fully master it.

- *The child's attention and learning focus evolve, of course, as the child advances the operational powers of their brain in both the cognitive and social realms.* In some older children, change progressions are generating more obvious operational distortions that will progress to mental illness, limitations in executive control and response control, struggles with attachment, poorly developed social cognition, a host of addictions, oppositional behaviours, and a negative self-evaluation. Paediatric medicine should direct a stronger focus towards monitoring and addressing issues of organic brain health that, as we shall briefly describe later, engender these negative brain plasticity-driven outcomes.

It is remarkable that the brain is capable of changing itself, at an older child-hood age—indeed, all across the span of an older adult life—to master the reception and the production of something (for example) as complicated as a second language, easily relabelling all of the things and actions and in-ternalized brain-generated ephemera of the child's or adult's world. Prof Michael Merzenich's (and others') laboratory's historical studies directed towards developing the modern cochlear implant showed that this can be achieved by the brain even when the sound inputs were encoded (by dif-ferent cochlear implant models) in a variety of highly unnatural ways, with all inputs coming from the extreme high-frequency end (not normal speech's low- to middle-frequency range) of hearing. With hearing recovery, the im-planted patient typically declares that the recovered language 'sounds com-pletely natural'.

Indeed!

Natural and cochlear implant second-language acquisitions are both crystal-clear demonstrations of the truly incredible powers of attention- and outcomes-guided older-age brain plasticity.

Brain health impacting body health

Regular physical exercise is important for the child's brain. After all:

- The brain is the control centre for voluntary movement.
- Exercise-driven hormonal and modulatory neurotransmitter expressions have positive impacts on neurological processes.
- The acquisition of, and progressive improvement at, any physical skill or ability is (of course) brain plasticity in action. In that acquisition phase, that brain master-switch is 'on'.
- Note that aerobic (repetitive, stereotypic) movement exercise has less value for the brain.
- Note that physical exercise cannot, by itself, ever fully generate the brain remodelling required to strengthen or refine most neurological abilities. *While it is valuable for the brain and its health, physical exercise does not substitute for exercising the attention, social, perceptual, cognitive, or executive control levels of brain operations.*

Recent studies have provided a growing body of evidence revealing a major impact of brain health on general physical health.

- *In a positive direction*, studies in adults have now recorded a direct impact of intensive brain training designed to rejuvenate neurological functionality on body health (autonomic nervous system function; immune response regulation; hypothalamus-based hormonal regulation; sleep regulation).
- *In a negative direction*, we now know that a brain that is substantially functionally degraded in a child because of the impacts of an intense epoch of stress or fear in their young life is a virtually certain contributor to their predicted higher incidence of a rich variety of somatic medical problems, and to a very substantially shortened lifespan.
- *The integrity and powers of the 'salience network' in the brain*—which integrates sensory information from body organs with behavioural status information from the brain, and projects to the brainstem and hypothalamic areas that dynamically control homeostasis and impacts hormone regulation—is a key index of these powerful brain-to-body impacts.

Who's surprised? The child with a healthy brain is, with high probability, a child with a healthy body. And vice versa.

Evaluating and managing brain health in an individual child

Our final concern here is practical:

- What can go wrong with these brain remodelling progressions in a child?
- What specific 'failure modes' are built into this change-progression machinery?
- How are the resulting neurological weaknesses or distortions actually expressed as a disability or a 'disease' in the child?
- How could we know how effectively or how appropriately the brain is progressing in its advances across childhood?
- How can we know if a brain is, or is not, organically healthy?
- What can we do to recover or improve neurological performance—and to sustain it?
- What strategies might we deploy to *manage* the organic brain health of a child?

A book or two or ten could be written in answer to any one of these questions. Moreover, in your paediatric training, you have heard a lot about child benchmarks and 'warning signs', and we're going to avoid focusing on the valid entries on those extensive lists. Our focus here is limited to a brain plasticity perspective about what can go wrong, and what can (should) be done about it. You should understand that the treatment of these complex subjects is necessarily far from complete.

Prenatal and early postnatal factors impacting plasticity progressions

From the perspective of the plastic brain, a modern childhood is a mine-field. Many factors can impact the prenatal and early postnatal epochs of brain plasticity—and a large proportion of them apply far more strongly for contemporary than for historic human life. A few among many potential factors that have been cited are:

- *The mother's gene expression.* High stress during pregnancy throws the mother's 'plasticity switch' (the regulation of the hundreds of associated genes) in a down-turned direction, which negatively impacts the initial developmental epoch in the fetus and infant.
- *Antidepressant and other prescribed medications, and 'recreational' drugs.* Prof Merzenich and others have documented the long-enduring negative impacts of antidepressant and antipsychotic drugs on neuromodulator status (and thereby, on progressive positive plasticity) in animal models. Many studies have documented the negative impacts of recreational drugs on fetuses and on nursing infants.
  - The recent discovery that selective serotonin reuptake inhibitor (SSRI) treatment for major depressive disorder in mothers results in a fourfold increase in the incidence of autism is a case in point. In animal models, SSRI exposure has major impacts on the development of the plasticity-enabling neuromodulatory machinery in the immature brain of animals.
- *Heavy metal and toxic organic chemical exposures.* Prof Merzenich and others have directly documented impacts of the polychlorinated biphenyl (PCB) class of organic chemicals (or polybrominated diphenyl ethers (PBDEs), a breakdown product of flame-retardant chemicals) and of lead and other heavy metal exposures in late fetal and early postnatal animal models, and in children. There are many other suspect chemicals that fetuses and infants are exposed to in modern environments. Again, impacts are long enduring.
- *Early umbilical cord clamping; any significant perinatal epoch of oxygen deprivation.* A rush to clamp the umbilical cord has been the norm over most of the past several decades. A consequence is a less than complete transfusion of blood (and iron) from the mother to infant. Because the iron required for red blood cell/haemoglobin genesis over the first months of postnatal life comes from the mother, the infant's brain can be consequentially oxygen deprived over a significant epoch in that first postnatal year. Simulations (in animal models) of extended, moderate oxygenate deprivation recorded large-scale impacts on progressive plastic brain remodelling.
- *Continuous auditory (or visual) noise exposure in the child's postnatal environment.* In contrast to early human histories, modern babies commonly grow up in the din. Astoundingly, many obstetricians and paediatricians prescribe noise machines for infants and toddlers, and premature infant and early at-home environments are often thoughtlessly noise loaded. Because the 'plasticity switch' in the infant is 'always on', meaningless stimuli could drive competitive plastic changes

at the expense of the brain organizing itself to represent what shall become meaningful sounds (like the phonemic elements of their native languages). Note that this applies uniquely for the baby in sleeping as well as in waking periods. The hearing brains of animals who endure extended daily epochs of noise have to wait until someone turns off the 'noise machine' before they can make any real progress in developing their neurological processing of environmentally important stimuli. As long as the noise exposure continues, the cortex is slowed in its advance to a level of brain-based plasticity control.

It is important to distinguish structured sounds (human voices, music, natural environmental sounds) from unstructured or repetitive noise (from a 'noise machine', fan noise, etc.). *Normal infants* require a rich exposure to natural structured sounds.

- A limited period of continuous noise exposure in waking periods at an older age can also destructively degrade neurological processing machinery.
- In parallel with its positive values resulting from exercising neurological operations and decision-making at speed, heavy exposure to media and computer 'games' has two important negative impacts. First, as with all other heavily engaged rewarding behaviours, it can distort the reward machinery to exaggerate the values of the computer game rewarding, reducing the values of 'rewards' associated with the home and natural physical environment. Second, it results in real-world deprivation. Computer games are a special problem because they are mythology and avatar and rule based, operating to control the child's responses and actions in that 'world' through their fingers. The real world, on the other hand, is loaded with real people and real surprises, and you continuously operate in that very real and dirty, often-smelly, and cold, hot, noisy, or sunny world with every part of your body and mind, very often in the company of your peers and the other real animals and plants that inhabit it.
- A stress or fear-loaded childhood. There is a long history of studies highlighted by the Adverse Childhood Experiences and the Dunedin Study (New Zealand) that have documented the devastating consequences of a stress- and fear-loaded early life on neurological and general physical health outcomes. The explanations of cause usually focus on the extended impacts of a hormonally (cortisol) and neurotransmitter- (noradrenaline) signalled stress response, but that explanation has not generally acknowledged the crucial neurological derailing of the normal progression of neurological development— paralleled by the neurological exaggeration of triggers of stress and fear. Sexual abuse is an especially strong form of stress- and fear-engendering trauma that arises in the life of one in seven female children (and in about half as many males), most frequently between the ages of 10 and 16 years.
- Bullying, both from adults and from peers. Sadly, bullying is a more common experience in a child that is already neurologically struggling. It can come from hypercritical and insensitive adults (family members, teachers, coaches, etc.), of course, as well from peers. Bullying can

initiate a high-stress, neuroplasticity-hijacking epoch at any time in any child's life—again, 'throwing that plasticity switch' in a downward direction.

- Impoverished language exposure; experiential neglect. Scientists have repeatedly documented the statistical variations in childhood experiences as a function of family income, employment, parental health, addiction, incarceration, instability and divorce, internal and external support, and many other factors. Differences can be astounding. In the US, just differentiating children on the basis of household income results in a sevenfold difference in spoken-word exposure in childhood hours spent at home (with a corresponding variation in vocabulary and phraseology) comparing the highest to the lowest family-income quartiles. To add to the child's stress burden, the majority of interactions directed from the parent to the child in the economically struggling family are corrective. By contrast, the great majority of interactions from parent to child when the family is thriving are affirmative.

- The grand result of a less-than-perfect or really struggling (fear and stress-loaded and/or experientially impoverished) childhood?
  - A brain that has engendered relatively weak executive agency, is operationally less reliable, and will have greater difficulty forming strong extra-personal attachments.
  - A brain that is sluggish and relatively imprecise in its operation, and has relatively sparsely and crudely generated its coded representations of its world.
  - A brain that will have not strongly advanced—and does not strongly exercise and sustain—the machinery that enables facile learning and sustains health, and that underlies critical learning-support faculties (attention, motivation, confidence, etc.).
  - A brain that is at high risk for engendering a negative self-evaluation— a common enduring, self-generated source of chronic cortisol and noradrenaline release, of a weaker and less elaborated evolution of social cognition and control, and of a rich variety of oppositional, angry, and withdrawal behaviours.
  - A brain that at an older age is at significantly higher risk of a progression to older age struggles—addictions, psychiatric illness, academic withdrawal and failure, oppositional behaviours, psychopathy, etc.
  - A brain that may (without correction) be enduringly distorted about what it *can* respond to and physically interact with in strongly emotional and aesthetic terms and operational terms, out in the real world.
  - An organically unhealthy brain.

It is important to understand that the physical and functional limitations in the environmentally challenged brain are strongly inter-related. A brain that is inaccurate and slow is stuck in a relatively primitive physical–chemical state, myelination to higher brain levels is behind schedule, and the brain's poorly coordinated cell assemblies at 'lower' system levels are not as highly coordinated or as reliable in their signalling and do not as strongly engage those higher-level processes that generate the child's executive powers. Remember that plasticity at all system levels is coincident-input dependent. The generation of the sustained neurological activities that so crucially support higher-level working memory and association *require* that they be fed highly coordinated inputs. All of these factors frustrate the generation of that requisite level of coordination. The result? The generation of a weaker 'self', and of more limited powers of 'executive control'.

This is, of course, a very incomplete list and account of those land mines out there in the modern child's world potentially slowing, degrading, misdirecting, or derailing the normal positive neurological progression of a modern child.

A note on genetics and brain plasticity

Almost all genetic mutations that have been associated with neurological health or ability impact plasticity-related processes in the brain. The majority of those faults therefore impact the overall grand progression of change that we associate with advancing neurological ability in a child. When we consider the origins of commonly identified neurological struggles that we label with terms like 'autism', 'dyslexia', 'dyscalculia', 'dyspraxia', or a dozen or more other functional labels, dozens to hundreds of genetic variations appear to contribute to their origins, and overlapping neurobehavioral expression is commonplace.

At the same time, *we have yet to identify a survivable neurological condition that profoundly disables brain plasticity*. Even in the case of genetic faults like DS (which can profoundly disable the expression of a key enabler of brain plasticity, acetylcholine), large-scale improvements in neurological ability result from the appropriate forms of intensive brain training.

A major goal of current scientific studies should be to identify neurological weaknesses or limitations in *all* children independent of their clinical and genetic labels—then apply strategies that amplify the brain-change powers of the brain and that advance their brain powers and brain health at all due speed.

Neurodevelopmental disorders and neurodisability

Please refer to Chapter 8 for further discussion of the topics discussed in this chapter

Introduction to neurodisability

Neurodevelopmental disorders are conditions involving the developing nervous system that have or are likely to have an impact on the future course of the child's development. Children with a neurodisability have a range of impairments; many have complex and continuing needs and as a result are frequent users of the health service at all levels—community care, primary care, and inpatient and outpatient settings in secondary and tertiary care.

The field of neurodisability has made massive progress in the last two decades. This progress is due to many factors.

Firstly, there has been a change in the attitude and approaches to childhood disability. In the past, the 'medical model' to disability was predominant and the 'focus' was to treat the diseases. Now these disorders are addressed by multidisciplinary and multiprofessional teams. Hence, children and families have access to a much broader range of interventions in all dimensions of health, i.e. holistic care.

Secondly, services are increasingly becoming 'child and family centred'. Families of children with a disability are being encouraged to participate actively in their child's enablement plan. Professionals now talk in terms of 'development goals' rather than medical goals. The physical, social, psychological, educational, emotional, and financial needs of the entire family are discussed and appropriate information, support, and advice are provided.

Moreover, changes in legislation such as the Disability Discrimination Act 1995 and 'Every Disabled Child Matters' have played a part by increasing awareness and accessibility for these children.

Adoption of evidence-based medicine in childhood disability is gradually changing the repertoire of interventions offered to children. Many therapists and professionals are gaining postgraduate degrees or diplomas in childhood disability and all this is driving up the quality of care provided. Guidance from institutes such as NICE on conditions such as CP, ADHD, and ASD are influencing the availability of resources to manage these conditions.

In addition, advances in neurosciences have furthered our knowledge and understanding of these conditions. Risk genes for complex neurodevelopmental disorders are being identified. Advances in pharmacokinetics have led to increased availability of medications for treating seizures, hyperactivity, spasticity, sleep disorders, depression, etc.

Spectacular technological advances have helped in the development of 'intelligent aids'. Assistive devices are helping to overcome functional impairments and enable these children to participate in daily activities such as accessing a computer, communication aids, independent feeding, living skills, mobility, postural stability, nutrition, etc.

Cerebral palsy

Introduction

Cerebral palsy

Introduction

- Cerebral palsy (CP) is an 'umbrella term' and can be defined as a disorder of movement and posture arising from injury or interference to the developing brain.
- A revised definition in 2005 stressed the importance of acknowledging comorbidities which can equally affect overall function of the child.
- These comorbidities include disturbances of sensation, perception, cognition, communication and behaviour, epilepsy, and secondary musculoskeletal problems.

In recent years there has been a shift in focus of CP management and key areas include:

- Accurately establishing the aetiology of the CP.
- Early identification of CP.
- Early intervention for CP.
- Use of functional classification systems in CP.
- A focus on function and participation in CP rather than medical management alone.
- Establishing an evidence base for interventions in CP.

This shift in emphasis helps us understand the causes of CP, its natural history, and which interventions will result in a functional improvement for the child.

Epidemiology, risk factors, and prevention

- Currently the prevalence of CP is ~2.1 per 1000 live births in well-resourced countries. In countries such as Australia, evidence shows the incidence is decreasing, with improved neuroprotective strategies accounting for some of the change (Table 3.1).
- As well as less overall CP, there is a reduction in the overall severity of survivors in terms of motor disability, rates of epilepsy, and severity of intellectual impairment.

Table 3.1 Neuroprotective strategies to help reduce the incidence of cerebral palsy

Magnesium sulphate	Recent trials show CP is reduced by ~30% in premature infants if mothers receive magnesium sulphate during labour
Antenatal steroids	Steroids given to mothers at risk of preterm birth help fetal lung maturation so there is less risk of brain perfusion issues related to postnatal lung pathology
Postnatal steroids (stopped)	The use of postnatal steroids is now not recommended for ventilation weaning due to the risk of neurodevelopmental impairment
Brain cooling	Brain cooling for term infants with hypoxic ischaemic injury improves outcomes by reducing the level of ongoing neuronal loss after the initial insult

- In the UK the prevalence is reported as 2–3 per 1000 live births with the lower estimates around 2.45 per 1000 live births. Coding may contribute to some variation in reporting.
- Prematurity remains the most common risk factor for CP; however, ~60% of children with CP are born at term. The risk of CP is ~50% more if born before 28 weeks of gestation compared to being born at term. Other risk factors may be targets for prevention of CP (Table 3.2).
- Low-resource countries may have slightly higher prevalences but aetiology patterns are different with prematurity being much less common due to reduced survival. Other pathologies are more prevalent such as rhesus disease and perinatal hypoxia.

Aetiology, pathophysiology, and diagnosis of cerebral palsy

- The definition of CP assumes the brain injury has occurred any time *in utero* to 2 years of age. There is no international agreement of the upper age limit but commonly 1–2 years is seen as a cut-off. Above this age, the diagnosis is better described as acquired brain injury (see ➋ pp. 108–9) as the pattern of injury and resultant disability is very different.
- Around 80% of CP is caused by an *in utero* event and it is increasingly being recognized that genetic and epigenetic factors contribute to CP. This may be due to genes which cause direct maldevelopment of the brain (*LIS1* gene in lissencephaly) or may be related to causal pathways such as prothrombotic risk (*COL4A* mutations).
- Timing of brain injury can largely be divided into four main time periods and injury during each time period typically gives rise to a particular phenotype of CP (Table 3.3).
- The diagnosis of CP is based on clinical history and examination, but international guidelines recommend the aetiology of CP can be established with neuroimaging.

Table 3.2 Risk factors for cerebral palsy

Prenatal risk factors	*Maternal factors*: TORCH infection (toxoplasmosis, other (syphilis, varicella zoster, parvovirus B19), rubella, cytomegalovirus, and herpes simplex virus), maternal hypothyroidism, iodine deficiency, thrombotic disorders (including factor V Leiden), chorioamnionitis
	Fetal factors: teratogen exposure, genetic and metabolic disorders, multiple births, prematurity
	Social factors: low socioeconomic status
Perinatal risk factors	Birth asphyxia and trauma, non-vertex presentation, placental abruption, rupture of the uterus, prolonged or obstructed labour, post-maturity
Postnatal risk factors	Hyperbilirubinaemia, neonatal sepsis, respiratory distress, early-onset meningitis, intraventricular haemorrhage, acquired brain injury <2 years of age

Table 3.3 Patterns and causes of brain injury at different stages

Timing of brain injury	Aetiology of brain injury	Cerebral palsy classification
Early brain injuries resulting in brain maldevelopment (usually before 20 weeks of gestation) Maldevelopment due to interference of migration and normal development of brain cells. Can be as a result of hypoxia, hypotension, infection, stroke, or genetic causes	• Maternal infection—cytomegalovirus, polymicrogyria • *COL4A1* genetic mutations—porencephalic cysts, schizencephaly • *LIS1* genetic mutations—lissencephaly • *GPR56* gene—polymicrogyria	Often bilateral spastic dystonic motor pattern affecting trunk, arms, and legs Frequently severe motor disability Increased associated comorbidities, e.g. dysphagia, epilepsy, ID
Injuries in early/mid-pregnancy (24–32 weeks of gestation) White matter disease of prematurity Periventricular leukomalacia	Blood supply is compromised preferentially to the periventricular area due to hypoxia, hypotension, infection, or as a result of intraventricular haemorrhage and venous haemorrhagic parenchymal infarction Leg motor fibres from the homunculus pass closest to the periventricular edge so are preferentially affected	Usually, bilateral spastic motor pattern Leg dominant distribution (spastic diplegia with arms less affected) Comorbidities are dependent on the extent of brain injury
Late injuries to the developed brain (injuries around term) Perinatal difficulties include hypoxia or hypotension due to placental abruption, cord prolapse, or shoulder dystocia Dyskinetic patterns are more common as the basal ganglia is preferentially injured due to its relatively higher energy demands Embolic strokes are as a result of clots in the venous circulation entering the fetal arterial circulation and then often embolizing to the middle cerebral artery Often no specific risk factor is identified but there may have been perinatal difficulty including maternal infection	• Peripartum hypoxia • Maternal infection • Stroke (embolic stroke)	Global hypoxic injuries usually result in bilateral dyskinetic motor patterns affecting arms and legs Prolonged injuries are associated with significant comorbidities affecting feeding, cognition, and communication Embolic strokes usually result in unilateral spastic dystonic motor patterns

Table 3.3 (Contd.)

Timing of brain injury	Aetiology of brain injury	Cerebral palsy classification
Post-neonatal brain injuries These injuries can take many forms and the upper age of brain injury for classification as CP is usually 1–2 years old	• Meningitis/encephalitis • Stroke • Trauma—accidental/non-accidental • Hypoxia—near drowning	Motor pattern and comorbidities dependent on the specific aetiology and severity of brain injury

- Approximately 50% of all CP arises from high-risk neonatal cases and they may have had neuroimaging in the early neonatal period; cranial ultrasound or magnetic resonance imaging (MRI). Of the remaining 50%, the aetiology may not be clear, and neuroimaging will help establish the aetiology of the movement disorder.
- Brain MRI is the imaging modality of choice, but early scans may sometimes be inconclusive and will need repeating after 2 years of age when brain myelination is more developed.
- Around 10% of CP has been shown to have normal neuroimaging. This percentage may change in the future, however, with newer, more detailed imaging techniques or indeed alternative genetic diagnoses being identified for these 'MRI-negative' cases.
- Any unexpected deterioration in function is an indicator for repeat neuroimaging.
- An accurate diagnosis and functional classification of CP allows the clinician to understand the natural history of each phenotype of CP. This is essential to enable meaningful discussions with families regarding management and prognosis (Box 3.1).
- Identifying an alternative diagnosis to CP is paramount as this has implications for deterioration in function, recurrence risk, and identifying treatment options.
- It is not essential to know every differential neurometabolic diagnosis, but the clinician should have an inquisitive mind and know when to question the diagnosis of CP (Table 3.4).

Box 3.1 Key steps to diagnosing cerebral palsy

- Detailed history and examination.
- What is the antenatal, perinatal, and postnatal history? When did a possible brain injury occur?
- What is the child's developmental progress? Have there been difficulties from the start?
- What is the predominant movement type, distribution, and functional level? Do the clinical signs fit with the clinical history?
- Does the neuroimaging fit with the clinical history and physical signs?
- If the history, clinical signs, and neuroimaging do not correlate, then question the diagnosis of CP.

Table 3.4 Red flags to question the diagnosis of cerebral palsy

No obvious aetiology on history or neuroimaging	Antenatal, perinatal, and postnatal history unremarkable MRI brain scan reported as normal
Family history of CP	Points to either a genetic risk factor for CP or an alternative genetic, neurological, or metabolic diagnosis
Fluctuating course of physical signs	CP follows a predictable pattern usually with signs from early development—be concerned if there is fluctuation in skills such as diurnal variation or loss of skills with age
Dysmorphic features	A child with a genetic syndrome may have CP as a co-diagnosis but frequently the clinical features are due to an isolated genetic diagnosis
'Pure' signs	CP is classified by its main motor type and distribution, but often there is a mix of hypertonia types and uneven limb distribution
	If signs are a pure motor type or just located to legs for example, then question other pathologies such as spinal lesions or metabolic conditions if the muscle tone is 'pure' dystonia

Early identification of cerebral palsy

- Early identification of CP has become a key theme of CP management in recent years. Not only is there a push from families to understand their child's difficulties more clearly at an early stage but it is also hoped that early identification will also allow early intervention to improve the natural history of the condition.
- Historically, CP has often been diagnosed between 12 and 24 months (average 19 months).
- The practice of simply watching and waiting is discouraged as this may miss a window of opportunity for developmental intervention.
- It is now encouraged to use the term 'high risk of CP' when there are concerns, but a formal diagnosis has not been made yet. This allows early intervention services to become involved earlier.
- Children may present with signs such as delayed motor milestones, asymmetry of movement, abnormal muscle tone, or difficulty feeding.
- About 50% of CP occurs in children with newborn risk factors. This population is likely to have enhanced high-risk neonatal follow-up and includes children who may have been born prematurely or suffered hypoxic ischaemic encephalopathy.
- About 50% of CP is identified through GPs or general paediatricians, so tools have been validated to help clinicians identify potential CP in high-risk populations.
- The General Movements Assessment (GMA) has a high sensitivity and specificity in the prediction of CP and can be used in children from birth to 20 weeks of age (corrected for prematurity).
- The best age to perform the assessment is 12–14 weeks after the baby's due date and it is therefore best suited to high-risk neonatal follow-up. The assessment is made from a 3–5-minute video of the child's movements taken in a standardized method.

- The Hammersmith Infant Neurological Examination (HINE) tool is promoted for use in high-risk infant follow-up programmes. It can be performed from age 2 months to 2 years and is fast to perform and score. This assessment helps identify children at risk of CP who do not have immediate infant risk factors.
- Training is required to use both tools. By using standardized neurological assessments, clinicians have a framework for monitoring, and this allows early identification of deviation from normal development, facilitating faster referral for diagnostic assessment and treatment.
- Both tools especially in conjunction with MRI neuroimaging have a high sensitivity and specificity for predicting CP, with defined cut-off scores corresponding to severity of potential CP (Table 3.5).
- The goal of early identification is to facilitate early intervention to improve motor and cognitive outcomes. There is evidence to suggest that therapy is most beneficial when goal directed and intensive. Early intervention studies are currently in progress.

Table 3.5 Tools for early identification of cerebral palsy

Tool	Test details	Predictive value to identify cerebral palsy
General Movements Assessment (GMA) Standardized assessment of writhing and fidgety movements	Fidgety movements assessed at 12–14 weeks post due date 3–5-minute video assessed (movements absent or exaggerated) (15 minutes to perform test)	Absent movements sensitivity 95–100%, specificity 85% (in high-risk population) Abnormal movements worrying but not as clear prediction
Hammersmith Infant Neurological Examination (HINE) Standardized neurological assessment Allow identification of early signs of CP and other motor disorders	For infants age 2–24 months Assesses cranial nerve, posture, quality and quantity of movements, muscle tone, reflexes, and reactions—scores 0, 1, 2, 3. Sum score 0–78 (5–10 minutes to perform test)	HINE score <57 at 3 months—96% predictive of CP HINE score <73 at 6, 9, and 12 months— high risk of CP HINE score <40 at 6, 9, and 12 months— almost always indicates CP May be harder to identify unilateral CP under a year on HINE
MRI brain scan before 5 months corrected	Neonatal MRI before sedation required	80–90% predictive of CP
MRI brain scan after 5 months	May require sedation or general anaesthetic May need to repeat scan at 2 years	MRI (86–89% sensitivity)

Describing and classifying cerebral palsy

- CP is classified by its distribution, predominant motor type, and, importantly, the functional level.
- Without this subclassification, the term CP is too heterogeneous to be useful.

Distribution (topographical description)

- Terms such as monoplegia, diplegia, tetraplegia, and quadriplegia are not used as commonly now, and it has been simplified to unilateral or bilateral CP.

Motor type

- The motor type is described as spastic, dyskinetic (dystonia, chorea and athetosis), ataxic, and mixed pattern.
- Due to the pathophysiology of CP, there may be a predominant motor type but often the motor types coexist, such as spasticity and dystonia (Table 3.6).
- The main motor type is simply a classification and does not adequately describe the complexity of movement problems nor functional difficulties of the child.
- Children with CP often have difficulties with coordination, strength, selective motor control, and sensation (including vision) and may not have the same opportunities to develop motor patterns as typically developing children.

Table 3.6 Physical classification of cerebral palsy

Movement type	Description
Spastic (85–90% of CP is spastic) Approximately one-third is unilateral, two-thirds are bilateral	Spasticity is velocity-dependent 'clasp knife' increased tone (hypertonia) with hyper-reflexia and upper motor neuron signs
Dyskinetic (7% of CP)	Recurring, uncontrolled, and involuntary movements that may be stereotyped. Tone abnormality varies
Dystonia	Characterized by hypokinesia (↓ activity) and hypertonia (↑ tone) muscle contraction resulting in twisting or abnormal muscle postures
Choreoathetosis	Characterized by hyperkinesia (↑ activity) and hypotonia (↓ tone) resulting in uncoordinated writhing (athetosis) and fast jerky movements (chorea)
Ataxic (4% of CP)	Generalized hypotonia with loss of muscle coordination. Characterized by abnormal force, rhythm, and control or accuracy of movement
Mixed forms	No single tone abnormality and movement disorder predominates. The most common mixed type has a combination of spasticity with dyskinesia

Functional classification
- Several functional classification systems have been developed to standardized terminology and aid discussion in relation to prognosis.
- They facilitate communication with parents and other clinicians and enable objective comparison for research.
- Common classification systems include the Gross Motor Function Classification System—Expanded and Revised (GMFCS-E&R), the Manual Ability Classification System (MACS), the Communication Function Classification System (CFCS), and the Eating and Drinking Abilities Classification System (EDACS) (Table 3.7 and Fig. 3.1).

Table 3.7 Classification systems used in cerebral palsy

Level	GMFCS-E&R[a]	MACS[b]	CFCS[c]	EDACS[d]
I	Walks without limitations	Handles objects easily and successfully	Sends and receives information with familiar and unfamiliar partners effectively and efficiently	Eats and drinks safely and efficiently
II	Walks with limitations	Handles most objects but with somewhat reduced quality and/or speed of achievement	Sends and receives information with familiar and unfamiliar partners but may need extra time	Eats and drinks safely but with some limits to efficiency
III	Walks using a hand-held mobility device	Handles objects with difficulty; needs help to prepare and/or modify activities	Sends and receives information with familiar partners effectively, but not with unfamiliar partners	Eats and drinks with some limitations to safety; there may be limitations to efficiency
IV	Self-mobility with limitation; may use powered mobility	Handles a limited selection of easily managed objects in adapted situations	Inconsistently sends and/or receives information even with familiar partners	Eats and drinks with significant limitations to safety
V	Transported in a manual wheelchair	Does not handle objects and has severely limited ability to perform even simple actions	Seldom effectively sends and receives information even with familiar partners	Unable to eat and drink safely—tube feeding may be considered to provide nutrition

[a] Gross Motor Function Classification System—general mobility.
[b] Manual Ability Classification System—hand function.
[c] Communication Function Classification System—communication.
[d] Eating and Drinking Abilities Classification System—eating and drinking.

GMFCS E & R between 6th and 12th birthday: Descriptors and illustrations

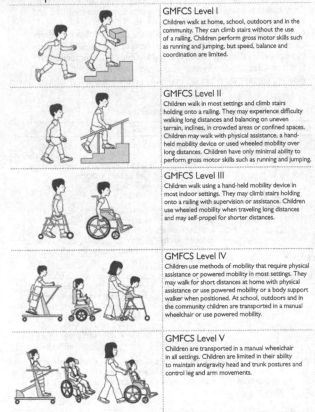

GMFCS Level I

Children walk at home, school, outdoors and in the community. They can climb stairs without the use of a railing. Children perform gross motor skills such as running and jumping, but speed, balance and coordination are limited.

GMFCS Level II

Children walk in most settings and climb stairs holding onto a railing. They may experience difficulty walking long distances and balancing on uneven terrain, inclines, in crowded areas or confined spaces. Children may walk with physical assistance, a hand-held mobility device or used wheeled mobility over long distances. Children have only minimal ability to perform gross motor skills such as running and jumping.

GMFCS Level III

Children walk using a hand-held mobility device in most indoor settings. They may climb stairs holding onto a railing with supervision or assistance. Children use wheeled mobility when traveling long distances and may self-propel for shorter distances.

GMFCS Level IV

Children use methods of mobility that require physical assistance or powered mobility in most settings. They may walk for short distances at home with physical assistance or use powered mobility or a body support walker when positioned. At school, outdoors and in the community children are transported in a manual wheelchair or use powered mobility.

GMFCS Level V

Children are transported in a manual wheelchair in all settings. Children are limited in their ability to maintain antigravity head and trunk postures and control leg and arm movements.

Fig. 3.1 Gross motor function classification system (GMFCS). E & R, expanded and revised.

Illustrations copyright: Kerr Graham, Bill Reid, and Adrienne Harvey, Royal Children's Hospital, Melbourne, VIC, republished with permission.

Function and participation in cerebral palsy

- CP historically was managed in a systems-based approach, in areas such as management of muscle tone, eating and drinking, respiratory difficulty, bone health, and epilepsy. This can be considered a body structure and function approach in terms of the ICF (see ➲ p. 20).
- The focus now is also to understand how interventions will help improve a child's activity and participation. Rosenbaum and Gorter have proposed a novel framework to help clinicians and families work jointly towards participation goals, the six Fs framework (Table 3.8 and Fig. 3.2).

Management of cerebral palsy

CP is best managed in multidisciplinary settings with involvement of the extended team (Table 3.9).

Systems-based approach to the management of cerebral palsy

See Table 3.10 and Table 3.11 for medical and surgical interventions.

Table 3.8 The 'F'-words framework in approaching childhood disability

Function	How a child performs an activity is not important, the goal is to allow them to try
Family	The family is the essential environment of the child and they know the child best; supports and resources for the whole family are vital to the child's health
Fitness	All children need to be physically active, regardless of the disability status; health promotion is more than a focus on remediating disability
Fun	Childhood is about fun, and it is incumbent upon caregivers to find out what the child wants to do
Friends	Social development is an important aspect of child development, regardless of ability; it is the quality of relationships that matters
Future	Child development is all about becoming, and this encompasses the other five Fs, the goals and expectations need to be considered in light of the present realities

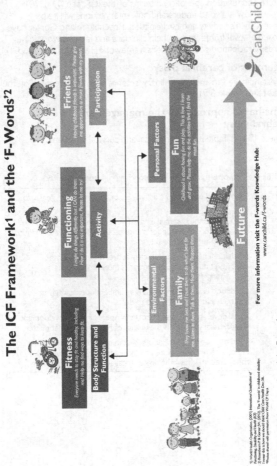

Fig. 3.2 The ICF framework and the F-words.

Reproduced from Rosenbaum P and Gorter J W (2012) 'The "F-words" in childhood disability.' Child Care Health Dev 38(4):457–63 with permission from John Wiley and Sons.

Table 3.9 The multidisciplinary team involved with the management of cerebral palsy

Specialist	Role
Physiotherapist	Physical therapy programmes, equipment to improve self-mobility (walking frames), assessment and monitoring of joint ranges, advice on static postural support equipment (see ➲ p. 374–6)
Occupational therapist	Classically more focused on arm function, upper limb splinting, involvement of seating and postural support equipment, adaptation of the environment to maximize function, improve independence of activities of daily living (feeding, dressing, toileting) (see ➲ p. 390–1)
Speech therapist	Assessment and management of eating and drinking (swallow function) and communication ability (see ➲ p. 402–3)
Psychologist	Behavioural management, adjustment of family and child to disability (see ➲ p. 412–13)
Educational specialist (SENCO)	Ensure engagement and adaption in school when necessary, so the child can be included socially and academically (see ➲ p. 656)
Neuropsychologist	Cognitive assessment. Assess for intellectual disability. Similar assessments may be performed by an educational psychologist (see ➲ p. 414)
Gastroenterologist	Assessment and management of GI disorders such as reflux, gastrostomy feeding, and constipation
Dietician	Ensuring adequate nutritional and fluid intake for children with eating and drinking difficulty or those on enteral tube feeding (nasogastric tube, percutaneous endoscopic gastrostomy tube)
Neurologist	Often involved with the initial diagnosis of CP and then later in the event of complex epilepsy management or management of complex motor disorders (see ➲ p. 234–7)
Neurosurgeon	Management of hydrocephalus and shunts or in the management of epilepsy surgery and complex motor disorder management; selective dorsal rhizotomy, deep brain stimulation, and intrathecal baclofen (see ➲ p. 107)
Orthotist	Assessment and provision of splints such as an ankle–foot orthosis (AFO) and in-shoe orthotics. Spinal orthosis (thoracolumbar sacral orthosis (TLSO)) (see ➲ p. 424–6)
Orthopaedic surgeon	Management of upper and lower limb contractures and bone deformity. Ensure bony alignment for efficiency in walking. Hip surveillance and hip surgery. Spinal monitoring and scoliosis surgery (see ➲ p. 533–4)
Social worker	Psychological and material support to the child and family. Advocating access to benefits or funding for services. Safeguarding of vulnerable children (see ➲ p. 682–3)

Table 3.10 Systems-based approach to the management of cerebral palsy

Hypertonia	See Table 3.11 for medical and surgical interventions
Gastrointestinal (GI)	• Gastro-oesophageal reflux (GOR) as a contributor to regurgitation and pain (see ➔ p. 438–9) • GOR may be an exacerbator for hypertonia • Constipation is common especially in more severe physical disability
Pain	• Pain is commonly underestimated and can be difficult to identify in children with communication difficulties (see ➔ p. 458–9) • Treat the source of pain such as muscle spasm, GOR, bony deformity, joint subluxation, constipation, urinary retention, and pressure areas on the skin
Sleep	• Sleep is commonly disturbed so actively enquire about sleep onset, quality, duration, and frequent waking (see ➔ p. 466–8) • Does the child need turning overnight? • Treat identifiable exacerbators such as muscle spasm or GOR. Vision impairment may affect normal melatonin release (see ➔ p. 299)
Cognition	• In some children cognition may be difficult to assess (see ➔ p. 416) due to motor and communication difficulty • It is important to not simply assume a cognitive level but try to assess it formally. Communication aids (see ➔ p. 431) and educational placements (see ➔ p. 124) should be matched to the child's cognitive level
Communication	• Children can communicate in several ways including using their eyes, noises, signs or gestures, communication aids, and speech (see ➔ p. 212–14) • Communication is dependent on a child's cognitive level, vision, hearing, and motor function • Promoting communication development is often overlooked in the early years as the focus may be on motor development. It needs to be actively assessed and promoted
Hip and spine surveillance	• Progressive hip subluxation (see ➔ p. 532–5) is common in CP and the severity of subluxation is related to the functional motor level of the child • Weight bearing and stepping are somewhat protective, but all children should have hip surveillance in the form of regular hip X-rays and clinical assessment according to validated CP hip surveillance programmes (see ➔ p. 542–7) • Scandinavia and Australia have led guideline development that are readily available • Kyphoscoliosis is more common in CP and related to the severity of motor disability. Regular monitoring is essential, especially through the adolescent growth spurt

Table 3.10 (*Contd.*)

Psychiatric disorders	• Psychiatric disorders are under-recognized in children with CP especially when there is cognitive or communication impairment • Anxiety symptoms are being more readily identified but may need to be specifically asked for (see ➔ p. 338–40) • These comorbidities can affect school function, independence, and even exacerbate motor disorders especially dystonia
Vision and hearing	• Vision impairment (see ➔ p. 202–8) and hearing impairment (see ➔ p. 168–9) may be structural or cerebral in nature • Screen for hearing and vision impairment in relation to motor, cognitive, and communication development
Nutrition and growth	• Nutrition can be affected by adequacy of intake or restriction of dietary variety • As children with more severe forms of CP get older, their oro-motor skills may not be sufficient to maintain adequate nutrition • Low-volume fluid intake may lead to constipation and in severe cases may present acutely with dehydration
Bone health	• Bone health (see ➔ p. 556–7) is related to nutritional intake, sun light exposure, and weight bearing • Medications can also make it harder to absorb vitamin D such as sodium valproate • Children with low bone density are at risk of low-impact fractures • Ensure regular monitoring of vitamin D and calcium intake, and supplement according to national guidelines • Consider performing a dual-energy X-ray absorptiometry (DXA) scan if there are concerns about low-impact fractures or generalized bone pain • Bisphosphonates may be indicated if there is recurrent fracture risk in the presence of low bone density
Dysphagia and drooling	• Dysphagia is more prevalent in the more severe motor phenotypes of CP • It requires specialist assessment by a speech therapist and sometimes requires further investigation with video fluoroscopy (see ➔ p. 435) • Aspiration risk needs to be assessed and this can be managed through a multidisciplinary team (MDT) including advice on posture management, texture modification, and sometimes using tube feeding for high-risk textures or to maintain adequate nutrition • Drooling may be managed with advice on postural support and oromotor awareness, assessment of dentition, and discussion around developmental maturity • Medications can be considered such as glycopyrrolate or hyoscine but over drying of secretions needs to be considered • Advanced treatments include salivary botulinum toxin and salivary duct ligation or transposition

(*Continued*)

Table 3.10 (*Contd.*)

Epilepsy	• Epilepsy is more frequent in children with CP • A particular difficulty in CP may be differentiating seizures from movement disorder (see ➔ pp. 248–55) • Special consideration needs to be given to children with concerns around seizures and movement disorders such as dystonia, especially in the context of severe cognitive and communication impairment (see ➔ pp. 248–55)
Mobility and posture	• In high-income countries, three in four children will now walk (see ➔ p. 384) • Independent sitting at 2 years of age is a good indicator of later independent walking • The GMFCS classification system allows targeted intervention to improve function and set appropriate goals for the individual child • Generally, for functional improvement the motor practice must be task focused, intensive, and repetitive • Consider the use of orthotics or postural support equipment in more severely affected children
Respiratory disorders	• Children with CP are more at risk of recurrent chest infection due to a combination of factors including aspiration due to dysphagia or reflux, epilepsy, and immobility (see ➔ p. 448–51) • Respiratory compromise may also arise as a result of skeletal deformity such as kyphoscoliosis

Table 3.11 Medical and surgical interventions to manage hypertonia/spasticity

	Comments	Spasticity	Dystonia
Oral medications			
Baclofen		Yes	Yes
Diazepam	Best used intermittently but may be regular in severe cases	Yes	Yes
Tizanidine	Monitor liver function	Yes	No
Dantrolene	Rarely used in paediatrics due to hepatoxicity	Yes	No
Levodopa	Limited effectiveness in secondary dystonia such as CP	No	Yes
Trihexyphenidyl	Anticholinergic side effects	No	Yes
Gabapentin	Can also have an anxiolytic effect. Can help with pain and sleep	No	Yes
Tetrabenazine	Not commonly used in paediatrics due to effect on mood	No	Yes
Clonidine	Sedative and hypotensive side effects	Yes	Yes
Injectables			
Botulinum toxin A	Intramuscular in all muscle groups	Yes	Yes
Ethanol	Intramuscular in large muscle groups	Yes	Yes
Phenol	Nerve block for larger muscle groups—e.g. obturator nerve (leg adductor muscles)	Yes	Yes
Surgical procedures			
Orthopaedic	Muscle and tendon lengthening, transfers, and dissection	Yes	Yes
Intrathecal baclofen	Indwelling pump and catheter to deliver baclofen. Higher doses needed for dystonia	Yes	Yes
Selective dorsal rhizotomy	Dissection of afferent spinal nerves to reduce lower limb spasticity	Yes	No
Deep brain stimulation	Indwelling stimulator and electrodes implanted into the basal ganglia. Better effectiveness in primary dystonia	No	Yes

Acquired brain injury

The distinction between CP (usually due to brain injury prior to birth or within the neonatal period) and acquired brain injury in later childhood is a little artificial as brain maturation continues throughout childhood. Many of the principles of care that apply to children with CP also apply to children with ABI. However, there are benefits from the period of normal development prior to injury, which is why poorer outcomes are associated with earlier age of injury, despite the potential for greater brain plasticity.

Acquired brain injury has numerous causes, which include:
• Trauma (accidental or inflicted).
• Infection, e.g. meningitis.
• Hypoxic-ischaemia, e.g. following cardiac arrest or near drowning.
• Metabolic, e.g. profound hypoglycaemia.
• Stroke.
• Demyelination.
• Autoimmune encephalitis.
• Central nervous system (CNS) malignancy (due to the direct effects of tumour and indirect effects of medical therapies).

Traumatic brain injury (TBI)

The incidence of severe childhood TBI has steadily fallen in the UK over recent decades, although there is an increased focus on the larger volume of relatively minor (concussion type) injuries in relation to potential longer-term effects in adult life, including dementia.

The American Congress of Rehabilitation Medicine suggestions for boundaries for the severity of TBI in adults are shown in Table 3.12.

These parameters are useful to note in children, although may not be transferable to younger children, particularly in infancy.

Common complications during the acute intensive care setting include:
• Raised intracranial pressure.
• Autonomic storming.
• Cranial diabetes insipidus.

In the immediate post-acute stage of severe TBI it is common for children to demonstrate prolonged disorders of consciousness. The broad categories for description include coma, persistent vegetative state (PVS), and minimally conscious state (MCS). See Table 3.13.

Table 3.12 American Congress of Rehabilitation medicine boundaries for severity of traumatic brain injury in adults

	Mild	Moderate	Severe
Glasgow Coma Scale	13–15	9–12	3–8
Loss of consciousness	Up to 30 minutes	>30 minutes	>24 hours
Post-traumatic amnesia	Up to 24 hours	>24 hours but <7 days	>7 days
Retrograde amnesia	Not usually	Common	Common

Table 3.13 Post-acute prolonged disorders of consciousness in children

Coma (absent wakefulness and absent awareness)	Unrousable (cannot be awakened) Unresponsive to painful stimuli, light, or sound Lack of normal sleep–wake cycle Does not initiate voluntary actions
PVS (wakefulness with absent awareness)	Preserved capacity for arousal Preserved sleep–wake cycle Range of reflexive and spontaneous behaviours
MCS (wakefulness with minimal awareness)	Inconsistent, but reproducible, responses which indicate some degree of interaction with surroundings

It is important to distinguish these states from the locked-in syndrome, which usually results from isolated brainstem injury. Individuals with locked-in syndrome are conscious and largely paralysed, although can usually communicate using movements of the eyes or eyelids.

The distinction between PVS and MCS may be helpful in prognostication, and has been considered to have important legal implications.
- For both PVS and MCS, the likelihood of significant functional improvement diminishes over time.
- The cause of brain injury is a strong determinant of outcome for both PVS and MCS, with non-TBI patients having a shorter window for recovery and greater long-term severity of disability.
- For patents in PVS, the large majority of those who regain consciousness have done so by 12 months for TBI and by 3 months for non-TBI, but a smaller number of patients (12% in one study) may emerge between 12 and 24 months post injury.
- The prognosis for recovery is more heterogeneous for MCS than for PVS, although age and level of awareness may have some predictive value.
- In both PVS and MCS there are isolated reports of recovery even after many years, but these are a rarity, and inevitably those who recover remain severely dependent.

However, in routine clinical practice distinguishing between PVS and MCS can be very challenging. There are some standardized assessment tools (e.g. the Coma Recovery Score—Revised and the Wessex Head Injury Matrix), but they are best considered part of a continuum rather than discrete stages.

Rehabilitation

The art and science of rehabilitation has the aim to restore as close as possible the individual's previous level of physical and cognitive function. Where a deficit remains, holistic strategies to minimize the impact of the impairment to retain activity and participation are employed.

Evidence for specific interventions is generally weak, for multiple reasons including relatively small numbers, heterogeneity of mechanisms and severity of injury, pre-existing comorbidities, and different age at time of injury. Nevertheless, it is widely accepted that intensive multidisciplinary rehabilitation in the early stages improves outcomes.

A typical MDT's specialties are covered in Table 3.14.

A range of other specialist may be involved as needed including the following:
- Family worker (e.g. from Children's Brain Injury Trust).
- School teacher.
- Play specialist.
- Wheelchair services.
- Assisted communication (see ⮕ pp. 212–14).
- Social services.
- Housing officers.
- Orthopaedics.
- Ear, nose, and throat (ENT).

Table 3.14 Minimum specialties for the traumatic brain injury

Neurologist or neurodisability paediatrician	Pharmaceutical management of tone disorders, epilepsy, etc.
	Oversight of intercurrent medical concerns
Physiotherapist	Physical management of tone and posture
	Promoting relearning motor skills, with emphasis on standing and walking
Occupational therapist	As for 'Physiotherapist', with emphasis on upper limb function and aids and adaptations to promote independence in personal care
Speech and language therapist	Assessment and promotion of language skills and safe swallowing assessment
Neuropsychologist	Detailed cognitive assessment
Orthotist	Provision of orthoses

Management of abnormal tone and movement disorder

Motor disorders are common following ABI. When considering interventions, it is important to be reminded of the triad of upper motor neuron signs of abnormal muscle tone, weakness, and abnormal motor control. The majority of the currently available therapies are targeted at reduction of abnormally increased muscle tone, but the weakness and poor motor control may be a greater barrier to function.

Strategies to improve function, reduce pain, and therefore improve quality of life in young people with ABI can include:

• Tone reduction to reduce contractures, postural deformity, and discomfort (see ➜ Table 3.11, p. 107).
• Strength training to improve weakness.
• Improve coordination by better motor control or reduction of involuntary inserted movements.

Increased muscle tone is not immediately apparent, but will often emerge over the first few weeks following injury, and plateau in severity by ~3–4 months.

Two main types of hypertonicity are recognized, i.e. spasticity and dystonia, although the two commonly coexist. The former is often present when injury involves the motor cortex and descending (pyramidal) pathways, while the latter may occur following injury to the basal ganglia and thalami (extrapyramidal) connections. Both spasticity and dystonia involve co-contraction of agonist and antagonistic muscle groups, but differ in important ways. Spasticity is defined as a velocity-dependent increase in muscle tone, which leads to clinical signs including a spastic 'catch', clonus, and brisk deep tendon jerk reflexes. Dystonia is more fluctuant, not velocity dependent, and more likely to lead to twisting postures.

There may also be inserted involuntary movements such as chorea, ballismus or myoclonus, or reduced motor control, e.g. ataxia.

Before undertaking any interventions, it is essential to perform a detailed baseline physical assessment, including:

• Assessment of tone—the modified Ashworth score is a useful tool to quantify the degree of spasticity in individual muscles. In subjects with predominant dystonia this can be quantified with tools such as the Burke–Fahn–Marsden, Barry–Albright or Dyskinesia Rating Scale. Where spasticity and dystonia appear to coexist, the Hypertonia Assessment Scale can be considered.
• Careful documentation of fixed contractures (sometimes examination under anaesthetic is very helpful).
• Assessment of power (e.g. using the Medical Research Council (MRC) 5-point scale).

Once the decision is taken to attempt reduction of abnormally raised muscle tone, the main options are enteral medications, temporary neuromuscular blockade with botulinum toxin, or neurosurgical procedures such as intrathecal baclofen or selective dorsal rhizotomy.

In addition to the movement disorder, there are a number of other key areas of concern:
• Risk of epilepsy.
• Visual impairment.
• Cognitive and behavioural side effects.

Risk of epilepsy

(See ➜ pp. 248–55.) Individuals with TBI have an increased risk of epilepsy that persists even 10 years after the accident.

Visual impairment

(See ➜ pp. 202–8.) A range of visual disorders may arise from TBI, including disorder of eye movements, conjugate gaze, visual field defects, and severe cortical visual impairment.

Cognitive and behavioural difficulties

Although physical impairments may be substantial, it is cognitive and behavioural difficulties that may prove a greater long-term barrier to independence.

The full severity of difficulties is not always apparent in the younger child, who may appear to 'grow into a deficit' over time. This is partly because the gap with typically developing children widens with time, and partly as certain regions of the brain are still developing in early childhood.

Frontal lobe injury is common in TBI. Difficulties may include disinhibition or impaired executive function.

Future developments

There is much interest in regenerative therapies such as stem cell therapy, but disappointingly little objective evidence of benefit.

More promising in the short to medium term is the use of robotics and artificial intelligence to assist with rehabilitation and successful reintegration into society.

Autism spectrum disorder

- Autism spectrum disorder (ASD) is characterized by persistent qualitative impairments/deficits in social communication and social interactions, and by restricted and repetitive patterns of interests and behaviours (*Diagnostic and Statistical Manual*, fifth edition (DSM-5) and ICD-11) (Table 3.15).
  - Previously, the DSM and ICD classification systems included diagnostic categories such as autism, Asperger syndrome, atypical autism, and pervasive developmental disorder–not otherwise specified. These diagnoses and others are still used by some people who were diagnosed historically—clinicians should nowadays make a diagnosis of ASD, and also describe the presence or absence of other neurodevelopmental and coexisting conditions.
  - The DSM-5 classification system now allows categorization of severity. Severity level 3: requiring very substantial support; level 2: requiring substantial support; level 1: requiring support.
  - DSM also allows classification of other conditions: with or without accompanying intellectual impairment; with or without accompanying language impairment; associated with another neurodevelopmental, mental, or behavioural disorder; with catatonia; associated with a known medical or genetic condition or environmental factor.
  - ICD-11 allows classification of coexisting 'intellectual development', and 'functional language'.
- Some people with ASD have LD/ID. People without intellectual ability may still have significant difficulties with everyday activities ('adaptive functioning') and 'functional impairment'.
- In recent years, some young people and adults on the autism spectrum and their relatives and professionals stated a preference for using person-first language. Thus, some people now refer to autistic people, and autistic children.
- Clinicians should be aware of the view that some people consider autism to be a difference, not a disability, and part of neurodiversity (with a focus on strengths, rather than difficulties or deficits).

Prevalence

- The prevalence of ASD in children is between 1% and 2%. Many reports and epidemiological studies indicate an increase in the detected prevalence of ASD. Possible factors responsible include:
  - Changes in diagnostic criteria.
  - Different ascertainment methods.
  - Conceptualization to a spectrum rather than a core categorical condition.
  - Diagnostic substitution.
- ASD is 3–4 times more common in boys than girls; girls are possibly underdiagnosed due to phenotypic differences.
- ASD commonly coexists with other neurodevelopmental conditions.

Table 3.15 Common features of children with autistic spectrum disorder at different ages (seek information of autism-specific developmental history)

	Preschool	Primary school	Secondary school
Social communication and social interaction difficulties	Less readily to respond to name. May use gestures less frequently, e.g. less pointing or waving. There may be disordered speech, 'language delay', or regression of speech. Echolalia and stereotyped speech may be present. Verbal rituals may be present	Some preschool characteristics remain Flat or odd intonation; unusual prosody. Taking things literally. Limited social chat and conversation. Preference to speak about own interests. Repetition of set phrases	Some preschool and primary school characteristics remain Likely that social difficulties and limited relationships with peers are more pronounced. Clearer evidence of reduced quality friendships
	Less responsive to social smile. Less social use of eye contact. Preference for solitary play. Difficulties turn taking. Reduced pretend play	Reduced response to greetings and smiles. Long-standing difficulties in behaviour and social communication. Limited friendships; difficult relationships with peers. Lack of awareness of personal 'space. Difficulty with social situations and rules. Temper tantrums that may or may not be due to specific triggers	
Stereotyped and repetitive restricted behaviour	Repetitive behaviours. Possibly unusual attachment to objects, sensory sensitivity to textures, sounds, and other stimuli. Sensory interests. Motor stereotypies such as hand flapping, tip-toe walking	Preference for routines and structures. Preference for narrow and specific interests	Some preschool and primary school features may remain
Other neurodevelopmental, coexisting, and mental health conditions	Speech and language regression common age 1–2 years; uncommon from age 3 years onward (consider other causes) Developmental language disorder may be identified Sensory eating and drinking difficulties common; some children have dysphagia	ADHD and DCD may become more obvious. Note some children with ASD have attention/hyperactivity difficulties, or motor difficulties but do not have ASD Anxiety may emerge—including situation-specific anxiety/phobia, other anxiety subtypes, or intolerance of uncertainty	Mental health conditions more common, including anxiety disorders and depression/low mood, eating disorders Some young people show/express suicidal thinking

Diagnosis

- Diagnosis of ASD can be made from the second year onwards; however, most children receive a diagnosis at preschool or primary school age. Some young people are diagnosed at secondary school age, and some people in adulthood.
- The lack of a specific biological marker or a diagnostic test means that identification relies on the developmental and current history, and observations from clinicians and others.
- Home 'videos' of children can be helpful in diagnosis.
- Screening instruments show high positive predictive value, but modest sensitivity limits their use for general population screening.
- Potential benefits and disadvantages of early diagnosis are listed in Table 3.16.

Table 3.16 Potential advantages and disadvantages of early diagnosis of autistic spectrum disorder

Advantages	Disadvantages
Access to interventions specifically designed for children with autism, and families	Uncertainty of diagnosis at very young age
Reduction in symptom severity	Can lead to 'reproductive stoppage', where parents have fewer children than they planned due to fears about possible recurrence
Awareness and identification and treatment of coexisting conditions may be easier in the context of ASD (although see 'Disadvantages')	
Awareness and early identification of mental and physical health conditions that are more common in children and young people with ASD	Autism diagnosis means other neurodevelopmental conditions are sometimes not identified
Appropriate preschool and educational placement and support may be easier post ASD diagnosis	
Parental awareness of recurrence risk in subsequent children may lead to early intervention and diagnosis for siblings	
Parental recognition of possible ASD or milder related phenotypes in family members can lead to improved understanding, diagnosis, and/or interventions	
Timely access to community information, services, and support.	
Ability to specify ASD diagnosis on applications for financial and other support	
Additional time or support in exams if warranted	

Screening Tools for ASD
- The Checklist for Autism in Toddlers (CHAT) for children 18 to 24 months of age.
- The Modified Checklist for Autism in Toddlers (M-CHAT) for children 16 to 30 months of age.
- The Social Communication Questionnaire (SCQ) for children 4 years and older.

Interviews commonly used in ASD diagnostic assessment
- Autism Diagnostic Interview-Revised (ADI-R).
- Diagnostic Interview for Social and Communication Disorders (DISCO).
- Developmental, Dimensional, and Diagnostic Interview (3di).
- Childhood Autism Rating Scale (CARS).

Observational tools/opportunities commonly used in ASD diagnostic assessment
- Autism Diagnostic Observation Schedule-2 (ADOS-2).
- Naturalistic observation at education provision or another setting.

Criteria
International criteria are available for ASD, developed by the American Psychiatry Association (DSM-5) and WHO (ICD-11).

Associated neurodevelopmental/medical and coexisting conditions
- In addition to social and communication difficulties, children with ASD are at higher risk of various neurodevelopmental disorders (Table 3.17).
- Their identification and appropriate management is an important component of an autism spectrum assessment and overall intervention/ treatment/management strategy.

Aetiology
- Strong evidence of genetic predisposition; autism runs in families. Recurrence risk in siblings 10–20%; evidence that other siblings who do not meet criteria may have social communication difficulties (broader autism phenotype). Children of parents with ASD more likely to be diagnosed with ASD than population rate. Some relatives are diagnosed following a child's diagnosis.
- Autism also occurs more frequently than expected in children with many other genetic and neurodevelopmental conditions, including:
  - Fragile X syndrome (see ➔ pp. 516–17).
  - NF1 (see ➔ p. 260).
  - Tuberous sclerosis (see ➔ p. 262).
  - DS (see ➔ pp. 496–500).
  - Angelman syndrome (see ➔ pp. 517–18).
  - Williams syndrome (see ➔ p. 507).
  - Congenital rubella syndrome.

Table 3.17 Common neurodevelopmental/mental health conditions, coexisting conditions, and their management

Common neurodevelopmental/mental health conditions	Treatment/management
Developmental coordination disorder (see ➲ p. 146–9)	Occupational therapist advice and strategies for home and school
ADHD. NB: many children with ASD have difficulties with attention, and with hyperactivity but may not meet the full criteria for ADHD (see ➲ p. 126–34)	Behaviour therapy and/or medication
Anxiety disorders (e.g. phobia, social anxiety) (see ➲ p. 338–40)	
Depression (see ➲ p. 330–2)	
Obsessive–compulsive disorder (see ➲ p. 340)	
Tics or Tourette syndrome (see ➲ p. 304–5)	Cognitive behaviour therapy (CBT) (see ➲ p. 366) that is modified for C&YP with ASD to make it appropriate for them. Consider medication (see ➲ p. 305) when appropriate
Epilepsy (see ➲ p. 248–55)	Electroencephalography (EEG). Consider medication to treat epilepsy when needed (refer to neurologist when needed)
LD/ID (see ➲ p. 136–41)	Investigation. Appropriate educational placement, and support
Common coexisting conditions	**Management**
Eating and drinking difficulties (see ➲ p. 436–7)	Dietetic assessment. Consider multivitamin. Refer for dysphagia assessment (see ➲ p. 436–7) when indicated
Sleep difficulties (sleep latency and difficulty staying asleep) (see ➲ p. 466–8)	Sleep hygiene measures. Consider medication

- Untreated phenylketonuria (PKU).
- Cytogenetic abnormalities such as maternal duplication of 15q1–q13 and deletion and duplication of 16p11.

Assessment

- An appropriate, comprehensive assessment is required to:
  - Make an accurate diagnosis of ASD or not, and if not ASD identify the cause of a child's difficulties.
  - Identify any coexisting conditions and diagnoses.
  - Formulate a treatment/intervention plan with the family.
- Local areas should all have a clear, well-publicized, and established referral pathway to allow easy and prompt access to specialized assessment services.

- Many countries have guidelines that underpin the pathway for recognition, referral, and diagnosis of C&YP with possible ASD (e.g. National Institute for Health and Care Excellence (NICE) and Scottish Intercollegiate Guidelines Network (SIGN guidelines)).
- An assessment by the MDT may require expertise and assessments from the following professionals:
  - Educational psychologist (see ➲ pp. 666–7).
  - Specialist teacher or an early year professional (see ➲ p. 23).
  - Community or neurodisability paediatrician (see ➲ p. 149).
  - Child and adolescent psychiatrist (see ➲ p. 288).
  - Clinical psychologist.
  - SLT (see ➲ pp. 402–3).
  - OT (see ➲ pp. 390–1).
  - PT (see ➲ pp. 374–6).
  - ASD family support worker (see ➲ pp. 682–3).
  - Social worker (see ➲ pp. 682–3).

Key components of diagnostic assessment of ASD
- Assessment teams should make efforts to adjust the diagnostic assessment for C&YP, and parents who may have ASD and/or ID and/or mental health conditions themselves, to maximize the acceptability and success of the assessment.
- Information already available from various settings should be collated and used to inform the assessment and conclusions.
- Detailed history from carers including information about birth, developmental history, family history, and current level of everyday functioning (see ➲ p. 120). See Box 3.2.
- Detailed ASD-specific history taking account of change over time (Table 3.15). Using a semi-structured interview can provide a framework to improve accuracy and reliability of diagnosis.
- Physical examination (see ➲ p. 128 and p. 235) should include a focus on dysmorphic features, neurocutaneous stigmata (including Wood's lamp examination), and neurological assessment (keeping in mind the sensitivity of some children to touch and personal space) in addition to routine paediatric assessment.
- Routine vision (see ➲ p. 204) and hearing tests (see ➲ p. 176).
- Observations: observation in education setting. Diagnostic teams should have access to assessments using a semi-structured standard observation tool (e.g. Autism Diagnostic Observation Schedule (ADOS)). The ADOS allows the administrator to rate social communication, play and repetitive, stereotyped behaviours. Not all children require ADOS assessment. Teams should undertake ADOS assessments when needed, record the ADOS where possible, and maintain interrater reliability.
- There is increasing interest in video observation/similar techniques in clinical and home settings; evidence about whether these contribute positively to assessment is needed.
- Communication, speech, and language assessment should include communication strategies, social interaction, and joint attention, as well as receptive and expressive ability.

Box 3.2 Autism-specific history
- Poor eye contact.
- Emotional inappropriateness.
- Inappropriate social responses to smile/hello.
- Repetitive, stereotypic routines/behaviours.
- Any loss of language or social skill.
- Hypersensitivity to noise, texture, and other stimuli.
- Lack of pointing to share interest (pointing for needs may be present in children with ASD).
- Difficulty sharing/playing with other children.
- Unusual hand/body movements and mannerisms.
- Lack of nodding/shaking of head for 'yes/no'.
- Use of gestures, facial expressions, and tone of voice during communication.
- Lack of pretend/imaginative play.
- Do they enjoy peek-a-boo/hide-and-seek games?
- Insight into social relationships and understanding of emotions/empathy.
- Turn taking in conversation and social chit-chat.
- Any insistence on routines and/or any rituals?

- Cognitive assessment should focus on preferred learning style, cognitive profile, including differences in abilities, and parent reported adaptive skills. For older children and young people an assessment of attainments might be helpful (see ➲ p. 418); standardized tests are available.
- Occupational therapy assessment especially if coordination difficulties (possible DCD) and sensory issues (see ➲ pp. 390–1).
- Behaviour and mental health assessment, especially to identify coexisting disorders (Table 3.17).

Investigations
- Identifiable medical disorders are present in about 10–15% of children with ASD; additional children will have relevant findings on microarray/genome-wide genetic testing.
- Investigations should be informed by the presence or absence of ID/LD, dysmorphic features, neurodevelopmental history, and neurological examination findings (Table 3.18).

Differential diagnosis (note: many conditions can coexist with ASD)
- Social communication difficulties and repetitive behaviours not reaching diagnostic threshold (in relatives of children with ASD can be conceptualized as broader autism phenotype); neither are a DSM or ICD diagnosis, but the concept is an important explanation for young people and families, and can be used as a justification for support.
- Social (pragmatic) communication disorder (DSM-5).
- LD (see ➲ pp. 136–41).

Table 3.18 Suggested investigations for autistic spectrum disorder

Investigation	Indication/rationale
Full blood count (FBC) including film	Restricted diet; exclude iron-deficient anaemia
Neurodevelopmental genetic testing (microarray or genome-wide testing) (see ➔ p. 490–4)	NICE guidance suggests genetic testing when there is congenital anomaly, dysmorphism, or ID/LD. However, some clinicians test a broader group of children
Testing for fragile X syndrome (see ➔ p. 516–17)	Fragile X syndrome is not identified through microarray testing
Thyroid functions and PKU screening	If not tested at birth
Metabolic investigations	None routinely. Consider if clinical presentation is suggestive (see ➔ p. 152–7)
EEG	Only if clinical features suggestive of epilepsy (see ➔ p. 253–4)
Brain imaging (MRI)	Only if neurodevelopmental history or examination suggests this is required

- Language disorders. Children with receptive language problems may also have imaginative play and social interaction difficulties (see ➔ pp. 402–3).
- ADHD (see ➔ pp. 126–34).
- Anxiety disorder(s) (see ➔ pp. 338–40).
- Attachment disorders (see ➔ pp. 324–5).
- Sensory impairments (see ➔ pp. 167–216); although note blindness, visual impairment, and deafness can all lead to an ASD phenotype.
- Acquired aphasia with epilepsy (Landau–Kleffner syndrome) (see ➔ pp. 252–3).
- Selective mutism (see ➔ p. 339).

A note on 'pathological demand avoidance' (PDA)
- PDA is not an ICD- or DSM-defined diagnosis.
- Children conceptualized as possibly having 'PDA' are most appropriately considered to be within the autism spectrum if they meet ASD criteria.
- High anxiety with feeling of losing control leads to avoiding or refusing demands made by others.
- Strategies used for children with ASD, and those with anxiety are most likely to be effective.

Post-diagnostic advice and support

Post-diagnostic support from a MDT is helpful for parents and young people; however, many diagnostic teams have limited capacity to deliver post-diagnostic appointments and advice. Those who cannot provide follow-up appointments should, as a minimum, provide clear and comprehensive advice at a post-diagnostic feedback session. Advice might include:
- Information about ASD; signposting to high-quality information in leaflets, online, or in other reading materials.

- Discussing the diagnosis with a child or young person, and the timing of this (if the health team has not already done this).
- Interventions regarding ASD, and interventions/treatments for other identified conditions.
- Appointments with or support from other MDT health professionals.
- Involvement from social care, including the possible need for daytime support or overnight provision.
- Involvement from education professionals or specialist teachers.
- Applying for benefits such as DLA.
- Advice about local post-diagnostic support from autism groups (voluntary/funded).

Interventions for core symptoms of ASD

- Interventions, not medications, are recommended to treat core characteristics of ASD.
- Many interventions have been evaluated through research, but sample size and replication are limited.
- While the evidence base for some interventions is stronger than others, some are in use in international healthcare systems.
- Some interventions require significant parent and young person time; some are costly. Interventions may take parents and children away from other activities; possible gains should be considered in relation to possible disadvantages.

Approaches, therapies, and interventions

Parent-mediated interventions
Preschool Autism Communication Treatment (PACT): parents are coached by a therapist using video feedback of parent–child interactions. Supported to recognize and respond to social communication and joint attention-based opportunities for interaction.

More Than Words (Hanen)
Used with preschool and early school-age children. Parents learn strategies with the aim of improving their child's social communication.

Early interventions
- Applied behaviour analysis:
  - Teaching linguistic, cognitive, behavioural, and self-help skills by breaking them down into small tasks.
  - Usually with young children.
  - Parent mediated with support from helpers and professional consultants.
  - Involves intensive therapy for long periods of time (up to 40 hours per week).
  - Research suggests possible benefits, but concerns about the amount of child, parent, and professional time needed for delivery, and health economics.
  - Behaviour interventions address a wide range of behaviours (e.g. self-injury and aggression) and may improve adaptive skills (see p. 412–13).

Other interventions

Social stories

- May improve social understanding.
- Might help to see things from other's perspective.
- Involves short description (using photos or images) of a particular situation, event, or activity including information about what to expect and why.

Social skills groups

There is some evidence of modest effects of group-based social skills 'training'; many schools provide groups for children with and without ASD diagnoses.

Communication approaches

- A total communication approach should be used by professionals working with children with ASD (the use of gesture, sign, sounds, words, and, where needed, augmentative and alternative communication (AAC) strategies) (see ➔ p. 212–14).
- AAC might include the picture exchange communication system, or tablet/computer-based equipment. Note that developing a shared understanding of communication goals with parents is essential; most children with ASD use AAC to express their wants and needs, rather than for spontaneous social communication.

Service-based interventions

- TEACCH: help to prepare people with autism to work more effectively at home/school/community.
- SPELL framework: structure, positive, empathy, low arousal, and link.

Pharmacotherapy

General considerations

- Assessment of child's environment (both at school and at home), daily routine (e.g. sleep), and triggers for behaviours that challenge should be made, and non-pharmacological interventions used before considering pharmacological intervention.
- Medication may be useful to address coexisting conditions and as an adjunct to educational, behavioural, and developmental interventions (Table 3.19).
- Potential benefits and risks from medications should be carefully considered before starting treatment.
- Clear goals and end points should be agreed with parents/young person to stop treatment.
- Pharmacological treatment should only be undertaken by clinicians with appropriate experience and expertise.
- Some of the medications used are not licensed for use in children.
- The principle of starting at a low dose, monitoring effect and side effects, and slowing increasing dosage when appropriate should always be followed.

Table 3.19 Medications that are considered for children with autism

Medications	Indications
Risperidone or aripiprazole	Short-term use for aggression, tantrums, and self-injury (see ➔ p. 299)
Stimulant or non-stimulant medication	ADHD (see ➔ p. 126–34)
Melatonin or other medication	Sleep problems persisting despite behavioural interventions (see ➔ p. 299)

Education
(See ➔ pp. 656–8.)
- Appropriate educational placement and provisions should be planned according to their ASD, intellectual ability, needs, and strengths to optimize the child's functioning.
- Children may attend mainstream or specialist schools; secondary mainstream school with expertise in ASD, or autism resource centres should be considered for young people for whom specialist schooling is not appropriate.
- Teaching strategies and techniques should be tailored to individual children taking account of their difficulties with social communication, repetitive behaviours and routines, attention, their cognitive, speech and language, motor ability profile, and any other neurodevelopmental disorders or mental health conditions.
- Should be taught in a structured way with predictable routines and timetables. Visual calendars and visual timetables are helpful.

ASD in adulthood
- Parents frequently ask about long-term and adult prognosis. ASD is a lifelong neurodevelopmental disorder. Outcome can be difficult to predict in individual cases, especially during early childhood.
- Across the ASD and cognitive ability spectrum, ~25% live independently as adults. Some autistic adults have jobs and families.
- Around 25% of UK autistic adults are in employment.
- More positive outcomes are seen in those without LD and adults with fluent speech.
- Ongoing difficulties in the areas of communication, social relationships, and independence may remain. Mental health conditions are common. Most people need some ongoing support.

Additional practice points

Second opinion assessments: some parents may disagree with diagnostic findings, or request a second opinion. Occasionally there is disagreement between professionals or within teams. Second opinion assessments are usually helpful to resolve diagnostic uncertainty or disagreement (consider referral to tertiary services).

Professionals sometimes have safeguarding concerns, and concerns about fabricated or induced illness (FII) (see ➔ pp. 580–3) regarding children with

ASD and their families. It is important to involve appropriately experienced professionals in discussions from an early stage.

Some parents may have ASD, and/or ID, and/or mental health conditions; these should be taken into account during any safeguarding process, with reasonable adjustments put in place to maximize opportunities for effective communication and discussion, and to reduce misunderstandings.

Counsel parents that online materials about ASD are of variable quality; some less reputable websites provide inaccurate information about various aspects, and 'cure'.

Further resources

Parents should be signposted to appropriate materials about children and young people with ASD. These should be made available by clinical teams at diagnosis.

Additional information is available from national organizations.

Local organizations commonly provide information about support and facilities for individuals and families available locally.

Autism Education Trust: https://www.autismeducationtrust.org.uk/

Local services for children with ASD: http://www.childrenintouch.org.uk/

National Autistic Society: http://www.autism.org.uk

Attention deficit hyperactivity disorder

Background/definitions

- A neurodevelopmental disorder.
- ADHD is characterized by inattention, hyperactivity, and impulsivity that are inconsistent with a child's or adolescent's developmental level.
- Children and adolescents with ADHD may manifest varying degrees and patterns of inattention, hyperactivity, and impulsivity.
- ADHD often persists into adulthood and is associated with increased risk for adverse long-term outcomes in all functional domains (educational/vocational, interpersonal, mental health, other—see ⯈ pp. 132–3).

Epidemiology

- Global prevalence among children is ~7%.
- Male:female ratio ~2:1.
- ADHD persists into adulthood for 30–40%.
- Adult prevalence ~4.4%.

Aetiology

ADHD is a neurobiological disorder with behavioural symptoms that can be influenced by the home, school, and community environment.

Genetic

- Twin studies indicate that this disorder is highly heritable. Genetics are a factor in about 75% of cases.
- May arise from a combination of various genes which affect dopamine transport, such as *D2, D4, DAT1, DRD4*, etc.
- Numerous susceptibility genes, each of small effect size, contribute to the symptoms, but the genetics of ADHD are still not well understood.
- Often, a parent or sibling will also have ADHD.

Other aetiologies

- Prematurity/low birth weight/late preterm birth, alcohol or tobacco use during pregnancy, lead poisoning, and brain injury all increase risk for ADHD.
- Poor parenting does not cause ADHD, but adverse factors in the home environment can influence expression of behavioural symptoms.

Neurobiology

- Neurochemical:
  - Recent pharmacological, imaging, and neuropsychological studies suggest that attention problems are due to dysfunctions of ventral catecholaminergic (dopaminergic and noradrenergic) pathways projecting to the prefrontal and frontal cortex.
- Neuroanatomical:
  - Structural and functional neuroimaging studies of the brain have implicated the prefrontal cerebral cortex and its innervations of subcortical regions such as caudate-putamen, nucleus accumbens, and amygdaloid complex in the pathophysiology of ADHD.
  - MRI studies have revealed that the more severe the symptoms of ADHD were, the smaller the frontal lobes, caudate nucleus, and cerebellum were likely to be.

- Neuropsychological theories to describe ADHD symptoms:
  - Failure of behavioural inhibition, with associated deficits in executive function.
  - Deficits in non-striatal function including state regulation, delay aversion, and performance variability.
  - Deficits in the reward system, with preference for 'smaller sooner' over 'larger later' rewards.
  - Temporal processing deficits.
  - Overall, no single theory captures the heterogeneity of ADHD symptom presentation at the individual level.
- Unproven:
  - Diet (e.g. sugar, food additives) is often blamed for ADHD symptoms, but there is no convincing evidence of a major role for diet in causing ADHD symptoms.
  - Parenting practices can contribute to the development of adverse behaviours, but do not cause ADHD.

Diagnostic criteria

- The child or adolescent must meet the DSM-5 or ICD-10 criteria.
- The ICD-10 provides lists of nine specific symptoms of inattention (six or more required for diagnosis), five specific symptoms of hyperactivity (three or more required for diagnosis), and four specific symptoms of impulsivity (one or more required for diagnosis).
- In contrast, the DSM-5 provides lists of nine specific symptoms of inattention and nine specific symptoms of hyperactivity/impulsivity. Six or more symptoms of *either* inattention *or* hyperactivity/impulsivity are required for diagnosis.
  - The DSM-5 allows for diagnosis of three different 'presentations' of ADHD: combined, hyperactive/impulsive, or inattentive.
  - The 'combined' diagnosis requires that the child meets both the inattention and hyperactivity/impulsivity criteria.
- These criteria specify that symptoms should cause significant functional impairment in two or more settings (home, school, peers, community).
- The DSM-5 introduced the concept of reduced number of symptoms for diagnosis in adolescents over 17 years of age.
- Age of onset prior to age 12 for DSM-5 versus prior to age 7 for ICD-10.
- Severity is judged clinically, based on degree of functional impairment.
- Boys are more likely than girls to manifest hyperactive/impulsive symptoms.
- Girls may be more likely than boys to present with just inattentive symptoms.

Coexisting conditions

The *majority* of children and adolescents with ADHD also have one or more of the following coexisting conditions:
- Developmental learning disability (DLD) in reading, maths, and/or written language (see → pp. 142–5).
- Autism spectrum disorder (Asperger syndrome, ASD) (see → pp. 114–25).
- LD/ID (see → pp. 136–41).

- Tics/Tourette syndrome (see ➜ pp. 304–5).
- Substance-related disorders (see ➜ pp. 360–1).
- Internalizing disorders (anxiety, depression).
- Disruptive behaviour disorders (oppositional defiant disorder, conduct disorder, bullying).
- Sleep disorders (e.g. delayed sleep phase syndrome (see ➜ p. 466)).
- DCD (see ➜ pp. 146–9).

Note: conditions that coexist with ADHD are often confused with primary symptoms of ADHD (e.g. children with language-based LD may appear inattentive in a classroom setting).

Diagnostic approach

History
- ADHD manifests differently at different ages.
- A comprehensive history should include the following:
  - ADHD symptoms and related functional impairment.
  - Developmental, educational, and mental health history.
  - Medical review of systems, with special attention to sleep, neurological, and cardiac history.
  - Family history, with focus on neurodevelopmental, neurological, and mental health conditions.
  - Social history, including adverse childhood experiences and family function.
  - Routine medical history.
- Review of supplemental information:
  - ADHD rating scales completed by parents/caregivers and teachers (e.g. Conner's TRS/PRS, Vanderbilt Parent/Teacher Rating Scales) are essential, but not sufficient.
  - Reports of any prior assessments, including psychological or educational testing.
  - Information from schools (school records, special services provided by school).

Physical examination, interview, and observation of the child or adolescent to include
- Age-appropriate interview.
- Growth parameters.
- Vital signs (blood pressure, pulse).
- Observation of behaviour.
- General physical and neurological examination.
- Careful observation for signs of other disorders (e.g. neurological, neurocutaneous, dysmorphic features).
- Gross and fine motor examination.

Note: child behaviours during medical encounter may not be representative of child's typical behaviour and should not be overinterpreted.

Investigations
- Guided by the history and physical examination and identification of coexisting conditions.

- Formal psychological and educational testing if history suggests cognitive delays or DLDs.
- Lower threshold for psychological and educational testing for children who are <6 years or adolescent age at time of presentation.
- Medical investigations (e.g. MRI head, EEG) are rarely helpful, and should be performed only if indicated by medical history and physical examination.
- Screen for substance use and abuse in all children age 9 or older given high risk.
- Lead levels, if indicated by history.

Diagnosis

- There is no definitive 'diagnostic test' for ADHD.
- Diagnosis of ADHD requires documentation of core ADHD symptoms that fulfil diagnostic criteria and that cause functional impairment.
- Diagnosis also requires exclusion of other possible causes of ADHD symptoms:
- ODD (see ➜ pp. 306–8).
- CD (see ➜ pp. 306–8).
- Autism/ASD (see ➜ pp. 114–25).
- Hearing impairment (see ➜ pp. 168–9).
- Vision impairment (see ➜ pp. 202–8).
- Sleep impairment (see ➜ pp. 466–8).
- Child abuse (see ➜ pp. 560–1).
- Epilepsy (see ➜ pp. 248–55).
- Anaemia.
- Thyroid problems.
- Lead poisoning.
- Substance misuse (see ➜ pp. 360–1).
- Anxiety/mood disorder (see ➜ pp. 338–40).
- Learning difficulties (e.g. global LD/DLD causing 'secondary inattention' (see ➜ pp. 142–5)).
- Final diagnostic conclusion requires clinical judgement based on the foregoing information.

Differential diagnosis

- The key concept is that conditions that often coexist with ADHD (e.g. cognitive impairment, DLD, sleep disorders) may also be the primary cause of 'ADHD symptoms' (see list of conditions under 'Diagnosis').
- *Secondary inattentiveness*: in certain situations, other conditions can cause children to appear inattentive or fidgety:
  - DLD, e.g. dyslexia, dyscalculia, dysgraphia, can give rise to inattentiveness.
  - Some children with high IQ will perform poorly or may become disengaged from schoolwork, demoralized, or depressed because the assigned class work is too simple, uninteresting, or unchallenging.
  - Hence it is important to evaluate the child's or adolescent's cognitive and learning ability, if necessary, with formal psychological or educational testing.

- • Children with borderline cognitive impairment or mild LD/ID may also appear inattentive.
- ADHD may be diagnosed in children with ASD, but only if the child or adolescent clearly has impairing ADHD symptoms in addition to core symptoms of ASD; combined diagnoses typically require more extensive, formal testing by a psychologist.
- Psychosocial stresses such as poor family function or other adverse childhood experiences (e.g. abuse) may lead to behaviours that resemble ADHD.
- Other conditions such as:
  - • Fragile X (see ➲ pp. 516–17).
  - • Tuberous sclerosis (see ➲ pp. 513–14).
  - • Neurofibromatosis (see ➲ p. 260).
  - • Smith–Magenis syndrome (see ➲ pp. 493–4).

Treatment

General principles
- Psychoeducation about ADHD provided to the parent and child or adolescent is the foundation for treatment.
- The clinician should obtain information about baseline symptoms and their functional impact.
- Treatment goals should be established through shared decision-making with the parents and child or adolescent.
- Treatment should focus on the conditions (whether ADHD or any identified coexisting conditions) that are causing functional impairment.
- The paediatric clinician should facilitate the transition to adult services to ensure continued monitoring and treatment in adulthood (see ➲ pp. 470–2).

Behavioural and educational treatment
- Behavioural and educational treatment are the foundation and first line of treatment for ADHD.
- Current practice guidelines recommend the following evidence-based treatment approaches:
  - • Behavioural parent training.
  - • Behavioural interventions in classroom provided by teachers.
  - • Social skills training (behavioural peer intervention).
  - • Organizational skills training for older children and adolescents.
- Behavioural parent training provides instruction to parents on how to apply behaviour modification approaches in the home setting:
  - • Focus is on positive reinforcement of desirable behaviours.
  - • Use of appropriate consequences for maladaptive behaviours.
- Behavioural classroom management should consist of:
  - • Clear rules and expectations.
  - • Positive reinforcement of appropriate behaviours.
  - • Consequences for rule violations.
  - • Principles can be applied for the entire class, and can be individualized for the child with ADHD.
  - • Monitoring of target behaviours and daily feedback provided to the child and parents are highly effective.

- School interventions:
  - General supports (e.g. individualized attention, reinforcement of appropriate behaviours, preferential seating).
  - Note: extended time on tests is often suggested, but there is little evidence to support this accommodation.
- Additional services based on meeting criteria for SEN:
  - Small group or individual support.
  - Modified curriculum.
  - Accommodations such as alternate format or alternate administration of tests.
- Interventions for older children and adolescents:
  - Organizational skills training.
  - Motivational interviewing.

Medications

- Should be used for children who have had an inadequate response to behavioural and educational treatment *or* whose ADHD symptoms are causing moderate to severe impairment.
- Decision to use medication should respect family preferences and shared decision-making.
- Children with additional mental health needs/complex needs should preferably be reviewed and followed up in close collaboration with colleagues in CAMHS.
- Before starting medications:
  - Review history (mental health, social/family circumstances, coexisting conditions).
  - Physical examination (height, weight, blood pressure, and heart rate. FBC, liver function tests, and ECG if indicated).
- Start medications at low dosage and gradually increase the dose as required.
- Simulant medications (methylphenidate and amphetamines) are the first line of medical treatment for ADHD.
- Methylphenidate should generally be used first for younger children, usually in an immediate use formulation for initial treatment trials.
- Monitor response and side effects by reassessing both severity of core ADHD symptoms and associated functional impairment.

If poor response to treatment, consider the following:
- Increase the dose of the existing medication to the maximum tolerated level.
- Try other medication (i.e. amphetamine if methylphenidate has been tried).
- Check treatment adherence.
- Check parental/child motivation.
- Review the diagnosis.
- Consider and deal with coexisting conditions.
- Provide more intensive psychological/behavioural interventions.
- Referral to specialist/tertiary CAMHS.

Types of medication

See Box 3.3 for stimulants and Box 3.4 for non-stimulants.

Box 3.3 Stimulants

Methylphenidate
- For use in children over age 5 years.
- It is a controlled medication. Risks for stimulant misuse and diversion, especially for older adolescents and young adults and in college/ university settings.
- Recommended as first-line treatment for:
  - ADHD without significant comorbidity.
  - ADHD with conduct disorders.
- Sustained/modified-release preparations are preferred as:
  - Single dosing is convenient.
  - Compliance/adherence to treatment is better.
  - No need for administration at school, hence reducing stigma.
  - No need to store and administer controlled drug in school etc.
- Short-acting/immediate-release preparations could be considered during:
  - Initial trial and titration—helps determine correct dose.
  - Where increased flexibility in dosing regimens is required.
  - Occasionally as a top-up dose in the evening to enable homework etc.

Lisdexamphetamine
- Do not use as a first-line treatment (greater potential for side effects).
- Acts by blocking the reuptake of noradrenaline and dopamine.
- Used only after methylphenidate has been tried and failed.
- Use limited to experienced professionals (e.g. specialist/tertiary CAMHS).

Other medications
- These medications are rarely prescribed due to limited efficacy and high risk of side effects. Use should be limited to very experienced professionals such as tertiary CAMHS.
- Antidepressants (e.g. imipramine):
  - Inhibits reuptake of norepinephrine and 5-hydroxytryptamine.

Transition to adulthood
- ADHD persists from childhood to adulthood in ~30–40% of cases.
- Among those whose ADHD does not persist, there are still increased risks for other mental health disorders including anxiety, depression, and substance use disorders among others.
- Therefore, the paediatric clinician should facilitate transition to adult care for ongoing monitoring and treatment.

Long-term outcomes
- ADHD places children at risk for adverse long-term outcomes in multiple domains:
  - Lower educational attainment.
  - Vocational difficulties and limitations.

Box 3.4 Non-stimulants

Atomoxetine
- Selective norepinephrine reuptake inhibitor.
- Generally not as effective as stimulants.
- For use in children over age 5 years.
- Should be considered when:
  - ADHD is associated with tics, Tourette's, or anxiety disorders.
  - Risk of stimulant misuse or diversion is present.
  - Stimulants are ineffective at maximum tolerated dose.
  - Side effects of stimulants preclude their use.
- Monitor for side effects: agitation, irritability, suicidal thinking, self-harming behaviour, and rare idiosyncratic liver disease.

Guanfacine
- Centrally acting alpha agonist medication.
- For use in children over age 5 years.
- Consider when stimulants have been ineffective at maximal tolerated does or stimulant side effects preclude their use.
- May be more effective for hyperactive/impulsive symptoms than for inattention.
- Sometimes used in combination with stimulants for treatment of severe symptoms.

- Lower income.
- Interpersonal problems.
- Poor mental health.
- Substance use disorders.
- Legal problems.
- Accidents/injuries.
- Early death from suicide or accidents.
- Risk for adverse outcomes is greater in children with coexisting mental health disorders and/or substance use disorders.
- Multimodal treatment employing behavioural/educational and medical approaches can ameliorate these adverse outcomes.

Support groups/patient information
- Provide parents/carers and children/adolescents with information on:
  - Causation.
  - Therapeutic approaches to managing.
  - Medical information regarding medicines, controlled medications, storage, holidays, and airport laws.
  - Local and national support groups.
  - Support websites.
  - List of books/booklets for parents, teachers, and siblings.
  - Increased focus on direct patient education for adolescent age patients.

Further resources

Adders.org: ℘ http://www.adders.org

ADDISS (National Attention Deficit Disorder Information and Support Service): Tel.: 020 8952 2800; ℘ http://www.addiss.co.uk

Hyperactive Children's Support Group: ℘ http://www.hacsg.org.uk

Children and Adults with Attention-Deficit/Hyperactivity Disorder (CHADD) (leading US organization): ℘ http://www.chadd.org

Living With ADHD: ℘ http://www.livingwithadhd.co.uk

Key references

Barbaresi WJ, Campbell L, Diekroger EA, et al. (2020). Society for Developmental and Behavioral Pediatrics clinical practice guideline for the assessment and treatment of children and adolescents with complex attention-deficit/hyperactivity disorder. J Dev Behav Pediatr, 41 Suppl 2S, S35–S57.

Barbaresi WJ, Campbell L, Diekroger EA, et al. (2020). The Society for Developmental and Behavioral Pediatrics clinical practice guideline for the assessment and treatment of children and adolescents with complex attention-deficit/hyperactivity disorder: process of care algorithms. J Dev Behav Pediatr, 41 Suppl 2S, S58–S74.

NICE (2018). Attention deficit hyperactivity disorder: diagnosis and management. NICE guideline [NG87]. ℘ https://www.nice.org.uk/guidance/ng87

Wolraich ML, Hagan JF, Allan C, et al. (2019). Clinical practice guideline for the diagnosis, evaluation, and treatment of attention-deficit/hyperactivity disorder in children and adolescents. Pediatrics, 144, e20192528. [Erratum in Pediatrics, 2020, 145, e20193997.]

Intellectual disability

Background/definitions

- The terms used to describe impairment related to cognitive deficits can vary by country. While learning disability (LD) is used in the UK, intellectual disability (ID) is used in the US, Canada, and Australia.
- In some countries, including the US, the term 'LD' is used to describe what is known as a 'DLD' (e.g. dyslexia, dyscalculia, dysgraphia) in the UK.
- Please observe that the term 'mental retardation' is no longer accepted and is considered derogatory.
- The DSM-5 has termed this as 'intellectual disability' and placed this under 'Intellectual developmental disorders'.
- The ICD-11 has taken a developmental perspective and has termed this as 'Disorders of intellectual development' (DID), thus replacing the term mental retardation in the ICD-10 and has placed this condition under the category of 'Neurodevelopmental disorders'.
- The core features of 'disorders of intellectual development' in the ICD-11 are:
  - Significant limitations in intellectual functioning.
  - Significant limitations in adaptive behaviour.
  - With onset during the developmental period.
- Paediatric clinicians tend to use the term 'developmental delay' long after the age at which it is still applicable. It is important to use terms like 'developmental delay' and 'LD/ID' correctly in order to help families better understand their child's developmental trajectory and prognosis.
- The DSM-5 urges the use of the term 'global developmental delay' (GDD) for children under age 5 and to use the term 'ID' after age 5, for children who fail to meet expected developmental milestones in several areas of functioning (e.g. motor, language, social).
- The ICD-11 encourages the use of the term 'provisional DID' when formal or standardized assessments cannot be undertaken for a variety of reasons.

'Valuing People', the 2001 White Paper, defined LD as a condition characterized by:

- A significantly reduced ability to understand new or complex information, to learn new skills (impaired intelligence), with:
  - A reduced ability to cope independently (impaired social functioning).
  - Which started before adulthood, with a lasting effect on development.
- This definition of LD is largely consistent with that of the WHO's ICD-11.
- Approximately two-thirds of children with GDD will meet the criteria for LD/ID as an older child.
- After the age of 5 years, the use of 'developmental delay' or 'GDD' are no longer accurate. Children with intellectual deficits after the age of five may be more accurately described as having an LD/ID.
- Age at which cognitive deficits are first suspected usually correlates with the severity of LD/ID. Children with more significant deficits present

for assessment of developmental concerns during early childhood while children with subtler deficits may present much later.
• Earlier recognition of cognitive deficits allows for optimization of supports in the school, community, and home settings.

Epidemiology

About 1–3% of children have LD/ID.

Aetiology

LD/ID can result from a number of causes, including:
• Genetic syndromes and inborn errors of metabolism (IEMs) (e.g. DS, fragile X syndrome, Rett syndrome, Williams syndrome, Angelman syndrome, and Prader–Willi syndrome).
• Environmental causes (e.g. prenatal alcohol exposure, TORCH infections, and significant caregiver under-stimulation or neglect, especially during the first 2 years of life).
• CNS disorders/malformations (e.g. lissencephaly, TBI).
• Nutritional (e.g. malnutrition or chronic iron deficiency).
• Unknown: for many individuals with LD/ID, a clear cause cannot be identified.

Diagnostic criteria

The definition of LD/ID refers to intellectual and adaptive deficits in three domains: cognitive, social, and practical. Examples of skills in each of these three domains include:
• Conceptual skills include skills related to academics, abstract thinking, reasoning, planning, organizing skills, executive functioning, and short-term memory.
• Social skills include skills related to communication, conversation, language, emotional and behavioural regulation, and social judgement.
• Practical skills include skills needed in self-care, domestic chores, grocery shopping, transportation, home organization, employment, recreation, and money management.

LD/ID severity can be classified as mild, moderate, severe, or profound.
Prior to the DSM-5/ICD-11, levels of severity were classified by intelligence quotient (IQ) score ranges. However, both the DSM-5 and ICD-11 mark a transition to severity level being based on adaptive functioning (and not just intellectual abilities) as these skills determine an individual's required level of support and are more closely tied to functional outcome.

Coexisting conditions

Individuals with LD/ID can experience a wide range of coexisting conditions:
• Medical (e.g. seizures, GI disorders, obesity, dental problems).
• Behavioural (e.g. ADHD, ASD, aggression, self-injury).
• Psychiatric (e.g. anxiety disorders, depressive disorders).
• For children with LD/ID, their coexisting condition can be a source of significant functional impairment.
• Children with cognitive, language, and communication challenges can have difficulty accurately reporting their symptoms, requiring vigilance regarding changes in functioning caused by a new-onset comorbidity.

Diagnostic approach

Clinical presentations

Mild LD/ID

- Present later than children with more significant deficits.
- Tend to think concretely and can have difficulty grasping more abstract concepts.
- Seem socially immature as compared to typically developing peers.
- Require intermittent support of their adaptive functioning.

Moderate LD/ID

- Conceptual skills lag significantly behind those of same-age peers throughout development.
- Social judgement and decision-making abilities are limited.
- Require limited support of their adaptive functioning.

Severe LD/ID

- Limited understanding of written language or numerical concepts.
- Speech may be single words or phrases.
- Require extensive support of their adaptive functioning.

Profound LD/ID

- Skills like matching and sorting may be learned.
- Wants and emotions are expressed through non-verbal forms of communication.
- Require pervasive support of their adaptive functioning.

Psychological assessment of LD/ID

- The diagnosis of LD/ID requires assessment of a child's intellectual and adaptive functioning by a psychologist.
- Intellectual functioning is measured using a standardized, individually administered intelligence test.
- Examples of intelligence tests include:
  - Wechsler Intelligence Scale for Children—Fifth Edition (WISC-V).
  - Wechsler Abbreviated Scale of Intelligence (WASI-II).
  - Wechsler Preschool and Primary Scale of Intelligence (WPPSI-IV).
  - Stanford–Binet Intelligence Scales 5 (SB-5).
- Intelligence tests typically have a SD of 15 and a mean of 100.
- Children with LD/ID have IQ scores ~2 SD or more below the mean, including a margin for measurement error of +5 points.
- Children with LD/ID therefore have IQ scores at least below 65–75.
- Examples of measures of adaptive functioning include the Vineland Adaptive Behavior Scales-3 (Vineland-3) and the Adaptive Behavior Assessment System—Third Edition (ABAS-3).
- If a child has a sensory or physical impairment like blindness or prelingual deafness, locomotor disability, severe problem behaviours, or co-occurring mental disorder, assessment of the degree of ID may be difficult or even impossible. In these cases, the diagnosis of *unspecified ID* can be used.

- Unspecified ID should only be used in situations like those previously mentioned. Children with this diagnosis require reassessment in the future.
- The term borderline intellectual functioning refers to intellectual skills between the low average range and those of a person with an LD/ID.

Medical assessment of LD/ID

The medical assessment of a child with LD/ID should include:

- A detailed developmental history that includes information regarding onset of developmental concerns, developmental trajectory over time, current functioning, and prior and current interventions.
- A medical history that examines prenatal and perinatal history, and past medical history (regression, seizures, head injuries, CNS disease).
- Physical and neurological examination focused on observation of growth parameters and possible neurocutaneous lesions or dysmorphic features.
- A family history with a specific focus on developmental and learning challenges or genetic disorders.

Investigations

- If a specific genetic cause of LD/ID is suspected, laboratory assessment should be targeted to confirm the suspected cause (i.e. karyotype for trisomy 21, metabolic testing).
- If neither history nor physical exam is suggestive of a particular aetiological cause, laboratory assessment of a child with LD/ID should include a chromosomal microarray (CMA).
- Recent estimates of the diagnostic yield of a CMA range from 16% to 28% in patients with congenital anomalies, developmental delay, or LD/ID.
- There is less consensus regarding whether or not to obtain fragile X testing in children with LD/ID:
  - Some experts recommend obtaining fragile X testing for boys and girls with ID and clinical features of fragile X syndrome or for children with unexplained GDD or LD/ID in the setting of a family history of ID.
  - Some geneticists recommend obtaining fragile X testing only if a microarray result is within normal limits.
- However, some experts recommend obtaining a CMA, fragile X testing, and a karyotype as first-line testing.
- Exome and genome sequencing studies are emerging technologies that have the capacity to detect a wider array of genetic variations. However, they are not yet widely available or routinely recommended, although this is likely to change in the near future.
- Brain MRI is not routinely indicated for children with LD/ID but can be considered in a child who presents with non-syndromic LD/ID with macrocephaly, microcephaly, or a focal neurological sign.

Treatment

School

- School programming should be focused on maximizing the child's academic abilities.

- SEN supports should be tailored to meet the child's areas of vulnerability.
- Children with LD/ID should have opportunities to interact with typically developing peers during the school day.
- School programming for older children with LD/ID should focus on acquiring vocational and daily living skills.
- Older children with LD/ID should also have access to developmentally appropriate sexual education.

Home
- Safety management is key. Goals may include appropriate boundaries with strangers, how to get help when needed, and caution with knives or the stove.
- Instructions should be clear and concrete.
- Families should focus on strengthening adaptive skills, as possible.

Community
- Children with LD/ID should have opportunities to engage in community life (i.e. recreational and social activities).
- Basic understanding of safety concepts, as described previously, can allow for more meaningful community involvement.
- Disruptive behaviours can be a limiting factor in community involvement.
- In vocational settings, individuals with LD/ID can benefit from job coaching.

Behavioural
- Behavioural intervention should be focused on addressing disruptive or externalizing behaviours that negatively impact a child's functioning.
- Behavioural expectations should be commensurate with a child's developmental level.

Medical
- Clinicians should be vigilant regarding children with LD/ID being at risk of abuse, obesity and nutrition concerns, dental problems, and challenges with pain management.
- Coexisting conditions should be managed effectively.
- Consultation with a geneticist can be helpful in determining the cause of a child's LD/ID. This information can guide prognosis and surveillance for associated conditions and family planning in some cases.

Systems
Clinicians should be aware of local and national supports available to children with LD/ID.

Transition
- During the early adolescent years, clinicians should begin to discuss transition planning with the adolescent and their family/caregivers.
- Transition planning should focus on vocational skills, social supports, housing, and finance management.

- According to the UK Mental Capacity Act, individuals with LD/ID should be presumed capable of making decisions until proven otherwise.
  - It also recommends that individuals with LD/ID receive appropriate supports to make and communicate their decisions.
- If an individual with LD/ID does not have decision-making capacity, decisions can be made by a parent, a person who has a power of attorney of the individual with LD/ID, or a deputy appointed by the Court of Protection.

Long-term outcomes

- Individuals with LD/ID have great potential to lead meaningful lives in which they work, maintain social relationships, and remain well.
- Disruptive or externalizing behaviours can negatively impact an individual's functioning in home, educational, and vocational settings.
- Adults with mild LD/ID generally require intermittent support and reach academic abilities up to year 7 or age 11–12 in the UK (the sixth-grade level in the US). They are more likely to live independently, work, marry, and have children, and maintain financial independence as compared to adults with moderate or severe LD/ID.
- Adults with moderate LD/ID generally require limited support and reach academic abilities up to year 3 or age 7–8 in the UK (the second-grade level in the US).
- Adults with severe LD/ID generally require extensive support and reach academic abilities up to the preschool level.
- Adults with profound LD/ID require pervasive supports across areas of functioning.

Further resources

ENABLE Scotland: ℬ https://www.enable.org.uk/
Mencap: ℬ https://www.mencap.org.uk/

Developmental learning disorders

Background/definitions

- Developmental learning disorders (DLDs) in the ICD-11 (previously known as specific learning disorders in the ICD-10) are more widely recognized by alternative terms:
  - DLD with *impairment in reading* is also known as *dyslexia*.
  - DLD with *impairment in mathematics* is also known as *dyscalculia*.
  - DLD with *impairment in written expression* is also known as *dysgraphia*.
- Early identification of a DLD is critical to a child being able to access evidence-based interventions which can improve academic outcomes.

Epidemiology

- The prevalence of DLDs, across the domains of reading, writing, and mathematics, is 5–15% of school-age children.
- DLD with impairment in reading is the most common LD, occurring more commonly than DLDs with impairment in mathematics or writing.
- Estimates suggest that one in ten people in the UK experience some degree of DLD in reading.
- DLDs in reading, writing, and mathematics often co-occur.
- DLDs are more common in males versus females.

Aetiology

- Environmental risk factors for DLDs include prematurity, very low birth weight, and prenatal nicotine exposure.
- DLDs are also thought to be heritable conditions.
- Some candidate genes associated with DLD with impairment in reading have been identified. Research regarding DLDs in mathematics and writing is emerging.
- Recent research also suggests that the brains of children with DLD with impairment in reading are notable for subtle neuroanatomical differences as compared to the brains of typically developing children.
- DLDs can also be associated with particular genetic syndromes (e.g. Klinefelter syndrome, Turner syndrome, and neurofibromatosis type 1 (NF1)).

Diagnostic criteria

DLDs occur when an individual's academic abilities are significantly lower than would be expected, based on the individual's cognitive ability.

In the reading domain, examples include

- Impaired single-word reading.
- Difficulty with phonological processing.
- Impaired reading comprehension.

In the written expression domain, examples include

- Difficulty with spelling.
- Impaired use of grammar and punctuation.
- Difficulty formulating sentences or, for older children and adolescents, organizing paragraphs.

In the mathematics domain, examples include
• Poor number sense.
• Impaired basic calculation skills.
• Impaired understanding of mathematical concepts.
• Impaired ability to solve 'word problems'.

Diagnosis of a DLD requires persistence of the impaired academic skills despite exposure to appropriate education for age.

The World Health Organization's (WHO's) *International Classification of Disease*, 11th edition (ICD-11), describes 'Developmental learning disorder (DLD) as a condition characterised by significant and persistent difficulties in learning academic skills, which may include reading, writing, or arithmetic. The individual's performance in the affected academic skill(s) is markedly below what would be expected for chronological age and their intellectual functioning, and results in significant impairment in the individual's academic or occupational functioning. DLD is not due to a disorder of intellectual development, sensory impairment (vision or hearing), neurological or motor disorder, lack of educational opportunity, lack of proficiency in the language of academic instruction, or psychosocial adversity.'

Coexisting conditions
Children with neurodevelopmental conditions like ADHD, autism, and language disorders and children with mental health disorders are at increased risk of DLDs.

Diagnostic approach
Clinical presentation
• In very young children, signs concerning for emerging learning challenges include delays or deficits in pre-academic skills: letter or number recognition, letter–sound correspondence, and counting with one-to-one correspondence.
• School-age children with learning disorders may present with:
  • Signs of increased learning effort: complaints that school is boring, school anxiety, 'class clown' behaviour, or spending more time on academic tasks than peers.
  • Signs of school distress (see ➲ pp. 650–1): failing grades, frequent school absences/detentions/suspensions, social disengagement, or bullying.
  • Signs of school failure: grade retention, expulsion, and/or dropping out.

Medical assessment of developmental learning disorders
• The medical assessment of a child with a potential learning disorder requires a detailed developmental history that includes:
  • Acquisition of developmental milestones.
  • Current school day routines: sleep schedule, possible ADHD symptoms, and degree of learning impairment.
  • A past school history: possible grade retention, behavioural challenges in school, teacher feedback, and academic progress to date.

- A past medical history: prenatal and birth history, potential genetic disorders, sensory deficits, seizures, chronic conditions that may affect school attendance, and medications that can impact cognitive functioning.
- A social history.
- A family history focused on a potential history of relatives with learning challenges.
- Clinicians should also rule out vision and hearing deficits as potential causes of learning impairment by performing hearing and vision testing in all cases.

Psychological assessment of developmental learning disorders
- The diagnosis of a DLD requires assessment of a child's intellectual and academic functioning by a psychologist.
- Intellectual functioning is measured using a standardized, individually administered intelligence test.
- Examples of intelligence tests include:
  - Wechsler Intelligence Scale for Children—Fifth Edition (WISC-V).
  - Wechsler Abbreviated Scale of Intelligence (WASI-II).
  - Wechsler Preschool and Primary Scale of Intelligence (WPPSI-IV).
  - Stanford–Binet Intelligence Scales 5 (SB-5).
- Academic functioning is similarly measured using a standardized, individually administered test of academic ability.
- Examples of academic tests include:
  - Wechsler Individual Achievement Test (WIAT-IV).
  - Woodcock Johnson IV Tests of Achievement (WJ-IV).
  - Kaufman Test of Educational Achievement—Third Edition (KTEA-3).
- A child's intellectual ability and academic achievement should be commensurate.
  - For example, a child with high average verbal intelligence should demonstrate reading skills in the high average range.
- If a child's academic functioning falls far below the level of achievement predicted by their intellectual ability, this discrepancy can be best explained by the presence of a DLD.
  - For example, testing that revealed that a child with high average non-verbal intelligence scored in the low average range on a test of mathematics ability is suggestive of a DLD with impairment in mathematics.

Treatment
- Treatment of DLDs centres upon the use of evidence-based reading curricula.
- Individuals with DLD in reading should receive access to audio and digital versions of textbooks, extended time to complete tests and quizzes, and should engage in daily independent reading practice.
- Due to the lack of robust research regarding DLDs in mathematics and writing, the associated interventions are more 'common sense' than evidenced based, and may include access to a calculator, extended time, breaking problems into smaller steps, use of graphic organizers, frequent check-ins with the teacher, and visual supports.

- Supports for children with DLD in writing include explicit and incremental writing instruction, explicit spelling instruction, use of graphic organizers, and access to assistive word processing programs or speech-to-text technology.
- Interventions are primarily delivered in the school setting.
- However, some families may hire a tutor to supplement school-based instruction.
- Some schools may recommend grade retention or 'holding a child back' when they are struggling with an academic domain, like reading. However, this is not a helpful intervention and may in fact be harmful.

Transition

Teenagers with DLDs who are transitioning to post-secondary education can reach out to their college or university's office of disability services regarding educational supports for which they may be eligible.

Long-term outcomes

- Children with DLDs are at risk of school failure as characterized by grade retention, expulsion, or dropping out of school.
- These risks can be mitigated by early identification of learning difficulties and intensive instruction using evidence-based curricula.
- Longitudinal studies of children with DLD with impairment in reading are suggestive of persistent reading difficulties into young adulthood.
- However, with appropriate supports, individuals with DLDs can achieve educational and vocational goals.

Further resources

British Dyslexia Association: ℘ https://www.bdadyslexia.org.uk/
LD Online: ℘ http://www.ldonline.org/

Developmental coordination disorder

- Historical terms associated with DCD:
  - Dysfunction of attention, motor function, and perception (DAMP).
  - Clumsy child syndrome.
  - Hand–eye coordination problem.
  - Apraxia.
  - Ideomotor dyspraxia.
  - Developmental dyspraxia.
  - Minimal neurological dysfunction.
  - Mild CP.
- Basically, DCD means an impairment or difficulty in planning, organizing, and executing movements in the absence of a neurological or intellectual impairment. This has an impact on schooling and social functioning secondary to the difficulties in carrying out activities of daily living.

Diagnostic criteria

- DCD is a neurodevelopmental disorder characterized by motor impairment that negatively impacts a child's functioning across settings.
- Importantly, this motor impairment is inconsistent with age and opportunity.
- Examples of DCD-related motor impairment include slowness in motor functioning, clumsiness, poor handwriting, balance and gait challenges, vulnerable motor planning, and fine motor difficulties.
- DCD-related motor challenges cannot be better explained by a LD (or ID), visual impairment, or a condition that impacts movement, like CP, a myopathy or a neuropathy.

Prevalence

- Approximately 5–6% of children may qualify for a diagnosis of DCD.
- The prevalence ranges from 5% to 15% in all the studies.
- About 2–3% are likely to be more severe and the rest are on a continuum.
- Boys are 3–4 times more likely to be affected than girls.

Risk factors

- Family history.
- Preterm birth.
- Extremely low birth weight.
- Exposure to teratogens in pregnancy, e.g. alcohol.
- Negative sociodemographic factors and environmental disadvantages may further compound the problem and/or worsen chances of enablement.

Factors underpinning motor function

- Attention.
- Executive function (e.g. impulse control).
- Memory and cognition.
- Praxis (refers to planning and sequence necessary to perform the action).
- Vision (visual tracking, visual perception).
- Proprioception (reception of stimuli from muscles and tissues that results in a sense of body position).
- Sensorimotor feedback (aural, kinaesthetic, vestibular) impede or enhance the motor postures and movements.

Impairment or dysfunction in any of the listed areas will cause motor/coordination difficulties.

Common comorbidities

- Attention deficit disorder (ADD)/ADHD.
- Dyslexia/reading disability.
- ASD.

Presenting features

Any of the activities of daily living could be affected. Commonly present with:

- Slow, laborious, and immature handwriting.
- Difficulty in playing ball games (i.e. poor catching/throwing).
- Ambidextrous.
- Difficulty with dressing, undressing. Left–right confusion, wear clothes inside out/back to front.
- Messy eating. Preferring to eat with hands rather than fork or spoon.
- Shy from sports or physical activity. Poor at running, jumping, and team sports.
- Significant emotional and behavioural problems. Refuse to go to school, physical complaints to avoid work, tearful, anxious, depressed, isolated, and withdrawn.

Assessment

- History and examination can rule out the presence of a physical or neurological condition causing incoordination.
- Neurodevelopmental testing can confirm the presence or absence of significant coordination difficulties by the ability to provide percentiles, motor quotient, and SD.

History

- Results of previous scans, metabolic tests, and genetic analysis, if any.
- Parent and teacher behaviour questionnaire (Strengths and Difficulties Questionnaire).
- Pregnancy (teratogens, complications, TORCH infections/screen).
- Birth history (gestation, complications, birth weight, resuscitation required, special care, etc.).
- Acquisition of developmental milestones usually delayed (e.g. age of walking).
- Has the child lost any skills?
- Personal–social/adaptive skills, e.g. dressing, eating, tying laces, self-care, etc.

Worsening of coordination difficulties and regression or loss of existing skills would be inconsistent with the diagnosis of DCD.

Physical examination

- Any dysmorphic features? Examine head to toe.
- Growth (height, weight, head circumference) and plot them on centile charts.

- Neurological examination (assess cranial nerves, posture, tone, muscle bulk, muscle strength, deep tendon reflexes, primitive reflexes, involuntary movements, cerebellar functions, stressed gait, etc.). Stressed gaits = walking on the toes, heels, sideways, and backward.
- Developmental soft signs (refer to fine motor and social skills milestones and plot child's attainment).
- Vision. Correction of any refractive error.
- Hearing. Confirm hearing thresholds. Treatment of otitis media with effusion (OME).

Presence of weakness, profound hypotonia, hypertonia, or ataxia would be incongruent with the diagnosis of DCD.

Investigations
- Movement Assessment Battery for Children-2 (MABC-2) is widely used to screen for movement difficulties in school and can be completed by teachers.
- Evaluation of a child with DCD may include the use of a measure designed to assess motor and visual perception like the Bruininks-Oseretsky Test of Motor Proficiency (BOTMP-2) or the Beery–Buktenica Developmental Test of Visual-Motor Integration (VMI).

Management
- Have a multifaceted and holistic approach to enablement.
- Treatments/therapies which incorporate the following are likely to be more successful:
  - Engage/motivate the child, i.e. child-centred.
  - Address functional activity, e.g. handwriting/drawing.
  - Are repetitive, i.e. practice and long term.
  - Goal directed, e.g. learning to ride bicycle.
  - Reward, i.e. SMART targets that give a sense of accomplishment.

Occupational therapy
The following approaches have been in use to address coordination difficulties, namely:
- Cognitive Orientation to Occupational Performance (CO-OP)—can result in significant improvements in motor skill acquisition.
  - The key feature is 'dynamic performance analysis' which looks into the difficulties the child encounters while performing an activity. Use a problem-solving approach.
  - 'Goal–Plan–Do–Check'—child is taught a framework for solving motor-based performance problems.
  - 'Domain specific strategies'—uses a number of motor-based, child-chosen activities such as cycling, using cutlery, handwriting, ball games, etc.
- Specific skills approach: one of the most effective approaches. Emphasizes repetitive training of specific motor skills/task-specific strategies.
- OTs can also give advice on seating, access, modifications to the cutlery/dressing/writing materials, work surface, etc. which is usually found very helpful by children and carers.

Physiotherapy

Can help with advice and modifications on posture, gross motor skills, and exercises.

Neurodevelopmental paediatrician

Identify and address comorbidities which compound the difficulty and impact on the treatment given, e.g. methylphenidate use for children with ADHD and DCD is shown to improve coordination and ADHD symptomatology.

School

- Educational/occupational interventions, e.g. teachers and teaching assistants can provide daily exercises as shown by the OT which would be effective in the majority of children.
- Provide scribe for important work or exams.
- Giving extra time for completing examinations.
- Actively encouraging and involving the child in team sports.
- Career counselling etc.

Psychologists

Counselling to address low self-esteem, shyness, and provide coping strategies.

Educational psychologists/neuropsychologists

Can identify associated comorbidities such as dyslexia, mild LD, etc. and give advice on appropriate interventions/modifications to the curriculum.

Adaptations to the environment

- Access to keyboard/laptop for work.
- Velcro fasteners instead of shoe laces.
- Fasteners instead of buttons.
- Rubber grip holders for pencils, chunky crayons, and modified forks/spoons.
- Adjustments to chair/desk height, inclination, etc.

Prognosis

- DCD usually persists into adulthood (i.e. lifelong). Hence likely to lead to poor social and occupational outcomes.
- Children with DCD are more likely to show social isolation, emotional and behavioural problems, and low self-esteem compared to their peers.
- Children with DCD are also more likely to have an aversion to physical exercises, have higher body fat, be obese, and suffer from poor cardiorespiratory fitness.
- With early identification followed by early multidisciplinary intervention, the prognosis for social integration, self-esteem, emotional adjustment, and educational achievement is likely to be good.

Support groups

- Provide information about support, run courses, activity camps, advice on activities to practice, advocacy, and raising awareness.
- Dyspraxia Foundation: ℘ https://dyspraxiafoundation.org.uk/

Inborn errors of metabolism

- IEMs are also known as congenital or inherited metabolic diseases.
- IEMs are conditions characterized by:
  - A lack of a specific enzyme, a cofactor, or a transport protein.
  - Leading to either toxic accumulation or deficiency of an end product.
  - Causing disruption of energy production, energy utilization, or progressive damage to organs due to disruption of normal physiological and biochemical pathways.
- Approximately 500 IEMs have been identified. Moreover, many of these conditions vary in their onset, severity, and in the way they are inherited. Hence a detailed summary of IEMs is beyond the scope of this book!
- Also, many of these IEMs present in neonatal period or infancy. Some could present anytime till adulthood.
- Most IEMs present to neonatologists, neurologists, or acute paediatricians. A smaller proportion present to community paediatrics masquerading as developmental delay or regression.
- Approximately 1–5% of developmental delay cases may have an IEM as an underlying cause.
- Worsening developmental delay, developmental regression, and/or ID is likely to occur in many IEMs.
- Professionals should be able to suspect IEMs and make onward referrals to tertiary centres for further investigations, specific therapy, genetic counselling, and for more precise prognosis.
- Specific treatment is available for an increasing number of IEMs.

Incidence

- Individually rare, ~1:100,000. Collectively ~1:1000 to 1:2500.
- PKU ~1:13000, mitochondrial disorders ~1:5000, lysosomal storage disorders ~1:5000, medium-chain acyl dehydrogenase deficiency (MCADD) ~1:8000.

Inheritance

- IEMs are generally single-gene disorders.
- Most common mode of inheritance for the IEMs is autosomal recessive (AR). Hence higher incidence/prevalence in populations with high consanguinity.
- Modes: AR (e.g. galactosaemia), X-linked recessive (XLR) (e.g. Hunter syndrome, ornithine transcarbamylase deficiency, Menkes syndrome); autosomal dominant (AD) (e.g. familial hypercholesterolaemia); or mitochondrial (e.g. myopathy, encephalopathy, lactic acidosis, and stroke (MELAS); myoclonic epilepsy with ragged red fibres (MERRF)).

Types of inborn errors of metabolism

Disorders of:
- Carbohydrate metabolism, e.g. glycogen storage diseases.
- Fatty acid oxidation, e.g. MCAD.
- Amino acid, e.g. PKU.
- Purine metabolism, e.g. Lesch–Nyhan syndrome.
- Urea cycle, e.g. ornithine transcarbamylase deficiency.
- Mitochondria, e.g. pyruvate dehydrogenase deficiency.

- Peroxisomal, e.g. Zellweger syndrome.
- Lysosomal storage disorders, e.g. mucopolysaccharidosis (MPS), Tay–Sachs disease, Niemann–Pick disease.
- Metal, e.g. Wilson disease and Menkes disease (copper); pantothenate kinase-associated neurodegeneration (PKAN) (iron).
- Others, e.g. hypothyroidism.

Clinical presentation

- IEMs can present in any age group. Severe variants present in the neonatal period or early infancy. Less severe cases could present anytime until the seventh decade.
- Clinical presentation depends on the severity of enzyme deficiency, the nature and rate of the accumulating toxic metabolite, and the severity of disruption of energy metabolism.
- Presentation also depends on timing of the insult/trigger in many cases. Illness, change in dietary habits, fasting, unaccustomed exercise, trauma, certain medications, childbirth, or surgery could trigger a decompensation and uncover IEMs.
- Neurological and GI manifestations are the most common way of presentation for IEMs.
- However, IEMs can present in the following ways:
  - *Neurological*: developmental delay, LD, acute encephalopathy, weakness, abnormalities of tone, ataxia, peripheral neuropathy, paraparesis, delirium, hallucinations, agitation, coma, seizures, and neuropsychiatric manifestations (e.g. self-injury in Lesch Nyhan disease, ADHD in Sanfilippo syndrome).
  - *Dysmorphic features*: lysosomal storage disorders (coarse facial features), homocystinuria (marfanoid body habitus), and peroxisomal disorders (high forehead, epicanthal folds, high-arched palate).
  - *Dermatological*: skin rashes (biotinidase deficiency), photosensitivity (porphyria), and hypopigmentation (untreated PKU).
  - *Ophthalmological*: manifestations may include cataracts, corneal opacities, cherry-red spots, etc.
  - *Gastrointestinal*: failure to thrive/poor growth, poor feeding, vomiting (e.g. organic acidurias), jaundice, hepatomegaly (e.g. glycogen storage disease), and hepatosplenomegaly (e.g. lysosomal storage disorders).
  - *Haematological*: neutropenia (e.g. glycogen storage disease), pancytopenia (e.g. Gaucher disease), and megaloblastic anaemia (e.g. disorders of vitamin B_{12} metabolism).
  - *Renal*: nephrolithiasis (e.g. cystinuria) and renal tubular acidosis (e.g. mitochondrial disorders).
  - *Musculoskeletal*: such as exercise intolerance, muscle pain, and cramps in metabolic myopathies.
  - *In infancy*: as sudden infant death syndrome, apparent life-threatening event (e.g. MCAD deficiency) or as critically ill neonate.
  - *Biochemical*: hypoglycaemia, ketosis, hyperammonaemia, metabolic acidosis, lactic acidosis, etc.

Abnormal biochemistry could accompany any of these system disorders or these biochemical abnormalities could be found unexpectedly in a child with a mild illness.

Neurodevelopmental disorders and inborn errors of metabolism

- IEMs account for ~1–5% cases of developmental delay.
- Developmental delay in IEM is:
  - Usually global, not specific or isolated skill delay (see ➔ p. 30).
  - Usually progressive.
  - Usually associated with 'developmental delay plus', i.e. central/peripheral nervous system disease, cardiomyopathy, dysmorphology (see ➔ p. 483), etc.
- Have a low threshold to investigate those children where developmental delay presents with other features in history or examination.
- Since IEMs span such a vast array of presentations, one could use a Boolean search process of electronic resources such as OMIM, using keywords (presenting signs and symptoms) with operator words (such as AND, OR) to broaden or narrow the search results and to produce a shortlist of the possible conditions/differential diagnosis.
- When there is a strong possibility of an IEM, a referral, or a discussion with a tertiary specialist centre, should be considered.
- There are >200 IEMs which could result in developmental delay.
- IEMs could present as developmental delay, regression, mild to profound LD, or autism (see ➔ pp. 114–25).
- Conditions causing developmental delay include lysosomal storage disorders, urea cycle disorders, peroxisomal disorders, and mitochondrial disorders.
- Prompt diagnosis may avoid progressive neurological damage, arrest developmental regression, and ameliorate the degree of ID or LD.
- Prognosis is likely to be better with earlier identification of signs and symptoms, prompt investigations, and referral to a specialist tertiary centre with expertise in metabolic disorders for further evaluation and management.
- Keeping the above-mentioned points in mind, a brief overview of the evaluation of IEMs and the associated neurodevelopmental disorders is covered here, as a detailed overview is beyond the scope of this book.

History

- Pregnancy: decreased fetal movements, e.g. Zellweger syndrome, non-immune hydrops, prolonged labour, previous miscarriages, HELLP syndrome, and neonatal encephalopathy could all be a signs of IEMs.
- Perinatal history of many IEMs could be normal since the metabolic error in the fetus is generally well compensated by the mother.
- Past medical history: lethargy in mornings, hospitalization for recurrent vomiting or dehydration, recurrent hypoglycaemia, failure to thrive/poor growth, developmental delay, developmental regression, seizures, abnormal movements, and stepwise deterioration.
- Triggers: specific triggers such as ingestion of certain carbohydrates/proteins, use of complementary foods, infections, medications, fasting, anaesthesia, or surgery.

- Family history: consanguinity, thrombotic events, developmental delay/ disabilities, unexplained deaths in infancy or early childhood, and affected siblings.
- Enquire about growth, diarrhoea, sepsis, unusual odours (organic acidurias), and protein aversion (urea cycle disorders).

Examination

- Height (tall in homocystinuria, short in MPS disorders), occipitofrontal circumference (OFC) (small in untreated PKU, large in Canavan disease), and weight.
- Hair (sparse and kinked in Menkes disease).
- Skin (hirsute in MPS, eczema/alopecia in biotinidase deficiency, hypopigmentation in phenylketonuria).
- Dysmorphic features (marfanoid habitus in homocystinuria, coarse facial features in MPS, etc.).
- Eyes (cataracts, e.g. galactosaemia, cherry red macula in Tay–Sachs disease, Kayser–Fleischer ring in Wilson disease, corneal clouding in MPS).
- Ears (conductive hearing loss in MPS, sensorineural hearing loss in mitochondrial disorders).
- Mouth (gingival hypertrophy in MPS).
- Abdomen (hepatosplenomegaly in lysosomal storage disorders, hepatomegaly in glycogen storage disorders).
- Neurology (assess tone, power, reflexes, abnormal movements, cognitive development); e.g. dystonia in Lesch–Nyhan syndrome and organic acidaemias, hypotonia in mitochondrial and peroxisomal disorders, myopathy in mitochondrial disorders, peripheral neuropathy in leukodystrophies, etc.
- Behaviour (e.g. challenging in Sanfilippo syndrome, autistic in Smith– Lemli–Opitz syndrome, self-mutilation in Lesch–Nyhan syndrome).
- Skeletal (dysplasias in lysosomal and peroxisomal disorders, arthritis in purine metabolism disorders).

Investigations

- Good detailed history (milestones) is the single most important investigation (will differentiate static vs progressive).
- Investigations should only be undertaken after a detailed history and head-to-toe examination as previously described, especially in non-acute situations such as in neurodevelopmental practice.
- A stepwise approach to IEM investigations is advisable, beginning with certain basic routine tests before undertaking specialized metabolic studies.
- Specialized metabolic tests should be undertaken in discussion with metabolic or genetic specialist.
- Results from specialized metabolic studies may benefit from a review/ interpretation by a specialist in IEMs from a tertiary centre.

Why investigate?
- Identify treatable condition (urea cycle defects, aminoacidurias, biotinidase deficiency, dopa-responsive dystonias, pyridoxine deficiency, Wilson disease, Refsum disease, etc.).
- Genetic implications and offering genetic counselling.
- Information and support group from self-help groups.
- Leverage with resources.
- An explanation to parents, siblings, and family.

Baseline

- Initial investigations to be considered for chronic clinical presentation and developmental delay are presented here. Investigations for acute/emergency presentations of IEM are outside the scope of this book.
- The possibility of an IEM and the need for appropriate tailored investigations needs to be considered periodically in a child with developmental arrest or regression as clinical signs may manifest over a period of time.

Consider undertaking following baseline investigations in a child with developmental delay with a suspected IEM:
- FBC.
- Blood gas (to check for metabolic acidosis and respiratory alkalosis).
- Ammonia (do not use tourniquet. Transfer bloods to laboratory on ice.).
- Urea and electrolytes (to calculate anion gap).
- Liver function tests.
- Thyroid function tests.
- Serum uric acid (high in Lesch–Nyhan syndrome).
- Plasma amino acids.
- Lactate (no tourniquet, transfer bloods on ice).
- Serum phytanic acid and very long-chain fatty acids (peroxisomal disorders).
- Serum creatine kinase.
- Blood glucose.
- Urine (amino acids, organic acids, glycosaminoglycans).
- Dilated fundoscopy from an ophthalmologist to detect retinal changes and atrophy.
- Brain MRI scan to look for basal ganglia changes (lysosomal storage disorders, mitochondrial disorders) and leukodystrophy.

See Table 3.20.
Interpretation of the results from the baseline tests should take the following guidance into account.

Further investigations

- These are guided by history, examination findings, and baseline tests.
- They are best done in a specialist/tertiary setting where there are facilities for ordering these tests and interpreting them appropriately.
- If specific clinical features are present then discuss with IEM team at a tertiary centre before ordering tests.

Table 3.20 Interpretation of baseline tests

Test abnormality	Comments and possible causes of abnormal results	
↑ Creatinine kinase	Muscle injury. Muscular dystrophy. Fatty acid oxidation disorders	
↑ Lactate	Excessive screaming, tourniquet pressure. Gluconeogenetic disorders. Disorders of pyruvate metabolism. Mitochondrial disorders	
	Is urine lactate ↑? Is plasma alanine ↑?	If yes suggests elevation of lactate.
↑ Ammonia	Sample contamination. Sample delay in transport/processing. Specimen haemolysed. Urea cycle disorders. Liver dysfunction	
Urate	An abnormally high or low result is significant. Glycogen storage disorder ↑. Purine disorders ↑. Molybdenum cofactor deficiency ↓	

Reproduced with permission from 'Best Practice Guidelines for the Biochemical Investigation of Global Developmental Delay for Inherited Metabolic Disorders (IEM)', Green A (2006) The National Metabolic Biochemistry Network, http://metbio.net

- Consider perusing the guidelines for investigations from an IEM specialist group/IEM society in your country, such as ℘ https://www.bimdg.org.uk/site/guidelines (in the UK).
- Investigations undertaken at the time of presentation are likely to have better yields.
- There are 'profiles', i.e. a bunch of tests for each scenario, such as hepatosplenomegaly, hydrops, cherry-red macula, etc.:
  • Brain MRI scan. MRI abnormalities in IEMs are usually symmetrical.
  • Plasma amino acids (quantitative).
  • Very long-chain fatty acids, plasmalogens, and phytanic acid.
  • White cell enzymes for lysosomal disorders.
  • Plasma and urine creatine.
  • Lumbar puncture (glucose, protein, protein, glycine, serine, alanine, organic acids, neurotransmitters, lactate, pyruvate).
  • Echocardiography (cardiomyopathy in fatty acid oxidation disorders).
  • X-rays for skeletal abnormalities.

Diagnosis

- Reliant on having a high index of suspicion of IEMs in the earlier given clinical scenarios, ordering appropriate tests, and considering referral to units with specialist expertise in IEMs.
- Diagnosis will help in offering specific treatment, where available.
- Also helpful in counselling and enables clinicians to give a prognosis.

Management

- Early recognition of the IEM would lead to better outcomes.
- Having a high index of suspicion helps in recognizing IEMs.
- A good history and head-to-toe examination could provide specific clues to necessary investigations and earlier identification.
- Early recognition is likely to prevent progressive neurological damage in many cases.
- An increasing number of IEMs are being included in the newborn screening programmes, but these cannot be relied upon entirely.
- Correct management requires input from a specialist in IEMs and intensive care facilities, especially during acute decompensation. Mortality and morbidity are higher if poorly treated during acute illness.
- In the acute situation, the child might need:
  - Ventilator support.
  - Fluid resuscitation.
  - Treating of hypoglycaemia (intravenous (IV) 10% dextrose).
  - Hyperammonaemia (medications).
  - Acidosis (bicarbonate).
  - Reversal of catabolism (insulin infusion).
  - Renal replacement therapy (dialysis).
  - Empiric antibiotics until cultures are negative.
  - For emergency management guidelines, see ℰ https://www.bimdg. org.uk/site/guidelines
- Specific long-term treatments might include the following:
  - Dietary education and compliance are crucial. Special diets, e.g. phenylalanine free in PKU.
  - Provision of cofactors, e.g. pyridoxine in pyridoxine-dependent seizures.
  - Enzyme replacement therapy, e.g. MPS; correcting deficiency, e.g. thyroxine in hypothyroidism.
  - Stimulating alternative metabolic pathway, e.g. benzoate for urea cycle defects, penicillamine for Wilson disease.
  - Organ transplantation, e.g. liver transplant in glycogen storage disease, bone marrow transplant in metachromatic leukodystrophy.
- Close follow-up to monitor growth, cognitive development (see ➔ pp. 36–8), and physical health.
- Periodic assessment at a specialist/tertiary IEM clinic is helpful.
- Enablement:
  - Housing, e.g. adaptations for ramps, railings, hoist, downstairs toilet/ shower/bed (see ➔ pp. 392–3), etc.
  - Aids, e.g. wheelchairs, glasses, hearing aids, etc.
  - Appliances, e.g. orthoses (see ➔ pp. 424–6), splints, special mattress, etc.
  - Education, e.g. statement of SEN, home schooling (see ➔ pp. 656–8 and p. 668), etc.
  - Leisure, e.g. access to swimming, entertainment activities, etc.
- Social support, e.g. help with respite, transport, benefits, allowances, etc. (see ➔ pp. 682–3).
- Refer affected families to geneticists for counselling regarding recurrence risks (see ➔ pp. 490–4).

Further resources

Association for Glycogen Storage Diseases: https://www.agsd.org.uk
British Inherited Metabolic Diseases Group: https://www.bimdg.org.uk (for emergency management).
Inherited Metabolic Diseases: http://www.climb.org.uk
Metabolic Support UK: https://www.metabolicsupportuk.org
National MPS Society: https://www.mpssociety.org
National Society for Phenylketonuria: https://www.nspku.org

Developmental disabilities in the developing world: challenges, opportunities, and possible solutions

A brief overview

- Childhood disability affects millions of children around the world, most of whom are in low- and middle-income countries.
- It is claimed that up to 1 billion people or 15% of the world's population could have some form of disability.

Disability

Persons with disabilities include those who have long-term physical, mental, intellectual, or sensory impairments which in interaction with various barriers may hinder their full and effective participation in society on an equal basis with others.

Developmental disabilities

- These are disorders of the developing nervous system that present during infancy or childhood as limitation of function or delay in development in one or more developmental domains, like gross motor, fine motor, cognition, language, or social development.
- Developmental disabilities are a group of conditions resulting from impairments that affect a child's physical, learning, or behavioural functioning.
- Affected children could have sensory impairments (e.g. hearing impairment (see ➔ pp. 168–9) or vision impairment (see ➔ pp. 202–8)), epilepsy (see ➔ pp. 248–55), CP (see ➔ pp. 92–101), ADHD (see ➔ pp. 126–34), ASD (see ➔ pp. 114–25), ID (see ➔ pp. 136–41), or other learning disorders (see ➔ pp. 142–5).

ICD-11 classifies 'neurodevelopmental disorders' into

- Disorders of intellectual development (see ➔ pp. 136–41).
- Developmental speech or language disorders (see ➔ pp. 402–3).
- ASD (see ➔ pp. 114–25).
- Developmental learning disorders (see ➔ pp. 142–5).
- Developmental motor coordination disorder (see ➔ pp. 146–9).
- ADHD (see ➔ pp. 126–34).
- Stereotyped movement disorder.
- Other neurodevelopmental disorders.

DSM-5 classifies 'developmental disabilities' into

- Cognitive: intellectual developmental disability and DLDs.
- Motor: CP, muscular dystrophies, neuroinfections, epilepsy, movement disorders, and DCD.
- Vision: refraction disorders, night blindness (vitamin A deficiency), congenital cataract, and eye injuries.
- Hearing: conductive and sensorineural deafness (congenital anomalies, infections).
- Speech: articulation disorders, receptive and/or expressive language disorders.

- Behaviour: ADHD and ASD.
- Global developmental delay.

Some common characteristics of developmental disabilities
- Skills are substantially below the expected level for chronological age, measured intelligence, and age-appropriate education.
- Cannot be explained by any obvious neurological disorder or any specific adverse psychosocial or family circumstances.
- An onset that invariably appears during infancy or childhood.
- An impairment or delay in the development of functions that are strongly related to biological maturation of the CNS.
- A steady course that does not involve the remissions and relapses that tend to be characteristic of many mental disorders.

Prevalence
- Approximately 15% of the world's population could have some form of disability. The prevalence of disability is higher in developing countries.
- More than 85% of the world's population live in developing countries, which include China, India, sub-Saharan Africa, Latin America, Caribbean, and the Middle East countries.
- In the Global Burden of Disease study in 2016, out of 632 million children <5 years of age, 52.9 million had at least one of the six developmental disabilities (vision loss, hearing loss, ID, ASD, epilepsy, and ADHD).
- Among these children with developmental disabilities, only 2.7 million were living in high-income countries and 50.7 million were living in low- to middle-income countries (Table 3.21).
- Of children with developmental disabilities, 54% were boys and 46% were girls.
- In the Global Burden of Disease 2016 study, the number of cases of developmental disabilities per 100,000 population was highest in India with 10,308. It was up to 9000 in sub-Saharan Africa, ~8621 in Southeast Asia, ~7000 in Europe, ~4787 in Australia, and ~4090 in North America. This report clearly highlighted the higher risk of developmental disabilities in developing countries.
- Vision loss was the most prevalent disability, followed by hearing loss, ID, and ASD.

Table 3.21 Global prevalence of children with developmental disabilities

Developmental disability	Prevalence per 100,000 population
Vision loss	3991
Hearing loss	2445
ID	1983
ASD	723
Epilepsy	603
ADHD	141

- ID was the largest contributor to years of living with disability.
- The prevalence of CP has been reported to be around 2–2.2/1000 live births in well-resourced countries. With the limited data available from developing countries, the prevalence of CP has been estimated to be as high as 10/1000 in Africa.

Challenges

Lack of neurodevelopmental services

- Most of the developmental disabilities if diagnosed and intervened early, show better long-term prognoses.
- But in developing countries, the unavailability of trained professionals, especially in rural areas, makes early diagnosis difficult.
- The availability of neurodevelopmental services shows gross disparities among the WHO regions (Table 3.22).

Wait-and-watch policy

Developmental disabilities, such as speech delay and ASD, are often dealt with by a typical grandparental approach—'Let's wait, the child may talk later, his father also started talking late!' This delays diagnosis and thus reduces the chances of a better outcome.

Limited resources

Poverty, inadequate facilities, food insecurity, lack of technology, and limited education are some of the causes that interfere with getting the right intervention at the right time; e.g. a child with CP may benefit from assistive devices such as a walker/wheelchair, if offered at an early age.

Inconsistent policies

In low-income countries, the government policies prioritize the allocation of resources to develop a basic health infrastructure or employment opportunities. This leads to reduced facilities/resources for children with developmental disabilities.

Poor social awareness and support

Unfortunately, in low-income and low-education countries, society often looks at children with developmental disability with stigma, pity, neglect, and/or avoidance, which makes their life difficult. These children require a social and human rights approach.

Table 3.22 Availability of neurodevelopmental services across WHO regions

WHO region	Median per 100,000 population
Europe	9.0
Western Pacific	3.7
Africa	0.1
South-East Asia	0.3

Lack of inclusive and special schools
Most developing countries have inadequate infrastructure required for inclusion schooling, which includes untrained teachers, lack of teaching material, overcrowding (high student-to-teacher ratio), a lack of awareness of modifications or accommodations required for children with disabilities, and insufficient funds.

Low level of parental literacy
Success of early intervention for developmental disability lies in education of the parent(s), especially the mother. A less literate mother may not be able to follow instructions from the therapist or may not understand the seriousness of developmental disability.

Barriers, distance, and transportation
Children with motor developmental disabilities are deprived of education and social interaction because of the lack of availability of modifications required (e.g. ramps, disabled toilets, etc.) in public transport and in institutions. Long distance from schools is also a matter of concern for children from poor families.

Lack of recreational opportunities
Whether it is physical limitation or lack of social communication, children with disabilities are deprived of 'play'—which Montessori says, is the 'work of children!' Peers can keep children with disability away from interactive play.

Sex inequality
Even today, in many developing countries, some people still look at girls as a burden. This matters even more for girls with disabilities.

Disturbed families
Addictions, violence, maternal health issues, and overcrowding are just some of the issues that directly affect prognosis of children with developmental disabilities.

Infectious diseases of the nervous system
- Viral encephalitis, rabies, cerebral malaria, dengue fever, and tubercular meningitis are most common neuroinfectious disorders seen in developing and low-income countries.
- Neuroinfections are caused by vaccine-preventable diseases, e.g. meningitis caused by measles (subacute sclerosing panencephalitis, *Haemophilus influenza* type B, meningococcus).
- These preventable infections are thankfully rare in developed countries, but are still a cause of concern in developing countries.
- Fortunately, polio eradication programme, such as in India, have reduced the neurodisability due to poliomyelitis radically.

Opportunities
- In the last two decades, increasing numbers of children with developmental disabilities are being diagnosed worldwide.
- These developmental disabilities have long-term effects on the individual, family, community, and country and also at a global level.

- A four-pronged approach has been suggested to reduce this burden:
  - Early diagnosis of developmental disabilities.
  - Early intervention to minimize the level of disability.
  - Rehabilitation services to make the individual independent.
  - Preventive measures to avoid developmental disabilities.
- Even today, the ratio of developmental paediatricians, paediatric neurologists, and therapists to the volume of children with developmental disabilities is very low. There is a massive need and a huge scope for trained medical and rehabilitation professionals to bridge this gap.
- There is an ever-increasing need for taking diagnostic services (laboratory, imaging, genetic) from urban to rural levels. Cost-effective solutions in this area could generate a huge amount of employment at a local level.
- Keeping the needs of children with developmental disabilities in mind, there is tremendous scope for developing disability-friendly infrastructure and ecosystems. There is an opportunity for architects, engineers, and developers to be creative.
- Strengthening of education systems with provision for 'inclusion' is another enormous area with lots of prospects.
- Global thought and local production: WHO, UNICEF, and many global projects are providing innovative solutions to help children with disabilities. Translating them to locally available, affordable services is an opportunity.
- Use of digital technology such as telemedicine, online education, software solutions, etc. could make the lives of individuals with disabilities easier.
- Community participation, in any form—whether it is education, fund raising, infrastructure development, platforms to interact, or simple initiatives such as befriending children with developmental disabilities—could change the approach of society towards inclusivity and less discrimination.
- Focusing on developmental needs of children with special needs is an opportunity for the world to come together to tackle this noble cause.

Solutions

- Management of children with developmental disabilities could be tackled at multiple levels.
- It requires a multipronged approach, especially in resource-limited settings, utilizing local resources and at the same time tapping into global partnerships with developed countries.

At family level
- Parents play a key role in early diagnosis and intervention.
- Parental education and motivation for stimulation, early intervention, and community participation.
- Participation of wider family, especially grandparents.

Some examples of family programmes
- The Portage model for early intervention—now adopted in 90 countries and translated into >30 languages.

- Adoption of Portage model—e.g. by the non-governmental organization 'Samadhan' for the poorest areas of New Delhi, India.
- Los Pipitos—an active parental organization in Nicaragua; it uses dance, creative movements, arts, drama, and music to support people with disabilities. It has >14,000 families as members.

At community level
- Involvement of society in supporting families for better care of children with disabilities.
- Providing opportunities to children with disabilities to interact with people around them is important to establish an 'inclusive society'.
- This requires community education, with purposeful involvement of people around to include children with disabilities.
- Arranging unique programmes and festivals in such a way that the families of children with disabilities feel included in society.
- Encouraging participation of children with disabilities in vocational activities would allow them to be useful and productive members of the society.

Some examples of global programmes
- Disability and rehabilitation programme by the WHO.
- National Federation of Disabled Persons (KAMPI), Philippines— produce low-cost wheelchairs from material sourced locally.
- Projimo—programme of rehabilitation organized by disabled youth of Western Mexico.
- Jaipur foot/limb technology developed (and provided cost free) by Devendra Raj Mehta in India has benefitted >2 million people with disabilities.

At a global level: inclusive education
- The 'Convention on the Rights of Persons with Disabilities' guidelines devised by the United Nations (UN), ratified by a majority of countries in 2016, include a specific clause: to ensure that children with disabilities have equal access with other children to participate in play, recreation, leisure, and sport activities including those activities in the school system.
- The UN 'Education for All' initiative clearly highlights the importance of inclusive education, stating that schools must change to accommodate a much wider range of children.
- Some successful examples of inclusive education include the following:
  - The Italian government passed a law in 1977 and consequently about 98% of children with disability are now attending regular schools.
  - The Department of Special Needs Education and Career Guidance in Uganda has committed to free primary education for all children.
  - The Columbian 'Escuela Nueva' model of flexible education for rural areas provides an excellent opportunity to respond to individual learning abilities and needs. Peer instruction is practised with older students tutoring younger ones.
  - The child-friendly school model in Brazil is another successful model of expanding inclusive education.

At global/government level: laws and policies

The WHO and UNICEF have been developing many policies over the years to advocate supporting families of children with developmental disabilities, including:

- 'Promoting the Rights of Children with Disabilities' (UNICEF, 2007).
- 'Convention on the Rights of Persons with Disabilities' (UN, came into force in 2008).

A majority of countries have adopted these guidelines by laws, budget allocation, and national programmes.

In India, the Right to Education Act and the Rights of Persons with Disability Act, 2016 together are empowering children with disabilities for inclusive education. Two National programmes (Sarva Shiksha Abhiyan and Rashtriya Bal Swastya Karyakram) also focus on inclusive schooling.

At a global level: collaboration and partnerships

- Many partnership programmes directed and funded by the WHO, UNICEF, and the World Bank are helping developing countries access support and/or resources from developed countries.
- Interestingly, these partnership models are also benefitting children in the developed countries in multiple ways.

Summary

- As one can see, the size of the challenge is enormous, but there are also innumerable opportunities and solutions that could address this challenge.
- Childhood developmental disabilities, especially in developing countries, pose multiple challenges to many aspects of life.
- Early diagnosis and intervention are the way forward to reduce the burden of these developmental disabilities.
- Paediatricians, developmental paediatricians, and multidisciplinary therapists everywhere should take this as an opportunity to collaborate, coordinate, communicate, and share good practice ideas.
- Cost-effective actions at local levels with global partnerships would help these children with developmental disabilities live an independent and productive life.

References

American Psychiatric Association (2013). Diagnostic and Statistical Manual of Mental Disorders, Fifth Edition. Arlington, VA: American Psychiatric Association.

Beckman PJ, Abera N, Sabella T, et al. (2016). From rights to realities: confronting the challenge of educating persons with disabilities in developing countries. Glob Educ Rev, 3, 44–27.

Global Research on Developmental Disabilities Collaborators (2018). Developmental disabilities among children younger than 5 years in 195 countries and territories, 1990–2016: a systematic analysis for the Global Burden of Disease Study 2016. Lancet Global Health, 6. e1100–21.

Maulik PK, Darmstadt GL (2007). Childhood disability in low- and middle-income countries: overview of screening, prevention, services, legislation, and epidemiology. Pediatrics, 120(Suppl 1), S1–55.

Pandey S (2012). Challenges in neurological practice in developing countries. Indian J Public Health, 56, 2277–30.

Petersen R, Procter C, Donald KA (2020). Assessment and management of the child with cerebral palsy. In: Salih MA (ed) Clinical Child Neurology (pp. 175–203). Cham: Springer.

Récamier A, Delft E (2011). Designing Tools for Prosthetic Device Fabrication at Jaipur Foot. Delft: Delft University of Technology and Bhagvan Mahaveer Viklang Sahayata Samiti (Jaipur Foot Organization).

Solarsh G, Hofman KJ (2006). Developmental disabilities. In: Jamison DT, Feachem RG, Makgoba MW, et al. (eds) Disease and Mortality in Sub-Saharan Africa, 2nd ed (pp. 125–47). Washington, DC: World Bank.

Stein DJ, Szatmari P, Gaebel W, et al. (2020). Mental, behavioral and neurodevelopmental disorders in the ICD-11: an international perspective on key changes and controversies. BMC Med 18, 21.

Sunderajan T, Kanhere SV (2019). Speech and language delay in children: prevalence and risk factors. J Family Med Prim Care, 8, 1642–6.

Syed SB, Dadwal V, Rutter P, et al. (2012). Developed-developing country partnerships: benefits to developed countries? Global Health, 8, 17.

UNESCO (2020). Global Education Monitoring Report, 2020: Inclusion and Education: All Means All. Paris: UNESCO. Available at: ℘ https://unesdoc.unesco.org/ark:/48223/pf0000373718

UNICEF (2007). Promoting the Rights of Children with Disabilities. Innocenti Digest No. 13. Florence: UNICEF Innocenti Research Centre.

United Nations (2006). Convention on the Rights of Persons with Disabilities and Optional Protocol. New York: United Nations.

United Nations (2018). Disability and Development Report, Realizing the Sustainable Development Goals by, for and with Persons with Disabilities. New York: United Nations Publications.

World Health Organization (2017). Atlas: Country Resources for Neurological Disorders, 2nd ed. Geneva: World Health Organization.

World Health Organization, The World Bank (2011). World Report on Disability. Geneva: World Health Organization.

Sensory impairments

Hearing impairment

Definitions and classification

Definitions
- Hearing threshold: lowest intensity of sound that an individual can respond to.
- Decibel (dB): logarithmic scale to measure intensity of sound in relation to a reference value, e.g. dB HL for audiograms, dB HL for auditory brainstem response (ABR).
- Frequency: relates to pitch, measured as hertz (Hz) or kilohertz (kHz). Described as low: up to 500 Hz; mid: >500 Hz–2 kHz; high: >2–8 kHz; or very high >8 kHz.
- Audiogram: chart of hearing thresholds as a function of frequency.
- Air conduction (AC): hearing measured using headphones or earphones.
- Bone conduction (BC): hearing measured using vibration transducers that fit against the skull, bypassing the outer and middle ear.
- Permanent childhood hearing impairment (PCHI): permanent hearing loss (HL) with average hearing level at 0.5, 1, 2, and 4 kHz of ≥40 dB HL.

Classification of hearing loss
British Society of Audiology classification:
- Normal hearing level: 0–20 dB.
- HL is mild (21–40 dB HL), moderate (41–70 dB HL), severe (71–95 dB HL), or profound (>95 dB HL).

Origin
See Fig. 4.1.

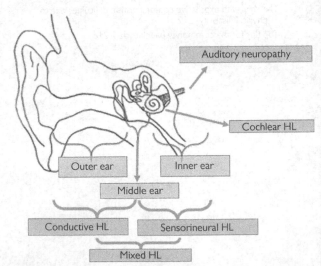

Fig. 4.1 Origin of different types of hearing loss (HL).

- Conductive HL: AC abnormal, BC normal.
- Sensorineural HL (SNHL): AC and BC abnormal, AC–BC difference <15 dB HL.
- Mixed (SNHL plus conductive HL): AC and BC abnormal, BC better than AC by ≥15 dB.
- Cochlear: from the outer hair cells of the cochlea (90% of SNHL).
- Auditory neuropathy spectrum disorder (ANSD): from inner hair cells, synapse, and auditory nerve (10% of SNHL).
- Central auditory dysfunction: from neural pathways beyond cochlear nerve until the auditory cortex.
- Symmetry and shape:
  - Unilateral, bilateral, asymmetric (bilateral HL with >10 dB HL difference between the ears at ≥2 frequencies).
  - Low-frequency, mid-frequency, or high-frequency HL.
- Progressive HL: drop in hearing of ≥10 dB at two or more adjacent frequencies between 0.5 and 4 kHz.

Epidemiology of permanent childhood hearing impairment

- The most common sensory impairment.
- Occurs in 1/1000 births; 50% moderate, 23% severe, 27% profound.
- Prevalence rises to ~2/1000 at age 9 years (because of late detection, late presentation, or progressive HL).
- In the UK, 800 children are born with PCHI each year.
- NICU babies are ten times more likely to have PCHI.
- The Joint Committee on Infant Hearing (JCIH) has outlined risk factors for early childhood HL (Box 4.1).

Box 4.1 Risk factors for early childhood hearing loss (JCIH Position statement, 2019)

Perinatal factors

- Family history of early, progressive, or late-onset PCHI.
- Neonatal intensive care of >5 days.
- Hyperbilirubinaemia with exchange transfusion.
- Aminoglycoside administration for >5 days.
- Asphyxia or hypoxic ischaemic encephalopathy.
- Extracorporeal membrane oxygenation.
- *In utero* infection such as cytomegalovirus (CMV), herpes, rubella, syphilis, toxoplasmosis, and mother positive for Zika.
- Birth conditions: craniofacial malformations including microtia or atresia, cleft, microcephaly, hydrocephalus, and temporal bone abnormalities.
- Syndromes with HL.

Postnatal factors

- Culture-positive infections associated with SNHL including confirmed bacterial and viral meningitis or encephalitis.
- Events associated with HL, e.g. significant head trauma and chemotherapy.
- Caregiver concerns regarding hearing, speech, developmental delay, and/or developmental regression.

Source: data from Year 2019 Position Statement: Principles and Guidelines for Early Hearing Detection and Intervention Programs. Journal of Early Hearing Detection and Intervention, 4(2), 1–44.

Causes of permanent childhood hearing impairment

The commonest cause of bilateral PCHI is genetic and unilateral PCHI is an anatomical abnormality of the inner ear.

Genetic: >50% of all PCHI

- Syndromic 30% (>400 syndromes identified):
  - *AR*: Jervell and Lange–Nielsen, Pendred, Usher, and Perrault syndromes.
  - *AD*: branchio-oto-renal, Waardenburg, Treacher Collins, Apert, and Crouzon syndromes.
  - *X-linked*: Alport syndrome and Norrie disease.
- Non-syndromic 70%:
  - *AR*: 76 genes identified. Commonest is *GJB2* (at DFNB1 locus).
  - *AD*: 49 genes identified.
  - *X-linked*: five genes identified.
  - *Mitochondrial*: m.1555A>G confers susceptibility to develop HL with aminoglycosides.

Congenital malformations

- Inner ear: Michel aplasia (absent inner ear structures), cochlear aplasia/hypoplasia, cochlea incomplete partitioning types I–III, common cavity, hypoplastic auditory nerve.
- Middle outer ear: microtia, atresia, ossicular anomalies.
- Other: cleft palate.

Antenatal causes

- Intrauterine infections—maternal transmission of:
  - CMV: causes 10–15% of all PCHI. Can cause progressive HL.
  - Rubella: HL occurs in 12–19%.
  - Toxoplasma, herpes, syphilis, lymphocytic choriomeningitis, Zika, HIV.
- Maternal drugs: alcohol, aminoglycosides, thalidomide.
- Maternal disease: diabetes, hypothyroidism.

Perinatal causes: causes 10–20% of PCHI

- Kernicterus: HL caused by deposition of bilirubin in cochlear nuclei and auditory nerve.
- Birth asphyxia, extreme prematurity with comorbidities. Often more than one causative factor involved including use of ototoxic medication, sepsis, birth trauma, neonatal jaundice, and/or intracranial haemorrhage.

Infectious causes

- Bacterial meningitis: commonest infectious cause (pneumococci, meningococci, *Haemophilus influenzae* type B). Can cause labyrinthitis ossificans. Urgent hearing assessment within 4 weeks of illness and early consideration of cochlear implant (CI) essential.

- Viral infections: measles, mumps, HIV, varicella, herpes.
- Bacterial infections: Lyme disease, tuberculosis.
- Labyrinthitis: viral, bacterial, can be due to spread of infection from otitis media.

Ototoxic treatment

Aminoglycosides, platinum-containing chemotherapy, cisplatin, loop diuretics, deferoxamine, radiotherapy.

Trauma

- Temporal bone fractures.
- Barotrauma.
- Noise-induced HL.

Tumours

Neurofibromatosis, astrocytoma, medulloblastoma, glioma.

Systemic causes

- Autoimmune causes: Cogan syndrome, systemic lupus erythematosus.
- Haematological causes: sickle cell disease.
- Endocrine: diabetes, hypothyroidism.

Unknown

- Otosclerosis.
- Meniere's disease.

Newborn hearing screening

Critical period for auditory development

- A time of heightened sensitivity and plasticity of the neural pathways to auditory stimuli, thought to occur in the first 2–3 years of life.
- Auditory deprivation during the critical period has an irreversible impact on auditory pathways and language development. Reintroducing auditory stimuli before close of the critical period allows development due to neural plasticity (see ➲ pp. 74–7).

Impact of hearing loss

- Delayed receptive and expressive speech and language.
- Reduced academic achievement.
- Social isolation and poor self-regard.
- Impact on vocational choices and independence.
- Even mild and unilateral HL can have an adverse impact.

Rationale for newborn hearing screening

- Early intervention for HL <6 months leads to better language outcome and social–emotional development.
- Delay beyond the critical period can cause an irreversible impact on development outcome.
- Sensitive tests are available to screen for HL in babies.
- Early detection and intervention of HL is cost-effective.

Newborn hearing screening programme (NHSP)

- Hearing screened for all babies born, implemented in England in 2006 (Fig. 4.2).
- Tests used: automated otoacoustic emissions (AOAE) and automated auditory brainstem response (AABR).
- Well babies have AOAE. Babies in neonatal intensive care unit (NICU) >48 hours additionally have AABR due to risk of ANSD.
- Exclusions from NHSP (referred directly to audiology due to the high risk of PCHI):
  - Microtia and external ear canal atresia.
  - Neonatal bacterial meningitis or meningococcal septicaemia.
  - Confirmed congenital CMV (cCMV).
  - Programmable ventriculoperitoneal shunts (risk of shunt malfunction with screening equipment).

Limitations

- Misses late-onset HL and ANSD in well babies.
- Can miss mild HL.

Continued hearing surveillance for babies who pass NHSP

Done at age of 8 months for:
- Syndromes associated with HL (including DS).
- Craniofacial abnormalities, including cleft palate.
- Confirmed congenital infection (cCMV, toxoplasmosis, or rubella).
- Special care baby unit or NICU >48 hours, with no clear response AOAE for both ears, but clear response AABR for both ears.

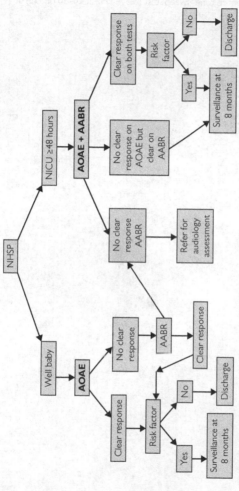

Fig. 4.2 Flow chart for babies having newborn hearing screen in UK.

School hearing screen
- Coverage in UK is 90%.
- Detects late-onset and progressive HL.
- Uses the pure tone 'sweep' test (0.5–4 kHz at 20–30 dB HL) at school entry.

Hearing assessment

Principles

- Take history of age-appropriate responses to sounds, i.e. toys, music, and voice.
- Do otoscopy to look for wax and infection.
- Choice of test/s depends on age, development, and cooperation (Fig. 4.3).
- Use British Society of Audiology guidance on test methodology. Tests should be done in a quiet room, with ambient noise levels below recommended standards.
- For 'difficult to test' children, repeat sessions, modification of test methodology, or objective testing may be needed.

Types of hearing tests

Subjective/behavioural hearing tests

- Based on child's response to sounds, auditory behaviour, attention, and cooperation.
- Preferred to objective tests.
- Take precaution to avoid visual clues during testing (e.g. shadows, reflection).
- Pure tone audiometry, >5 years (reliably from 7 years):
  - Frequency-specific sounds played through headphones or bone conductor and response given by child (e.g. raise hand, press button) is noted. Play-based responses used for younger children.
  - Usually needs single tester.
- Play audiometry, ≥2½–5 years:
  - Child conditioned to respond to frequency-specific sounds with an action (e.g. put man in a boat) by modelling. May need to change activity frequently to maintain attention. Can do AC and BC. May need two testers.
- Visual reinforcement audiometry, 6 months–2½ years:
  - Child's head turn in response to sound is reinforced with visual reward/reinforcer (animated toys, flashing lights).
  - Can do AC and BC. Preferred set-up is using two testers and two rooms, with specific reinforcer set-up.

Age ⟶	<6 months	6 months–2 years	>2.5 years	>5 years
Subjective tests				
Hearing threshold tests		VRA	Play audiometry	PTA
Distraction test				
Behavioural observation				
Objective tests				
OAE				
ABR	Test of choice	If unable to do subjective test		
ASSR				
CERA				
Impedance tests				
Tympanometry	1000 Hz probe		226 Hz probe	
Acoustic reflex				

Fig. 4.3 Selection of hearing test based on age. ASSR, auditory steady-state response; CERA, cortical evoked response audiometry; VRA, visual reinforcement audiometry.

- Distraction test, >6 months:
  - Does not measure absolute threshold of hearing, can only test down to 30 dB. Not recommended as sole test of hearing.
  - Needs two testers. One seated in front to capture and release child's attention and observe responses. Second tester presents stimuli (humming voice, Manchester rattle, 'ss' sound, frequency-specific stimuli) from behind. Response to the sound (head turn) is observed.
  - Infants should sit with minimal support and have good head control. Can be used in older children unable to perform other behavioural tests reliably.
- Behavioural observation audiometry:
  - Done <6 months and in developmentally delayed children unable to do other behavioural hearing tests. Does not measure absolute threshold.
  - Stimuli include music, Ling sounds, toy sounds, and frequency-specific sounds.
  - Responses seen are reflexive (startle, eye blink/flutter) or attention type (increase or decrease body movement, eye widening, searching, localization, quieting, vocalizations). Can be subject to tester and interpreter error.
- Speech-based tests:
  - Child asked to identify or repeat a word. Indicator of functional hearing.
  - McCormick toy test: >2 years.
  - Manchester junior word list: >6 years.
  - BKB sentence test: >8 years.

Objective tests

Done at any age, usually when child is unable to do subjective tests or to support subjective test results.

- Otoacoustic emissions:
  - Weak sounds generated by motility of outer hair cells of cochlea in response to presented sounds. Quick and simple test of outer hair cell function.
  - Response recorded as present/absent.
  - Absent in cochlear HL, with middle ear effusion.
  - Present in auditory neuropathy, mild HL.
- ABRs:
  - Electrophysiological response elicited by clicks, tone burst, or chirp acoustic stimuli and detected by skin electrodes.
  - Waves 1–7 generated by auditory pathway; hearing threshold is indicated by presence of wave 5. Although an objective test, interpretation of waveforms is subjective and peer review is done to make results robust. Correlates with pure tone audiometry thresholds with +/− 10–15 dB difference. AC and BC can be done. Cochlear microphonic done in suspected ANSD.
  - Used for referrals from NHSP, suspected ANSD, when subjective tests are difficult (i.e. developmental difficulty or non-organic HL).
  - Limitation: influenced by neurological abnormalities. Does not indicate hearing thresholds in ANSD. Requires child to be asleep or sedated.

- Auditory steady-state response:
  - Electrophysiological response elicited with frequency and amplitude modulated pure tones. Uses statistics-based mathematical detection algorithm to detect and define hearing thresholds. Used for hearing threshold estimation like ABR.
- Cortical evoked response audiometry:
  - Electrophysiological response (waves P1, N1, and P2) from higher regions of auditory pathways, including thalamus, hippocampus, internal capsule, and cortex.
  - Used for frequency-specific hearing thresholds. Can be done with speech stimuli.
  - Done in an awake and alert child, hence useful in older children.
  - Used in non-organic HL, assess response with hearing aids, and in ANSD.

Tests for impedance (all ages)

- Tympanometry:
  - Test of middle ear function. Quick and simple.
  - Place probe in the ear and pressurize ear canal briefly for a few seconds. Use 226 Hz probe >6 months of age and 1000 Hz probe <6 months.
  - Classification of responses by Jerger (Fig. 4.4).
- Acoustic reflex:
  - Checks stapedial muscle contraction in response to frequency-specific sounds, ipsilaterally and contralaterally.
  - Tests auditory pathway from the inner ear to the brainstem. Pattern of responses may indicate site of lesion.
  - Absent in conductive HL and ANSD.

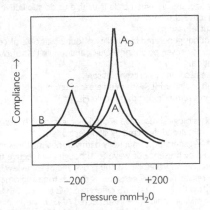

Fig. 4.4 Classification of tympanometry response: type A, normal; type Ad, disarticulation of the ossicular chain; type B, middle ear effusion, eardrum perforation, impacted wax; type C, negative middle ear pressure.

Source: data from Jerger J. Clinical experience with impedance audiometry. Arch Otolaryngol. 1970 Oct;92(4):311–24.

Aetiological investigations in permanent childhood hearing impairment

Rationale

- To answer the question 'Why is my child deaf?'
- Identify treatable conditions, e.g. congenital CMV.
- Give preventative advice for drop in hearing, e.g. avoidance of aminoglycoside in m.1555A>G mutation.
- Manage associated medical conditions, e.g. thyroid dysfunction in Pendred.
- Inform genetic counselling, e.g. Norrie disease.
- Inform communication choices, e.g. Usher syndrome type 1.

Guidelines

- Written by British Association of Audiovestibular Physicians (BAAP) to investigate unilateral, bilateral severe to profound, bilateral mild to moderate, progressive HL and auditory neuropathy (2015–19).
- Level 1 investigations are mandatory and level 2 investigations are done in some children depending on clinical features.
- A cause for HL is found in 50–60% of children after investigation. This may increase with advances in genetic testing. If no cause found, re-evaluate periodically as clinical features may evolve over time, e.g. visual difficulty in Usher syndrome. A number of 'unknown' causes may be genetic.

Level 1 investigations

History

- Of causes of HL detailed previously, e.g. meningitis, ototoxic drugs.
- Detailed antenatal and perinatal history.
- Developmental history, to identify systemic conditions and vestibular hypofunction. Three-generation family tree with history of genetic conditions, e.g. thyroid disease.

Examination

- Top-to-toe general examination to look for syndromic features, e.g. ear pits or tags, thyroid swelling, coloboma, epibulbar dermoid, spine, hands.
- Systemic examination, developmental assessment.
- Examination of parents.
- Clinical vestibular examination:
  - Babies <6 weeks: Farmer test.
  - Infants: Moro reflex, head righting reflex, parachute reflex, observation of vestibulo-ocular reflex on office chair.
  - Older children: postural tests (standing on one leg, jump, hop), head thrust test.

CMV

- CMV DNA polymerase chain reaction (PCR) in saliva swab or urine. Positive result <3 weeks age confirms cCMV. Positive result >3 weeks of age, could be acquired CMV and needs neonatal blood spot testing for CMV DNA to confirm cCMV.

- Important test, as ganciclovir/valganciclovir treatment in the newborn period prevents progression of SNHL.
- Child >1 year of age: do CMV immunoglobulin G (IgG) and urine CMV. If either is positive, request retrieval of neonatal blood spot to confirm cCMV.

Inner ear imaging
- High yield of abnormalities.
- MRI inner ears and brain for SNHL and computed tomography (CT) petrous temporal bone for permanent conductive HL.
- MRI best done in natural sleep <3 months of age. Older children may need sedation.

Ophthalmic assessment
- Important as 40% of children with hearing impairment have visual difficulty.
- Electroretinogram done in children with profound deafness and vestibular hypofunction to look for Usher type 1.

Blood test for GJB2 mutation
- Commonest cause of genetic HL.
- Informed consent required.
- Guidelines for genetic testing likely to change in the future due to availability of next-generation sequencing (see ➜ pp. 484–5) 'deafness panels' which allow testing for several genes at a time.

Family audiograms: for parents and siblings
- Electrocardiography (ECG) for QTc interval: in profound HL and vestibular hypofunction for Jervell and Lange–Nielsen syndrome.
- Urine dipstick: microscopic haematuria/proteinuria in Alport and brancho-oto-renal syndromes.

Level 2 investigations
- Serology: for congenital infection (syphilis, HIV, rubella, toxoplasma).
- Haematology and biochemistry: e.g. thyroid function tests in Pendred syndrome.
- Autoimmune tests: when systemic involvement, e.g. joint swelling, fever.
- Metabolic screen on blood and urine: when epilepsy or neurodegeneration.
- Renal ultrasound: if preauricular pits or sinuses, microtia, enlarged vestibular aqueduct, permanent conductive HL, or syndrome with kidney involvement, e.g. CHARGE (choanae, heart, anal, growth, and ear anomalies) syndrome.
- Chromosomal studies/comparative genomic hybridization microarray: if developmental delay or dysmorphic features.
- Further genetic testing (see ➜ pp. 484–5): for specific syndromes and ANSD. With availability of next-generation sequencing, these tests will be requested as a 'panel'.
- Vestibular testing: consider if motor milestones delayed, progressive deafness, post-meningitis, Pendred syndrome, inner ear malformations, or vertigo/dizziness.
- Specialist referrals: e.g. to neurologist for children with ANSD.

Middle ear disease

Causes
- Infections/inflammation (otitis media): common. Causes fluctuating hearing and is amenable to treatment.
- Anatomical: causes fixed/permanent conductive HL; due to ossicular abnormality, otosclerosis, craniofacial syndromes such as Apert, Crouzon, Treacher Collins, and Goldenhar syndromes.

Common middle ear inflammations

Acute otitis media
- Fever, earache, ear discharge, and red bulging tympanic membrane on otoscopy.
- Consider antibiotics if child systemically unwell, has underlying predisposing factor, bilateral infection, and <2 years of age.
- Potential to cause serious intracranial complications, mastoiditis, meningitis, intracranial abscess, and venous sinus thrombosis.

Chronic suppurative otitis media
- Chronic ear discharge from perforated tympanic membrane/grommet >2–6 weeks.
- Treated with aural toilet, topical antimicrobials, and sometimes surgery.
- Complications include intracranial spread of infection and cholesteatoma.

Otitis media with effusion (OME) 'glue ear'
- *Definition*: fluid in middle ear cleft, without acute symptoms. Called 'chronic' OME if lasts >3 months.
- *Cause*: postulated as eustachian tube dysfunction, bacterial biofilms, altered immune reaction in middle ear, or genetic factors. Horizontal orientation of eustachian tube in children predisposes.
- *Incidence*: peak at 1 year. Point prevalence at 2 years is ~20%, Up to 80% of children would have had OME by age 4 years.
- *Symptoms*: commonly asymptomatic. May cause temporary and fluctuating HL, speech delay, difficulties in attention and behaviour, and imbalance.
- *Risk factors*: passive smoking, bottle feeding, low socioeconomic group, attendance at nursery, allergy, and enlarged adenoids. Breast feeding is protective.
- *Predisposing conditions*: craniofacial syndromes (DS, Apert, Crouzon), cleft palate, and immunodeficiency.
- *Diagnosis*: otoscopy (appearance of tympanic membrane: dull, fluid level, bubbles, retracted), pneumatic otoscopy, and tympanometry (type B or C curve). Audiogram indicates mild–moderate conductive HL with fluctuation, more at low frequencies. Tuning fork tests may be difficult in young children.
- *Treatment*:
  - Depends on hearing level, predisposing factor, and duration of symptoms.

- Follow NICE guidelines (2008). Watchful waiting for 3 months as 50% will self-resolve. Use of Otovent® balloon. Antibiotics, nasal and oral steroids, and antihistaminics have no evidence base.
- Consider grommets or hearing aids for OME >3 months, particularly if underlying predisposing factor. Grommets cause short-term improvement in hearing, but long-term benefit on language is unclear. Adenoidectomy may help.
- *Complications*: related to long-standing HL, impact on language and behaviour, retraction pockets, cholesteatoma, and possibly development of auditory processing difficulty.

Auditory neuropathy spectrum disorder

Diagnosis

Caused by pathology between the inner hair cells to the brainstem (10% of PCHI).

Electrophysiological diagnosis which includes a heterogeneous group of conditions with common pattern of hearing test results characterized by:
- Absent or grossly abnormal ABR at high stimulus levels.
- Present otoacoustic emissions and/or cochlear microphonic, i.e. normal activity in the outer hair cells of cochlea.

Common features

- Variable results on behavioural hearing tests (normal hearing to profound HL) and hearing fluctuation.
- Speech development affected out of proportion to that expected for hearing level.
- Disproportionately poor speech recognition for the degree of HL.
- Absent stapedial reflexes.
- Difficulty hearing in noise and impaired temporal processing.

Risk factors

- Extreme prematurity, low birth weight, or intrauterine growth restriction.
- Severe hyperbilirubinaemia.
- Hypoxic ischaemic encephalopathy.
- Intraventricular haemorrhage.
- Prolonged assisted ventilation.
- Severe sepsis.

Hence, all NICU babies should have AOAE and AABR hearing screen.

ANSD picture can be mimicked by

- Anatomical anomalies: hypoplastic auditory nerve, hydrocephalus, and space-occupying lesions involving auditory nerve.
- Delayed auditory maturation: ABR and hearing level returns to normal generally by 2 years of age. Seen in preterm babies.

Aetiology

- Genetic non-syndromic: otoferlin, pejvakin mutations.
- Genetic syndromic: neurodegenerative, Charcot–Marie–Tooth.
- Metabolic: maple syrup urine disease.
- Mitochondrial: Mohr–Tranebjaerg syndrome.
- Riboflavin transporter deficiency: Brown–Vialetto–Van Laere syndrome.
- Other: cerebellar ataxia, areflexia, pes cavus, optic atrophy, and SNHL syndrome (CAPOS), NF2.
- Acquired: mumps, demyelination (Guillain–Barré), neoplasia, sarcoidosis.

Management

- Multidisciplinary approach with involvement of audiologist, speech therapist, and medical professionals.
- Aetiological investigations according to BAAP.
- ABR should be repeated at 8–10 weeks and at 12–18 months of age to look for delayed auditory maturation.
- Hearing aids offered only after behavioural hearing tests and not on basis of ABR test results.
- Early consideration of CIs.

Auditory processing disorder

Characterized by poor perception of speech and non-speech sounds due to impaired neural function. This may involve the afferent and efferent pathways of the central auditory nervous system, and neural processing systems that influence these pathways (e.g. cognitive functions of language, attention, executive function, and memory) (British Society of Audiology, 2018). Affects ~5% of school children.

Symptoms

Difficulties in listening, difficulty hearing in noise, mishearing speech, and poor attention to and poor memory of auditory instructions despite a normal hearing test.

Types

- Developmental: present in childhood, have a normal audiogram, and no other aetiology other than a family history of developmental communication and related disorders.
- Acquired: associated with a known cause, e.g. brain lesion.
- Secondary: as a result of transient or permanent peripheral HL.

Associations

- Language, attention, memory, and executive difficulties; ADHD (see ⊃ pp. 126–34), ASD (see ⊃ pp. 114–25), and dyslexia.
- Auditory processing disorder may contribute to childhood learning difficulties.

Diagnosis

- Made by history and battery of tests. Parent report questionnaires used.
- Diagnostic tests include speech perception tests in quiet/in noise/with speech maskers, spectral discrimination, temporal resolution, binaural interaction, and electrophysiological tests.

Management

- Modifying listening environment and improving listening skills (optimizing room acoustics, remote microphone technology/wireless communication device, teacher/speaker adaptations).
- Auditory training using interactive training devices and musical training.

Management of permanent childhood hearing impairment

Principles

- Start management as soon as possible after diagnosis. The 1–3–6 rule for babies diagnosed from NHSP (screen for HL by age 1 month, complete an audiologic evaluation by age 3 months, and start early intervention by age 6 months).
- Management should be holistic, multidisciplinary, and joined up (Fig. 4.5).
- Family education, counselling, and engagement are mandatory parts of management as they improve language outcomes.
- Long-term reviews are necessary until transition to adult services.

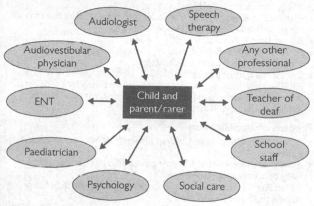

Fig. 4.5 Multidisciplinary professionals involved in management of a child with PCHI.

Hearing aids

Aims
- Provide audibility across speech spectrum.
- Avoid discomfort, distortion, and unsafe level of sounds.
- Maximize audibility of the desired signal and reduce undesired signals (i.e. noise).

Candidates
- Children with bilateral and unilateral PCHI, including mild loss.
- Long-standing HL due to middle ear dysfunction.
- Can be fitted at any age including in neonates.

Types
- Behind-the-ear: most common in children, robust, wide spectrum of fitting, compatible with FM systems.
- In-the-ear: cosmetic appeal. Unsuitable in infants/toddlers due to rapid ear growth, may not be suitable for severe HL.
- BC aid: used for conductive HL, e.g. glue ear.
- Bone-anchored hearing aid: used on a soft band in permanent conductive HL, e.g. microtia, aural atresia.
- Contralateral routing of signals (CROS): used with unilateral profound HL. The signal from the 'dead' ear is routed wirelessly by a receiver to a microphone in the 'good' ear. When the 'good' ear also has a mild/moderate HL, a BiCROS is considered.

Process of amplification
- Governed by Modernising Children's Hearing aid Services (MCHAS) guidelines.
- Accurate, frequency-specific hearing thresholds must be determined using behavioural or objective tests.
- All hearing aids fitted are digital. Selection of hearing aid depends on degree and configuration of HL.
- Ear moulds taken, with good fit. This is important to avoid feedback and deliver output of the aid. Different types of moulds available depending on type of HL and hearing aid.
- Hearing aid fitting using a recommended, threshold-based prescriptive procedure and features as appropriate, i.e. wide dynamic range compression, noise reduction, non-linear frequency compression, etc. Use of tamperproof battery drawer for safety.
- Hearing aid verification: takes into account the child's individual acoustic parameters. Done with real ear measures, either real ear to coupler difference or real ear-aided response.
- Hearing aid evaluation: done by aided testing, questionnaires of listening ability, common monitoring protocol, and communication development.
- Family counselling regarding aids and regular reviews.

Auditory implants

Cochlear implant

This is a surgically implanted device that stimulates the auditory nerve through electrodes placed in the cochlea (it bypasses the damaged hair cells in the cochlea).

It has internal and external parts. The external parts (microphone, sound processor, transmitter coil) are connected through intact skin by a magnet to the internal receiver–stimulator package that is implanted surgically in the mastoid bone. This is connected to an electrode array placed surgically within the cochlea.

Candidacy in children (NICE, 2019)

Bilateral CI indicated if:
- Hearing levels ≥80 dB HL at two or more frequencies (500 Hz, 1, 2, 3, and 4 kHz) bilaterally without hearing aids.
- Children do not receive adequate benefit from acoustic hearing aids, i.e. develop speech, language, and listening skills appropriate to age, developmental stage, and cognitive ability.

Assessment

Multidisciplinary assessment with ENT surgeon, audiovestibular physician, audiologist, speech therapist, teacher of deaf, and psychologist.

Trial of a hearing aid for at least 3 months.

Factors considered are those that affect outcome.
- Age (prelingual HL): ≤2 years best outcome, ≥4 years limited benefit.
- Duration of HL (postlingual): ≤5 years best outcome, ≥8 years limited benefit.
- Radiological anatomy: poor outcome with very abnormal CT or MRI, e.g. complete bilateral ossification, very abnormal middle ears.
- Medical concerns: issues affecting use of CI, e.g. mild such as visual loss, severe such as autism, and severe physical difficulties.
- Hearing levels: should be within NICE criteria.
- Hearing aid use: should use aids at least 50% of the time.
- Functional hearing: speech perception if not consistent with audiogram indicates a concern.
- Communication: a significant delay in speech (considering exposure), significant delay in prelinguistic skills, and primary sign communication are concerns for outcome.
- Cognition: severe global delay, struggle with new tasks is a concern.
- Behaviour: severe problems cause difficulty with rehabilitation.
- Supporting factors: family showing commitment, realistic about expectations, access to teacher of deaf, educational support, and speech therapist.

Following cochlear implantation

- Switch-on occurs 2–4 weeks after the surgery.
- A 'MAP' is an individual listening programme stored in the speech processor. Frequent appointments are needed to optimize the 'MAP'.
- Children need to participate in intensive rehabilitation to get optimum benefit from implant.

Bone-anchored hearing aids

- For permanent, predominantly conductive HL, e.g. microtia/atresia, chronic discharging ears with inability to use conventional hearing aids.
- Titanium prosthesis implanted into the calvarium connects with an external receiver/sound processor through an abutment, allowing BC of sound directly to cochlea.
- Recent development: magnetic bone-anchored hearing aid, where sound processor is attached to implant by subcutaneous magnetic plate through intact skin.

Middle ear implants

- Bypass the external ear canal, directly stimulate cochlea through coupling with the ossicular chain using mechanical vibrations.
- Not routinely offered to children.
- Initially developed for SNHL but now offered for conductive and mixed HL.

Auditory brainstem implants

- Surgically implanted prosthesis with electrodes stimulating cochlear nucleus directly.
- Indicated where CI is not an option, e.g. NF2, tumours of auditory nerve, and absent cochlea/cochlear nerve.

Medical management

Medical treatments

Medical treatments that need considering in some children with HL include:
- Intrauterine infections such as cCMV, toxoplasma, and syphilis.
- Sudden SNHL: oral or intratympanic steroids.
- Long QT syndrome: beta-blocker, pacemaker, advice to avoid certain medications that may precipitate a cardiac arrest.
- m.1555A>G: advice to avoid aminoglycosides to reduce risk of drop in hearing.
- Monitoring: Pendred syndrome—thyroid function, Alport syndrome—kidney function.
- Enlarged vestibular aqueducts: advice to avoid large pressure changes and head injuries to reduce risk of drop in hearing.
- Intracranial tumours: medical/surgical treatment.
- Control of underlying medical conditions, e.g. sickle cell anaemia is likely to limit the HL caused.
- Bacterial meningitis showing labyrinthitis obliterans on CT/MRI merit urgent consideration of CI.
- HL investigation may uncover neurodegenerative conditions such as mucopolysaccharidosis, in which early treatment is crucial to a better prognosis of the underlying disorder.

Specific medical advice

Vestibular hypofunction
- Associated in 30–70% of children with SNHL.
- Children present with delayed motor skills and balance difficulty. Age of walking is delayed beyond 18 months.
- Common causes include cochlear/vestibular anomalies, cCMV, and genetic syndromes.
- Advice about supervised swimming and risk of drowning with underwater swimming should be given.

Genetic counselling
- Counselling about recurrence of HL/associated systemic conditions (Norrie disease, mitochondrial disease) in future offspring. This may affect planning of further pregnancies including preimplantation genetic diagnosis, amniocentesis, *in vitro* fertilization (donor).
- A positive genetic test result may have implications for the extended family.
- Up to 40% of children with PCHI may have additional needs, requiring medical management.

Future medical options

Gene therapy for hearing loss

Attempts have been made to treat mouse models of human deafness with gene therapy with variable success. Issues to be considered are timing of therapy, mode of delivery, viral vectors, and stem cells. We remain optimistic that research will be extended to humans in decades to come.

Educational support

Optimize the listening environment

- Reduce background noise.
- Reduce distance to speaker.
- Allow lipreading.
- Optimize room acoustics: reduce reverberation, e.g. plaster ceilings and walls, linoleum, high ceilings.

Teacher of hearing impaired

- Qualified teacher with mainstream experience, plus postgraduate masters/diploma in audiology and deaf education.
- Support soon after diagnosis of HL in newborns until transition to adult services.
- They support hearing aid use, educate family, monitor listening, advise on early play, inform about choice in educational placements, and support and assess the child at school.

Assistive listening devices

- To facilitate optimal learning and communication, speech signal should be at least 20 dB above background noise (i.e. 20 dB signal-to-noise).
- Assistive listening devices improve signal-to-noise ratio, and convey speaker's voice directly to listener.
- Can be used through or without a hearing aid.
- Range of options based on:
  - Electromagnetic induction: e.g. 'loop system' used in public office, libraries, with phone and television. Induction coil fitted in a space and hearing aid used in the 'loop' setting.
  - Frequency modulation: e.g. radio aid, soundfield system. Teacher wears a transmitter. Receiver is fitted to the hearing aid to an amplifier/speakers placed around the classroom for soundfield system. Signals transmitted from transmitter to receiver through wireless carrier frequency.
  - Digital modulation: e.g. Bluetooth devices. Hearing aids can connect to multiple devices wirelessly. Devices can be used in class for the teacher's voice, for group discussions, and for music streaming. Increasingly popular with modern hearing aids.

Assessment of educational needs

- Indicated if child requires specialist support, e.g. speech therapy, learning support.
- Undertaken by educational authority, considering multiple professional opinions, and formulating a support package by an EHC plan (see ➔ pp. 656–7).

Educational choices

- Early nursery placements: help to form a routine, support language, and allow early assessment of educational needs.
- Mainstream schools: suitable for most children with PCHI. Advantage of integration with hearing children, and strong speech models.

- 'Partial Hearing Units' or 'Deaf Resource Base': attached to mainstream schools, have favourable acoustics, technology, and support from specialist staff. Children spend part of the day in the unit and part in the mainstream. Good mix of integration with mainstream and providing specialist support.
- Specialist schools for hearing impaired: only accept deaf children. They either follow auditory verbal approach, sign communication, or total communication (sign and speech). They have specialist expertise and equipment, and some are residential. Children have a strong deaf peer group, but are segregated from mainstream education.

Communication support

Requirements for normal language development
- Clear speech models by competent language users.
- Opportunities to hear, read, use, and practice; conversation, songs, TV.
- Clear explanations, definitions, support, and encouragement.

Impact of hearing loss on speech and language
- Reliance on gesture, visual cues, eye contact, body, and facial expressions.
- Slow vocabulary development. Gap in vocabulary as compared to normal hearing children widens with age, without intervention.
- Difficulty hearing word endings/quiet sounds such as 's', 'sh', 'f', 't', and 'k'. These are not included in speech, affecting intelligibility. Verb tense, pluralization, and possessives, are difficult. Phonological errors.
- Make shorter and simpler sentences.
- May not hear their own voice. Hence speech too loud/quiet/high-pitched/inadequate stress/inflection.
- Difficulty understanding words with multiple meaning, pragmatics (social use, context), semantics (meaning).

Factors affecting speech and language outcomes
- Auditory factors: degree/type of HL, age of hearing aid fitting/CI. Children born with profound bilateral PCHI unlikely to develop speech without early intervention. Mild and unilateral HL can also affect speech and language. HL due to OME can cause difficulties with attention, listening, tiredness, and speech delay.
- Child-related factors: cause of deafness, associated disability, and cognition.
- Environmental factors: social environment and professional support.

Improved language outcome
- Consistent use of hearing aids/CI.
- Maximizing auditory attention: using 'infant-directed speech', early joint attention and responsive two-way interactions with child, reduction of noise at home, and using an FM system during the early years.
- Using lip reading, visual support for language. Exposure to sign language in addition to speech does not delay speech acquisition in a deaf child.
- Optimizing parents' language input by training parent in communication skills.

Modes of communication
- Listening and spoken language: most common as 90–97% of deaf children are born to hearing parents.
- Visual/manual communication (e.g. British Sign Language, Signing Exact English).
- Total communication: oral plus manual communication.

Role of speech and language therapist
(Also see ➜ pp. 402–3.)
- Inform and support communication modes.
- Assess, diagnose speech and language difficulties and advice on management.
- Contribute to EHC plan (see ➜ pp. 656–7).

Psychosocial impact and support

Newborn
Diagnosis of PCHI may cause uncertainty, guilt, confusion, and helplessness in parents. Infant bonding is affected in deaf children of hearing parents (affecting empathy, socially competence). Deaf children of deaf parents develop attachment like hearing children with hearing parents.

Social emotional development
- 'Theory of mind' is delayed in deaf children with hearing parents, which impacts long-term social cognitive development.
- Children with PCHI have difficulty keeping up with the speed of conversations, understanding semantics and pragmatics, humour, and understanding the rules of games.
- Greater impulsivity and poorer emotional regulation, poor vocabulary of emotion, and emotionally immature.
- Restricted social sphere, lower social competence, psychosocial problems, and issues with identity development.
- Overdependence on family members for social modelling and role identification.

School
Bullying, teasing, lack of role model, social isolation, poor self-esteem, and low confidence.

Psychological difficulties
- Occur in 15–50% with preponderance of behaviour disorders.
- Depression (see ➜ pp. 330–2) and anxiety (see ➜ pp. 338–40) are 2.5 times more common than in the hearing population.
- Create difficulty with hearing aid use and in accepting professional support.

Learning
- Incidental learning reduced.
- Auditory deprivation impacts neurocognitive development.
- Low academic achievement. Poor literacy, reading, and mathematical skills.

Adulthood
High underemployment, social maladaptation (e.g. violence and drug and alcohol problems), psychological distress, and disorder.

Impact on family
Stress, overprotection, and difficulty with boundary setting.

Risk factors
- Parental negative attitude to deafness and lack of communication with child.
- Child's characteristics, e.g. associated disability, ADHD, and poor cognition and behaviour.
- Psychoeducational, socioemotional, and behavioural difficulties can also be seen with mild and unilateral HL.

Psychosocial, communicative, and cognitive outcomes
Improve with:
- Responsive and supportive families, parent–child interaction, and positive parenting.
- Early intervention to enhance competence of caregivers and access to stimulating resources at home.
- Early intervention of PCHI.
- Peer group and type of schooling.

Deaf community and culture

- Identify as culturally deaf and have a strong deaf identity, peer support, and role models.
- Do not regard deafness as a disability ('medical model' causing disability), but as a positive attribute, as signing allows free communication.
- Use sign language and are drawn together by a set of common beliefs, experiences, and events. They may meet in 'Deaf Clubs'.
- British Sign Language is a recognized language in the UK with its own grammar. Other countries have their own sign languages, e.g. Chinese Sign Language and American Sign Language.
- Use of eye contact, physical contact (patting, backslapping), and facial expression is common and accepted.
- Some members do not support CIs.

Further resources

British Association of Audiovestibular Physicians (guidelines on aetiological investigations for HL): ℰ http://www.baap.org.uk/documents-guidelines-pathways-and-clinical-standards.html

British Society of Audiology (for recommended hearing test procedures, Position Statements): ℰ http://www.thebsa.org.uk/resources/

Hereditary Hearing Loss Homepage (information on genetic causes of HL): ℰ http://hereditaryhearingloss.org

Joint Committee of Infant Hearing (risk factors for hearing impairment): ℰ http://www.jcih.org

National deaf children's society (for parent and professional resources): ℰ http://www.ndcs.org.uk/

National Institute for Health and Care Excellence (NICE) (guidelines for management of cochlear implant and glue ear): ℰ http://www.nice.org.uk/guidance

Modernising Children's Hearing aid Services (MCHAS) (guidelines for hearing aid fitting): ℰ http://research.bmh.manchester.ac.uk/mchas

Public Health England (guidelines for infants after hearing screening): ℰ https://www.gov.uk/government/publications/surveillance-and-audiological-referral-guidelines/guidelines-for-surveillance-and-audiological-referral-for-infants-and-children-following-newborn-hearing-screen#categories-of-babies-and-recommended-follow-up-related-to-the-newborn-hearing-screen

Visual Impairment

Visual impairment

The child with severe congenital visual impairment (VI)

Babies and young children with severe VI occurring as a primary condition due to an abnormality of the eye or optic nerve develop more slowly than fully sighted children. There is particular vulnerability in the toddler and preschool years. Severe congenital VI should be considered a neurodevelopmental disorder, rather than a 'sensory' disorder.

Developmental support and advice should begin as early as possible and should not be dependent on confirmation of underlying diagnosis (or completion of the certification/registration process). The key practitioner is the specialist teacher for VI who provides infancy, preschool, and school-aged support. Community paediatricians and therapists in the child development team can provide valuable input, enhanced by robust MDT working.

What is 'severe' VI?

- Visual acuity refers to clarity of vision—how 'in focus' things appear—and is the main criterion used to classify severity of VI.
- (Recognition) acuity is measured according to the smallest size of target that can be named or matched at specific distances.
- Most classification systems including the ICD-11 are based on WHO categories of mild/moderate/severe/blindness; these definitions depend on recognition acuity measured at distance and are difficult to apply to very young children. See Table 4.1.
- Functional classification of severe VI in young children as devised by Sonksen conceptualizes form vision—the ability to detect a non-light-reflecting object at a specified near distance—and is quantified with the Near Detection Vision Scale.
- Profound VI is defined as light awareness only and severe VI as the detection of visual form.
- A definition of severe VI relevant to early childhood development states: VI is considered severe when substantial adaptation of everyday materials and experiences is required to mitigate its potentially significant interference on development, interaction, and learning.

Table 4.1 Classification (WHO and ICD-11)

Category	Presenting distance visual acuity		
	Worse than	Equal to/better than	
No VI		6/12 (logMAR 0.3)	
Mild VI	6/12 (logMAR 0.3)	6/18 (logMAR 0.5)	
Moderate VI	6/18 (logMAR 0.5)	6/60 (logMAR 1.0)	
Severe VI	6/60 (logMAR 1.0)	3/60 (logMAR 1.3)	SI
Blindness	3/60 (logMAR 1.3)	1/60	SSI
Blindness	1/60 (logMAR 1.8)	Light perception	SSI

Causes of severe congenital VI in the UK

Most cases of severe VI are identified in the first year of life.[1] Conditions in which vision deteriorates in later childhood are rarer but do occur and include retinal dystrophies, which may be isolated and occur as part of a neurodegenerative condition such as Batten's disease.

- Retinal disorders (including retinopathy of prematurity and retinal dystrophies) and optic nerve disorders (predominantly optic nerve hypoplasia) each account for 25% of cases.
- Cataract, glaucoma, corneal abnormalities, globe malformations (e.g. anophthalmia/microphthalmia), and anterior segment anomalies cause 1% of cases.
- Genetic conditions (e.g. early-onset rod-cone retinal dystrophies and bilateral cataracts) cause up to about 33% of cases but diagnostic rates are increasing dramatically in many conditions.
- Cerebral abnormalities account for 40% of cases; additional problems arising from the underlying brain condition are common.
- Severe VI is rare (6 per 10,000 children by the age of 16) but is often associated with additional impairments; children from ethnic minority backgrounds and of lower socioeconomic status are over represented.
- Only 25% of cases are due to preventable or treatable causes.

logMAR, logarithm of the minimum angle of resolution; SI, sight impaired; SSI, severely sight impaired.How is severe congenital VI identified?

(See also British Childhood Visual Impairment Study, 2000[1].)

Routine screening done as part of the neonatal examination and 6–8-week check identifies 25% of cases. Specific screening for retinopathy of prematurity follows evidence-based guidelines and identifies most cases; early treatment limits disease progression.

- Inspection of the eye/red reflex examination is intended to identify any major structural abnormality and cataract.
- Children with a family history of eye disease (e.g. retinal dystrophy, cataracts, glaucoma, or retinoblastoma) should be referred promptly.
- Parental concern should prompt referral:
  - Abnormal eye appearance: pupil abnormality, white pupil in flash photos, squint, abnormal eye movements.
  - Concerns about poor vision (e.g. failure to develop responsive smile, abnormal fix/follow/visually directed reach).
- Mark referrals as urgent to avoid the distress of delayed diagnosis.

Diagnosing the underlying cause of severe VI

Ophthalmological evaluation for suspected severe VI should aim to identify the underlying cause, the presence of treatable components (e.g. refractive error) and the child's level of vision, if any.

- In some conditions, fundoscopy may be normal; specialist examination under anaesthesia or additional electrodiagnostic testing may be required via referral to the regional paediatric centre.
- An electroretinogram may be required to confirm serious retinal abnormality; usually only available in specialist centres.

- Genetic testing may be carried out by the paediatric ophthalmologist with genetic counsellor input or via referral to clinical genetics.
- Further tests may be required according to what is diagnosed, e.g.:
  - Optic nerve hypoplasia: brain MRI and pituitary baseline tests: is the optic nerve hypoplasia occurring as part of septo-optic dysplasia?
  - Some genetic subtypes of early-onset rod-cone retinal dystrophy: brain MRI to look for cerebellar vermis abnormalities (Joubert syndrome phenotype); renal investigations in case of renal cysts.

Eye examination and vision assessment: general guidance
- *Recognition acuity*: gold standard method of measuring visual acuity: determines smallest size letter/picture identified at specific distance; measures now in logMAR values; normal vision is logMAR 0.0 (Snellen 6/6), higher values indicate reduced vision (logMAR 1.0 is 10× worse than normal) (Snellen 6/60); recognition acuity cannot be measured in young children who cannot name or match.
- *Resolution acuity* can be measured instead; grey cards with black and white striped targets at one end, successive cards display stripes of decreasing width; may be called 'preferential looking' tests (child prefers to look at the contrast not grey blank); tester notes child's fixation responses and whether this corresponds to the location of the striped target; resolution acuity is measured in cycles/degree.
- *Squint (strabismus)* if present can cause diplopia (double vision), which if persistent will lead the brain to dampen the vision = amblyopia, treated by patching the stronger eye to make the brain use/improve vision from weaker eye.
- *Refraction* is the process of checking if the eye brings the image into focus on the retina; refractive errors can be corrected by spectacles:
  - Hypermetropia or longsightedness: image falls behind retina, convex lens corrects (makes eye look bigger).
  - Myopia or short sightedness: image falls in front of retina, concave lens corrects (edge of face has 'sucked in' appearance).
- *Nystagmus* is a repetitive, involuntary movement usually of both eyes; commonly occurs when an underlying eye problem causes severe VI (sensory defect nystagmus) and is thus a 'sign' but not a 'diagnosis'. (Idiopathic nystagmus is diagnosed if nystagmus occurs in the absence of any underlying eye condition; causes some acuity reduction but not usually severe in degree.)

Refraction and acuity assessment involve separate procedures and measure different things:
- *Ophthalmologists*: examine the eye to diagnose eye disease, can perform refraction and carry out surgery.
- *Orthoptists*: work alongside ophthalmologists to diagnose and treat squint; acuity assessment is key part of role as each eye's acuity measures are needed to identify amblyopia.
- *Optometrists*: examine the eye, perform refraction, and prescribe refractive corrections including contact lenses.
- *Eye clinic liaison officer*: provides information and guidance.

Paediatric vision assessment in the child with severe VI

Confirmation of underlying diagnosis will ideally be accompanied by vision assessment conducted by the ophthalmology team; look for descriptions in the letter of materials used, responses observed, refractive error identified, and correction issued.

Simple observations in clinic show what the child responds to and guides practical vision promotion activities. Specialist teachers usually also carry out functional assessment:

- Is there evidence of light awareness (lowest level of vision)?
- Is there evidence of form vision? What size object is detected/at what distance? (The Near Detection Scale uses items of 12.5 cm/6.25 cm/ 2.5 cm/1.25 cm/5 mm/3 mm/1 mm at 30 cm placed against a plain well-contrasted background on a table top.)
- Can the child recognize what is seen (no touch or sound clues)?
- Think about how the child can show a visual response—depends on skill level—this contributes to advice on vision promotion:
  - Can s/he turn towards a visual target?
  - Can s/he reach for it in space, or on a table top?
  - Can s/he understand a spoken instruction and visually locate a specific object?
- *Vision maturation*: occurs from birth onwards in those with a normal visual system; also occurs in many ocular/optic nerve conditions but from a lower baseline; maturation is particularly slow in some conditions (e.g. albinism, optic nerve hypoplasia).
- *Vision promotion*: research evidence indicates that simple activities designed to increase *active visual interest and use of vision* can lead to faster maturation of vision: a better level of vision available at a younger age is developmentally beneficial; activities and materials are described in the *Developmental Journal for Babies and Young Children with Visual Impairment* (DJVI) and can be carried out at home.

Impact of severe VI on child development

Vision is the most important human sense, driving many aspects of early development: severe VI is potentially very disruptive. Parent–child bonding is at risk: a young baby can appear unresponsive. With fewer or more subtle cues as to what interests the baby, parents can struggle to respond appropriately and early social interaction is affected. Early face-to-face social interaction may be limited or impossible. Development often progresses more slowly and somewhat differently than in the sighted child and needs support (Table 4.2).

- Parenting stress may be increased with greatest risk in profound VI; parents need support and reassurance to build up confidence.
- Specialist assessment using materials designed for children with VI (e.g. the Reynell–Zinkin scales) can indicate whether progress is as expected for the degree of VI.
- Early intervention support materials: the DJVI is an evaluated set of resource materials to support early intervention intended for use by professionals working in partnership with parents.

Table 4.2 Development in the child with visual impairment

Area of difficulty	Ways to support
Hearing: turning towards sounds is delayed, as object permanence develops later; baby 'stills' when listening and can appear unresponsive	Explain that child is actively listening when they 'still' to sound Support development of sound location skills—gently guide infant's arm by the elbow towards a sound played in front, then to side
Hands: some babies are reluctant to touch things and may withdraw their hands	Do not 'force' tactile exploration, may increase anxiety and cause further withdrawal
Movement: sitting may be delayed—baby cannot see the floor and does not learn saving reflexes and how to support with their hands	In supported sitting position rock infant from side to side so that their hand 'finds' the floor Good sound localization skills can encourage movement through space
Understanding sounds and words: may develop more slowly as source of sound or object described is not seen	Encourage use of very simple descriptive language by parent that describes what infant is hearing or touching
Communicating: expressive communication may develop more slowly and with unusual patterns. Echolalia common but copied phrases may also be used in communicative way	Encourage parent to identify meaningful communication and to shape this through responses Talk about the 'here and now': help child focus on current experience Avoid responding to echolalia if there is no clear meaning
Playing: early play actions such as banging and shaking may persist for longer	Model new play actions, use gentle hand under hand guidance, reinforce with verbal feedback
Social interaction: eye contact, triadic gaze, awareness of other's actions and interests may all be reduced or impossible	Support parent to observe infant to identify what interests them; encourage parent to convey to infant their presence/interest through body contact and simple verbal commentary; turn-taking activities, joint play at appropriate level

- The DJVI is available to relevant professionals for licensed usage and replaces previous versions in print and electronic circulation (ℜ https://xip.uclb.com/i/healthcare_tools/DJVI_professional.html).
- Shared use of the materials enables parents and professionals to track and understand the progress of children from 0 to 3 years of age (or equivalent developmental age), to identify areas of difficulty needing further support, and to promote interagency working.

Specialist teacher for VI

- Specialist teachers are trained teachers who complete additional training to become a qualified teacher for visual impairment (QTVI). Many teams include teaching assistants.
- VI teams also have habilitation specialists who support with daily living skills, mobility, and independence.
- Specialist VI teams will ideally begin working with children and families from the moment that severe VI is suspected; support is usually provided through home visiting; later advice is given to nurseries and schools as required.
- Specialist teachers are encouraged to introduce the DJVI to families.

Certification and registration

These processes were designed for adults but also apply to children. There are two levels: sight impaired (SI) and severely sight impaired (SSI) with acuity the key criterion (Table 4.1). Certification enables contact with social care (crucial for adults with acquired sight loss) and permits registration (helps service planning). The ophthalmologist completes a certificate, and sends it to social services who contact the family to ask if they wish the child to be registered.

- Certification is *not* designed as a referral route to the QTVI, but is misunderstood as such by some.
- The category of sight registration may be cited in clinic letters but is *not* a full description of vision level: the ophthalmologist has discretion in choice of category, and vision level may change. Acuity measures/ functional descriptions are more informative.
- If the only detail you have is the certification status, ask for more!

Developmental difficulties beyond infancy

Social communication is particularly vulnerable and characteristics which resemble those seen in sighted children with ASD may be evident (e.g. re-petitive play actions, limited interests, repetitive speech). Some children show developmental stasis with or without regression in the second year of life ('developmental setback'). Others move forward developmentally but show persistent difficulties in play, communication, and interaction. Assessment for ASD requires adaptation and specialist advice may be useful.

- The risk of ASD is higher than in sighted children,
- Some children show later catch up with learning at school age,
- Others do not; specific and general learning difficulties may occur,
- Braille learning presents additional challenges,
- During the primary years, high rates of fatigue are common; social relationships and general mental well-being require support.

The child with severe congenital VI: your community paediatric role

- Listen to parent concerns about eyes/vision: elicit information carefully as acceptance may be affected if understanding is not explored and information not given in ways most relevant to the family.
- Identify parent-friendly sources of information and family support groups; listen to parents' expressed fears and hopes.

- Make additional onward referrals as relevant; conditions may be rare but further information is readily available.
- Be familiar with the impact of severe VI on development.
- Liaise with other professionals involved to ensure comprehensive information sharing: link with the specialist teacher for VI, discuss the child's progress; contribute to goal-setting discussions as relevant; offer developmental reviews linking with therapists as relevant if there are particular difficulties to be addressed.
- Join or establish a MDT including VI teaching team to ensure the needs of all children with severe VI are addressed locally. Models of team work vary: joint assessment clinics, case discussions, Team Around the Child meetings.
- Make links with your local ophthalmology team: who is the lead for paediatrics? *Is a direct referral route to the specialist teaching team established?* Does the eye clinic liaison officer provide support to parents and children as well as adults? Is there an orthoptist with an interest in children with severe VI? Is there a low-vision aids clinic for children? Ask to attend a paediatric clinic: expand your knowledge of eye examination and vision assessment and strengthen links with community paediatrics.

Reference

1. British Childhood Visual Impairment Study 2000.

The child with a disability: identifying visual difficulties

- A child with a disability has an increased risk of ocular abnormality (e.g. squint, refractive error) and cerebral visual impairment (CVI).
- CVI is a broad-spectrum condition, defined as a verifiable visual dysfunction not attributable to disorders of the eye or optic nerve.
- CVI may result in reduced visual acuity which ranges in severity.
- Signs of severe reduction of visual acuity may be less obvious than in children with eye problems: eye appears normal; nystagmus less common; reduced body movements and communication limit the ways in which child can respond to visual targets.
- A number of other potential features of CVI are reported (difficulties with recognition of objects/faces; following moving targets, spotting things in busy environments, poor visually guided movement, visual field defects, weaknesses in visual attention, a tendency to visual tiring); however, these difficulties may not be evident in children with complex disability; measurement of acuity is important and should be actively pursued.
- Remember that atypical visual responses may be indicative of a non-visual problem (child is tired, uncomfortable, affected by seizures, developmentally unable to respond to visual materials presented); important not to diagnose any atypical visual response as CVI.
- Acuity assessment may be overlooked in the ophthalmology clinic or not fully reported; assessment by staff with skills in assessing children with disabilities in specialist school settings is advocated.
- Visual materials are used to support learning and communication in children with disabilities and acuity measures are crucial in guiding appropriate adaptation; an appreciation of the child's overall level of skill will also guide choice of such materials.

The child with expressive communication difficulties due to physical disability

Children with movement disorders such as CP may have bulbar involvement limiting speech sound production, causing expressive communication impairment. Difficulties with speech sound production may occur in other conditions for reasons that are harder to determine (e.g. autism, or genetic conditions such as Angelman syndrome) but the same principles of support can be applied. A first step is to recognize what a child currently understands (receptive skills)—this sets expectations for the level of expressive communication—and what, and how, a child currently communicates (expressive skills): other than at very early developmental stages most children communicate some basic messages via some means. From such a baseline we can determine the best ways of expanding the child's communicative repertoire.

- AAC is the shorthand for augmentative and alternative communication and refers to any form of communication other than speech or writing used to express needs, wants, and ideas.
- AAC includes facial expression, non-word vocalizations (e.g. tone of voice), gesture, sign, photos, or picture symbols.
- Remember that everyone uses some AAC, but people with speech limitations may rely on AAC.
- AAC may be useful for children who have physical limitations to developing speech, and children who have lost speech due to injury to the brain or bulbar area.

Who supports the child with AAC needs?

Therapists manage communication difficulties, but the community paediatrician should have a broad grasp of the child's overall communication profile and understand the management approaches used by therapists.

- SLTs (see 🔖 pp. 402–3) have a primary responsibility.
- OTs (see 🔖 pp. 390–1) also have a key role, through provision of supportive seating to enable the best physical position to use AAC materials and through advising on the best access method to use AAC materials.
- Teachers and school staff will need to understand how communication support materials are to be used.

What to discuss with parents and carers

- What are their hopes and expectations for their child's communication?
- Do they have any specific ideas about what might be useful for their child? (This could range from a piece of equipment to expectations for direct therapy input.)
- How does their child show what they understand (everyday situations, spoken language)?
- What does their child communicate now (*reasons*) and in what ways (*means*)? Reasons might include making requests for food or activities, means might include making vocalizations, reaching, and/or gestures. What communication *opportunities* are available to their child (making choices, giving news, expressing opinions, asking questions, and chatting)?

- What types of communication support have been tried so far, how useful are these at home?
- What other factors could affect communication—any concerns about hearing or vision, discomfort or pain, positioning, and nutrition; what does their child like to do or play with (we all communicate best about things we find interesting); and what about social motivation and social interaction?
- How confident are they about understanding their child—communication asymmetry between adult and child can commonly occur and parent–child interaction training can be helpful.

What to look for when you meet the child

- Social responsiveness and interest: how does the child respond to greetings and overtures?
- Look for evidence of receptive language skills: ask a simple question and observe how the child responds.
- Observe how the child makes a response from options offered—points/reaches, looks, or gives yes/no response when adult presents each option?
- Is the yes/no response clear, and repeatable? Is it easy to distinguish from other body movements or vocalizations?

Communication: therapy assessment should consider

- Receptive language skills: help set expectations for expressive language skills. Assessment may be *informal*—key word level, using objects or pictures—or *formal*, using standardized assessment materials (e.g. Peabody Picture Vocabulary Scale, preschool language scale).
- Expressive language skills, including the following if applicable: speech intelligibility, gesture and sign, yes/no/I don't know responses, and complexity of utterance.
- Communication reasons (functions): requesting more/finished, choosing an activity from options offered, initiating chat or comment, and requesting information.
- Tools such as the Communication Matrix can give a pictorial representation of the child's current overall communication skills.
- Assessment of receptive and expressive language skills will reveal the size of the *gap* between the two.
- What is the child's most reliable body movement for selecting options presented, and is positioning in supportive seating optimized?
- Low-tech communication options: these are non-electronic and do not require power. Options include objects, communication boards and books (photos or symbols), alphabet boards, and writing or drawing a message.
- High-tech communication options: these are electronic devices which allow for speech output. These include dedicated communication devices or tablets/iPads with communication applications installed onto them.
- Access method: this refers to how a person accesses AAC. A person with complex physical difficulties may not be able to use their hands effectively to point and might control their AAC using another part of

their body such as feet, eyes, or head. If direct access is not possible, indirect access methods may be required, e.g. switches, joystick, or a head mouse.
- Eye gaze access technology is a specific direct access method involving the use of a person's eyes to activate a computer device.
- Specialized services: there are 15 specialized AAC services in England, commissioned and funded by NHS England. Specific referral criteria must be satisfied. Their remit is to provide specialist AAC assessment and funding of high-tech AAC equipment for 10% of the AAC population, and to provide training and advice. Local services are responsible for supporting 90% of the AAC population.

Top tips for the community paediatrician

- Although speech limitations may be the most 'obvious' difficulty, avoid assuming that adding in an alternative to speech will solve all communication difficulties.
- The child who cannot speak is unlikely to be communicating nothing— consider what is communicated informally, e.g. through behaviour during interactions.
- A 'communication system' may include a piece of equipment (e.g. symbol board or book, or communication software) but communication partners are a key part of any 'system'.
- It takes two to talk—become a skilled listener in interactions with C&YP with physical disability: be patient if communication takes longer, don't guess at the meaning, ask for clarification or a repeat if you have not understood.
- When observing the child's responses, consider how confident you felt about what you saw: was the response intentional and correct, intentional and incorrect (remember children of any ability may give an incorrect response!), or difficult to distinguish from other vocalizations and body movements?
- Presume little about possible success with communication support provided, without thorough assessment: a lack of assessment could lead to inappropriate support and materials being provided.
- Receptive language level has been shown to broadly correspond to overall cognitive level.
- The risk of ID in children with CP is highest in those with the most severe movement restrictions, but children with severe movement restriction may have good cognitive skills and those with less severe movement restrictions may have cognitive impairment of varying degrees.
- Yes/no responses can be useful but require understanding of the options presented or question asked. If the question is 'Do you want this toy?' or 'Shall we sing?' then a positive response effectively means 'Yes please' (*acceptance* of what is offered), and a negative response effectively means 'No thanks' (*rejection* of what is offered).

Neurological disorders

Neuroanatomy and embryogenesis

- Early in the second week of gestation, the inner cell mass converts to a primitive ectoderm (epiblast) and a primitive endoderm.
- Starting at the third week of gestation, gastrulation begins and mesoderm appears. Gastrulation begins with the formation of the primitive streak at the caudal end of the embryo; the streak is a linear thickening on the dorsal surface of the epiblast in which cells of the epiblast form endoderm and mesoderm.
- A collection of cells at the end of the primitive streak forms the primitive node (Hensen's node)—epiblastic cells migrate anteriorly through the node to become the longitudinally running cellular rod called the notochord, which develops from the axial mesoderm. The dorsal ectodermal surface of the early embryo thickens and elongates to form the neural plate.
- At about 20 days of gestation, the neural plate becomes a neural groove. Rapid cell proliferation at the margins creates a midline neural groove between neural folds, which gradually deepens. The elevated margins of the neural folds grow towards each other and fuse to form a neural tube (Fig. 5.1).
- Cells lining the groove are neuroepithelial cells which ultimately give rise to all the cells of the CNS. The anterior end of the neural plate enlarges and will form the brain while the caudal portion of the neural plate

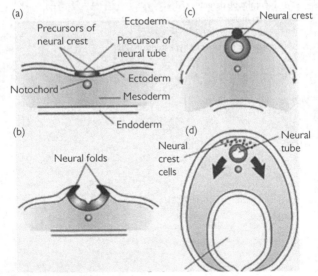

Fig. 5.1 Folding of the neural tube.

Reprinted from Goodlett C and Horn K (2001) 'Mechanisms of Alcohol-Induced Damage to the Developing Nervous System' Alcohol Res Health 25(3):175–184.

will form the spinal cord. The cavity of the developing neural tube is destined to become the ventricular system. Ectoderm at the margins of the neural folds becomes neural crest cells that will give rise to the main elements of the peripheral nervous system.

- Cells from the margins of the neural tube detach from the neural folds to form clusters of neural crest cells. These dorsally located cells migrate peripherally to become sensory ganglia of the cranial and spinal nerves, autonomic and enteric ganglia, Schwann cells, melanocytes, adrenal chromaffin cells, and the pia/arachnoid membranes (dura develops from mesoderm).
- After closure of the neural tube, the expanded rostral portion of the neural tube will differentiate and subdivide into three vesicles representing the forebrain, midbrain, and hindbrain.
- Further development of the CNS and peripheral nervous system continues but essentially the primary early development of the nervous system is already completed by 24 days of gestation. It is from this early embryonic nervous tissue that we see defects of the neural tube and neuroepithelial tumours. It also helps us understand the neurocutaneous syndromes.
- By the end of the 3rd week, the three-part brain begins to assume a 'C'-shape by the formation of a cephalic flexure at the level of the mesencephalon; at the end of the 4th week, a cervical flexure develops between the hindbrain and spinal cord. By the 6th week, the pontine flexure develops in the rhombencephalon which divides it into a metencephalon and myelencephalon (Fig. 5.2). The metencephalon forms the pons and cerebellum; the myelencephalon becomes the medulla. A depression develops in the prosencephalon which defines the telencephalon from the diencephalon. Subsequent growth of the telencephalon will cause it to expand dorsally, caudally, laterally, and inferiorly. The optic cup continues its development.

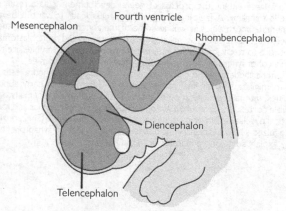

Fig. 5.2 Brain development at 6 weeks of gestation.

- As the spinal cord develops, neuroblasts of the neural tube's mantle layer proliferate in two zones. In cross section, the mantle layer develops a characteristic 'butterfly' shape of grey matter. Neuroblasts of the brainstem develop in a manner similar to the spinal cord.
- The ventricular system is established early. The prosencephalon separates into two expanding telencephalic vesicles (lateral ventricles) and a slit-like diencephalic vesicle (third ventricle). Thickening of its walls narrows the lumen of this segment to a vertical slit, the third ventricle. The lumina of the lateral and three ventricles connect just behind the lamina terminalis via the paired foramina of Monro. Expansion of the mesencephalon narrows its vesicle forming the cerebral aqueduct, which connects the third ventricle and the fourth ventricle of the rhombencephalon. The rhombencephalic roof is thin and covers the fourth ventricle which forms a shallow, diamond-shaped depression. The expansion of the cerebral hemispheres affects the shape of the lateral ventricles which become 'C' shaped.
- The eyes develop from (1) neuroectoderm of the diencephalon, (2) surface ectoderm, and (3) intervening neural crest/mesoderm. Neuroectoderm gives rise to the retina, epithelium of the ciliary body/iris, and optic nerves. Surface ectoderm gives rise to the lens and anterior surface of the cornea. The surrounding mesenchyme is of neural crest origin and contributes to the sclera, part of the cornea, choroid, ciliary body/iris, and blood vessels of the eye. Early in the 4th week, optic sulci appear and are transformed into hollow outgrowths of the diencephalon called optic vesicles which approach the surface ectoderm. The optic vesicle forms the optic cup which is connected to the diencephalon by the constricted, hollow optic stalk.

Understanding this process helps us understand the abnormalities of nervous system morphogenesis such as congenital hydrocephalus, cyclops, septo-optic dysplasias, anencephaly, hydranencephaly, holoprosencephaly, etc.

To a large extent, the process of neural development is as a result of genetic signalling. A fault in the signalling process leads to various developmental abnormalities as well as some of the abnormal cell proliferation processes. Examples of this include medulloblastomas and retinoblastomas. Exposure to toxins can cause underproliferation of cells. Examples are the fetal alcohol syndrome, fetal valproate syndrome, and thalidomide.

Genetically determined defects in cellular migration cause neural cells to fail to migrate to their final resting position. This results in early abnormalities with failure of gyration of the forebrain such as lissencephaly or a double cortex, or more subtle abnormalities such as heterotopias and focal cortical dysplasias. Similar migration abnormalities outside the CNS are also recognized such as Hirschsprung disease. Abnormalities of synaptogenesis may explain some of the features of fragile X syndrome and autism.

Neuroanatomy

An anatomical approach to neurological disorders is the crucial aspect of adult neurology. While neurological disorders in children tend to be more diffuse pathological processes due to underlying genetic and metabolic aetiologies, a secure understanding of the anatomy is always advantageous.

Central nervous system

The cerebral cortex consists of four lobes in each hemisphere with specific functions.

Frontal lobes

- Lie anterior to the central sulcus and superior to the lateral sulcus.
- Various functional areas are recognized such as:
  - Broca's area: expressive language centre in the inferior part of the dominant frontal lobe.
  - Precentral gyrus: the primary motor cortex controlling contralateral movements.
  - Supplementary motor area: controls contralateral head and eye turning.
  - Prefrontal area: controls personality and initiative, emotion, judgement, gait, praxis, etc.
  - Paracentral lobule: regulates cortical control over bladder and bowel voiding.
- Interpreting symptoms in the context of this anatomical knowledge is very helpful in localizing pathology.
- Frontal dysfunction presents with:
  - Failure of expressive language.
  - Motor deficit.
  - Apathy.
  - Akinesia.
  - Gait apraxia.
  - Disinhibition.
  - Loss of continence.
  - Head and eye deviation is often seen in frontal seizures towards the side of pathological focus.

Parietal lobes

- Lie posterior to the central sulcus with a rather indistinct boundary with the occipital and temporal lobes.
- Areas with specific identified functions are the:
  - Postcentral gyrus: the primary sensory cortex receiving afferent pathways for posture, touch, and passive movement.
  - Supramarginal and angular gyri: Wernicke's language area in the dominant hemisphere, an area where auditory and visual aspects of comprehension are integrated.
  - Visual pathways (optic radiation): pass deep through the parietal lobe, representing the lower visual field.
- Parietal dysfunction of the dominant or non-dominant hemisphere results in disturbance of:
  - Contralateral cortical sensation such as posture.
  - Localization of light touch.
  - Two-point discrimination.

- • Appreciation of size, weight, and texture of an object (astereognosis).
  - • Sensory inattention.
- • Wernicke's dysphasia produces non-sensical but fluent speech.
- • Characteristically, praxis is affected by affection of the non-dominant parietal lobe causing constructional and dressing apraxia.
- • Dominant parietal lobe dysfunction may produce confusion of right and left, acalculia, and agraphia.
- • Damage to the optic radiation can cause homonymous quadrantanopia.

Temporal lobes
- • Separated anteriorly from frontal lobes by lateral sulcus but less clear separation from occipital and parietal lobes.
- • Three main gyrations—superior, middle, and inferior temporal gyri—have specific functions:
  - • Auditory cortex lies in the superior gyrus buried in the lateral sulcus (Heschl gyrus).
  - • The dominant hemisphere is the primary auditory cortex responsible for hearing of language. The non-dominant hemisphere is important in hearing sounds, rhythm, and music.
  - • Middle and inferior gyri are concerned with memory and learning.
- • Limbic lobe: the inferior and middle portions of the temporal lobe including the hippocampus and parahippocampal gyrus. This is an important part responsible for sensation of olfaction but also complex emotional and affective behaviour. Along with the inferior frontal and medial parietal structures it forms the limbic system.
- • Visual pathways pass deep in the temporal lobe around posterior horns of the lateral ventricle.
- • Temporal dysfunction causes:
  - • Cortical deafness.
  - • Auditory and olfactory hallucinations.
  - • Disturbance of memory such as the phenomena of déjà vu and jamais vu.
  - • Learning problems and aggressive antisocial behaviour.

Occipital lobes
- • Medially separated from the parietal lobes by the parieto-occipital sulcus but more subtly merges with the temporal lobes.
- • Calcarine sulcus lying along the medial surface holds the primary visual cortex often called the striate cortex, above and below which lie the parastriate cortex, which is the association visual cortex.
- • An extensive bilateral striatal occipital lesion will cause cortical blindness (with preserved light reflex). Depending on where the lesion is, it will cause a central hemianopic defect involving the macula or a homonymous hemianopia without macular involvement.
- • Parieto-occipital lesions cause:
  - • Inability to direct voluntary gaze.
  - • Loss of visual recognition (visual agnosia).
- • Occipital seizures and migraine often give visual hallucinations which are typically unformed and in a hemianopic field (as opposed to temporal which are complex, well-formed, and filling the whole visual field) or visual auras such as micropsia and macropsia.

Circulation

The circle of Willis is the anastomotic connection of major arterial circulation in the brain. It connects the right and left circulations through the anterior communicating arteries and anterior and posterior circulations through the posterior communicating arteries.

The internal carotid artery gives off the middle and anterior cerebral arteries. The anterior cerebral artery follows the curve of the corpus callosum and supplies the medial surface of the hemisphere (cortical branches). Occlusion results in hemiplegia or paraplegia, sensory loss, and akinetic mutism by frontal infarction.

The middle cerebral artery supplies the anterior limb of the internal capsule (lenticulostriate branch) and lateral surface of the cerebral hemisphere (cortical branches). Occlusion causes dense hemiplegia, sometimes aphasia, apraxia, and hemineglect.

The vertebral arteries arise from the subclavian artery, supply the medulla and inferior surface of the cerebellum, and join to form the basilar artery. The basilar artery supplies the brainstem from the medulla upwards. Vertebrobasilar occlusion causes vertigo, ataxia, and cerebellar and brainstem signs.

Posterior cerebral arteries are terminal branches of the basilar artery supplying the posterior thalamus, choroid plexus, and midbrain. It also supplies the inferior aspect of the temporal lobe and the occipital visual cortex. Occlusion will cause cortical blindness, hemiplegia with third nerve palsy, and chorea or ballismus. The lateral medullary syndrome is caused by occlusion of the posterior inferior cerebellar artery which arises from the vertebral artery. It causes an ipsilateral Horner syndrome, vertigo, nystagmus, and ataxia and a mixed sensory loss involving the face on the same side and limbs on the contralateral side.

Lacunar strokes are caused by occlusion of the deep perforating arteries thereby sparing the cortex and cortical functions such as language, cognitive, and visual function.

Cranial nerves

- It is important to quickly visualize the anatomical location of the cranial nerve nuclei and their origins:
  - First and second—outside the brainstem.
  - Third and fourth—in the midbrain.
  - Fifth to eighth—in the pons.
  - Ninth to 12th—in the medulla.
- The functions and anatomical localization of the cranial nerves are as follows:
  - Olfactory: inferior frontal lobe—smell.
  - Optic nerve: enters brain at the lateral geniculate body—vision.
  - Oculomotor: midbrain—supplies medial, superior, and inferior rectus; inferior oblique; pupil and lid elevator muscle (levator palpebrae superioris).
  - Trochlear: midbrain—supplies superior oblique.
  - Trigeminal: pons—muscles of chewing, facial sensation, corneal reflex.
  - Abducens: cerebellopontine angle—supplies lateral rectus.
  - Facial: cerebellopontine angle—facial movements, tearing, salivation.

- Auditory: cerebellopontine angle—hearing and vestibular function.
- Glossopharyngeal: medulla—palatal sensation.
- Vagus: medulla—swallowing, autonomic supply to internal organs.
- Spinal accessory: craniocervical junction—sternomastoid and trapezius muscles.
- Hypoglossal: medulla—tongue muscles.

Midbrain

- Midbrain contains the third and fourth cranial nerves, the red nucleus, and connections of the visual pathways.
- Disturbance of the midbrain causes an eye movement palsy and squint with the third and fourth cranial nerves being affected.
- A lesion at the level of the superior colliculus causes failure of upgaze, convergence, and papillary light reaction (pinealoma).
- A tumour obstructing the aqueduct may cause these signs. Red nucleus lesion causes tremor. Substantia nigra affection causes Parkinsonian features.
- A fourth nerve lesion in this region often causes a compensatory head tilt. Pupillary light reflex may be impaired with preserved accommodation.

Pons

- Sixth–eighth nerve lesions are fairly easily diagnosed because of the signs and symptoms they produce.
- Vertical nystagmus may result from brainstem dysfunction.
- Lesions of the medial longitudinal fasciculus typically cause an internuclear ophthalmoplegia with failure of adduction in the same side eye and nystagmus in the opposite abducting eye. There may be a mixture of ipsilateral loss of sensation in the face and contralateral loss in the limbs.

Medulla

- Tongue fasciculation and deviation to the side of the lesion is seen with 12th nerve involvement whereas the other lower cranial nerves cause dysphagia and dysphonia. Horner syndrome may result from sympathetic fibres being involved. Mixed ipsilateral loss of pinprick and temperature with contralateral loss of position and vibration syndrome may occur.
- A lot of the syndromes are eponymously named (Wallenburg, Gradenigo) and although well described in adult neurology are rarely seen in children and very difficult to characterize and diagnose with confidence.

Spinal cord

- The spinal cord runs through the vertebral column with roots and nerves exiting from the foramina between the vertebral bodies. There are 31 pairs of spinal nerves. The cord ends between L1 and L2 levels in a tapered end called the conus medullaris. The final tuft of spinal nerves arising inferiorly from the conus is called the cauda equina.

- The grey matter of the spinal cord is divided into anterior, posterior, and lateral horns whereas the white matter forms the funiculi—ventral, dorsal, and lateral. Spinal nerves form dorsal and ventral roots and then emerge laterally as spinal nerves. Decussation of corticospinal pathways occurs in the pyramids at the level of the medulla.
- Upper motor neurons decussate in the pons and synapse at the anterior horn cell with lower motor neurons which then innervate the muscles. Ascending pathways carry sensation to the thalamus and thence to the sensory cortex.
- Injuries of the spinal cord between T1 and L1 cause paraplegia whereas injuries above T1 into the cervical cord cause quadriplegia. Transection causes total loss of sensory and motor function below the level of the injury.
- Because the dermatomal supply of the nerves is often below their level of exit from the vertebrae, there is a 'dropped' sensory level. Knowledge of the dermatomes is therefore important to localize the lesion. This may be very difficult to achieve with precision in children (Fig. 5.3 and Fig. 5.4).
- The anterior spinal artery supplies the entire cord except dorsal columns. Occlusion produces paralysis and loss of pain and temperature sensation with preservation of position and vibration sense.

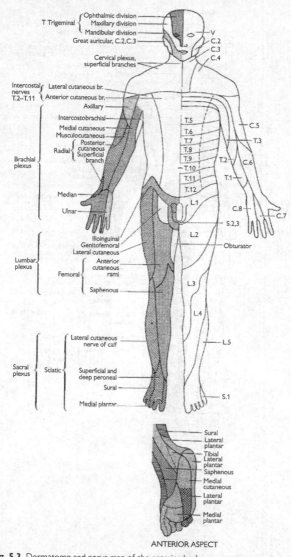

Fig. 5.3 Dermatome and nerve map of the anterior body.

Reproduced from Warman P et al. (2014) 'Regional Anaesthesia, Stimulation, and Ultrasound Techniques' Oxford University Press with permission from Oxford University Press.

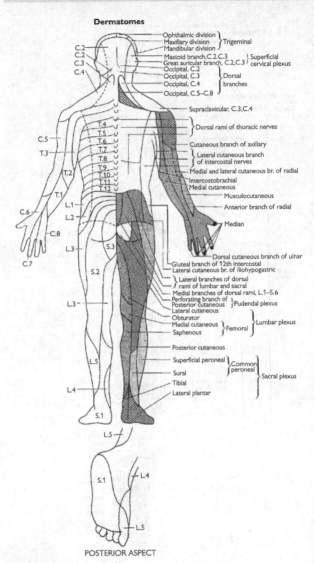

POSTERIOR ASPECT

Fig. 5.4 Dermatome and nerve map of the posterior body.

Reproduced from Warman P et al. (2014) 'Regional Anaesthesia, Stimulation, and Ultrasound Techniques' Oxford University Press with permission from Oxford University Press.

Neurophysiology

The main neurophysiological diagnostic tools are:
- Electroencephalography (EEG).
- Evoked potentials.
- Electromyography (EMG).
- Nerve Conduction Studies

Electroencephalography

- The EEG records electrical activity of the brain.
- Its main use is in the characterization of epilepsies but not as a diagnostic tool. In some epilepsy syndromes of childhood such as West syndrome (hypsarrhythmia) and childhood absence epilepsy (3 Hz spike and wave), the EEG can be diagnostic.
- An EEG can be recorded in wake phase or sleep. It can be a snapshot in time as in ictal EEG or interictal EEG or a prolonged continuous recording as in ambulatory EEGs.
- Continuous video recording often accompanies EEG recording where each paroxysmal event needs to be correlated with electrical abnormality and where lateralization and precise localization of the epileptogenic focus is needed (video telemetry).
- EEGs can also be useful in the diagnosis of encephalopathies and coma states.
- Electrodes are applied to the scalp in certain positions (montages) with glue. The EEG is then recorded on a hard drive or on paper. Video recording often accompanies it to catch any ictal activity.
- A standard wake EEG will be abnormal in 50% of patients with epilepsy. If an EEG is normal in the wake phase, another is repeated with natural sleep, sleep deprivation, or by using sedation. A sleep EEG increases the diagnostic yield to about 75%.
- As many as 15% of patients with epilepsy will have a normal EEG. Patients with frontal lobe epilepsy often have a normal EEG and will need several attempts at recording sleep EEGs to get a positive yield.
- The EEG is recorded with eyes open and closed and the patient is asked to hyperventilate. Photic stimulation is carried out by recording while a light is flashed at the patient at varying flash frequencies. These are all techniques to increase the sensitivity and gain additional information. An ECG is always recorded alongside.
- The interictal background rhythm and paroxysmal EEG changes are noted. Laterality or generalization of changes is commented on.
- When epilepsy surgery is being considered, special tools such as grid mats placed over the brain and ictal single-photon emission computed tomography (SPECT) scans etc. are used to identify the epileptogenic cortex as accurately as possible.
- It has to be emphasized that the diagnosis of epilepsy is a clinical diagnosis based on meticulous history taking and witnessing an event.

Evoked potentials

- Evoked potentials are a method of testing the integrity of sensory pathways from end organ to cerebral cortex.

- The most commonly used evoked potential studies in children are visual evoked potentials to ascertain their cortical visual function. They may be combined with an electroretinogram to measure retinal function and to localize the site of visual dysfunction, which may be difficult to assess in a child especially with learning difficulty.
- Recording is similar to scalp EEG electrodes with stimulus being delivered to the end organ and the EEG recorded being averaged, eliminating background activity and only recording stimulus-induced effects. The output is the latency of different waveforms.
- An evoked potential may be delayed as in demyelination or reduced in amplitude due to loss of axons.
- They need to be interpreted in conjunction with other investigations such as imaging and the clinical story.
- Other evoked potentials used are auditory and somatosensory evoked potentials. They are most useful in the context of cortical dysfunction, demyelination, and neurodegeneration.

Electromyography

- This is the recording of electrical activity from a muscle by inserting a concentric needle into it.
- The electrical activity is displayed on an oscilloscope and transduced to an auditory signal via a loudspeaker.
- Spontaneous activity at rest, motor unit analysis, and recruitment of motor units interference patterns give characteristics which help classify muscle pathology.
- Patterns seen are those of denervated muscle, myopathic muscle, or myotonic muscle. Normal muscle at rest is electrically silent. Fasciculations suggest denervation. Myotonic discharges can be seen and produce a 'dive bomber' sound.
- Recordings made as the muscle contracts help identify a myopathic process (full interference pattern with limited force) or a denervating process (fewer but larger motor units firing at high rates).
- Special EMGs such as stimulated single-fibre EMG are used to diagnose neuromuscular transmission defects along with repetitive nerve stimulation tests showing a decremental response in the amplitude of motor action potentials with a train of stimuli. An increased jitter on stimulated single-fibre EMG is also very suggestive of a neuromuscular transmission defect (myasthenia).

Nerve conduction studies

- These are used to study the motor and sensory function of large myelinated fibres of selected nerves that are easily accessible. The main values measured are the amplitude and conduction velocity.
- The nerve is stimulated at one point and a recording is made at a distant site. The conduction velocity can then be calculated. The amplitude of the action potential can be recorded.
- Motor studies involve stimulating the motor nerve at proximal and distal sites and recording the compound motor action potential (CMAP). Time from distal stimulation to onset of the CMAP is the latency. This measures the nerve conduction, neuromuscular transmission,

and muscle activation time. Motor nerve conduction velocities can be calculated by stimulating at two different points and calculating the time difference to onset of CMAP.
- Two main abnormalities can be detected:
  - Slowing of conduction times due to demyelination.
  - Reduction in amplitudes due to loss of axons.
- The patterns of nerve involvement such as focal, multifocal, or generalized can be worked out and whether the pattern is more axonal or demyelinating.
- It is not possible to detect abnormalities in small unmyelinated nerve fibres and autonomic nerves, in nerves that are deep and inaccessible, and in nerve root disease (radiculopathies) proximal to the dorsal root ganglions.

Taking a neurological history

Always listen to the parent and child. They are trying to tell you the diagnosis.

The key to neurological diagnosis is a meticulous history, good observation, and careful examination. One needs to keep an open mind and avoid bias.
- Ensure you have all available information about the child and the reason/s for the clinic consultation.
- A well-prepared clinician will gain the child and carer's trust and confidence with ease.
- Start observing the child from the waiting room as crucial clues may be noted which could guide your history taking and aid subsequent examination.
- Remember to include the child in the history taking process. Give them the opportunity to say what is bothering them. Drawing pictures can be an excellent alternative to a narrative story.
- A timeline for the history should be sought and will give clues as to whether the problem is static, progressive (acute or chronic), or paroxysmal.

Important components of a neurological history

In any child with a suspected neurological disorder, the history should be comprehensive and cover all aspects of a paediatric history.

Pregnancy and birth
- Drug use (prescribed and recreational), alcohol abuse.
- Significant illness, antenatal bleeding.
- Fetal movements (reduced in neuromuscular disorders, increased/jerky or hiccups suggestive of antenatal seizures).
- Ultrasound findings.
- Preterm or term birth, mode of delivery.
- Details of resuscitation, Apgar score.
- Neonatal period—infection, feeding difficulties, hypoglycaemia.
- Weight and head circumference at birth (review red book).

Development and social history
- Depending on the clinical concern, developmental history needs to be all-encompassing or concise.
- Loss of acquired skills always has a sinister connotation and needs to be actively teased out from history.
- Schooling—learning concerns at school (static or progressive).
- Family circumstances.
- In specific circumstances, exploring peer relationships, bullying, etc. may be required.

Family history
- Three-generation family tree including half siblings.
- Consanguinity and ethnicity.
- Extended neurological family history based on the clinical concern may need to include epilepsy, physical disability, learning difficulties,

migraine, etc. Common conditions such as heart disease, diabetes, hearing difficulties, thyroid problems, etc. also may be relevant, e.g. in mitochondrial disorders.

- Unexpected sudden deaths and recurrent miscarriages must be probed.

Medication, dietary history, toxins, and travel
- Regular medications.
- Diet deficiency: neonatal/infantile hypocalcaemic seizures due to maternal vitamin D deficiency, vitamin B_{12} deficiency due to maternal vegan diet presenting as hypotonia, developmental delay/regression, and megaloblastic anaemia.
- Substance abuse: peripheral neuropathy with glue sniffing and nitric oxide, strokes with cocaine use.
- Toxin exposure: peripheral neuropathy due to lead, arsenic, and mercury.
- Pets, travel may be relevant: Lyme disease, tick paralysis, tuberculosis, cat scratch disease.

Immunization history

For details on immunization schedule for health professionals, please access: ℘ https://www.gov.uk/government/publications/routine-childhood-immunisation-schedule

Recent and past medical history
- Any associations with current problem must be thought of.
- Child with developmental delay and history of inflicted head injury or severe meningitis in infancy.
- Ataxia, neuropathy in coeliac disease.
- Developmental delay/muscle weakness in hypothyroidism.

Examination

A meticulous examination should be endeavoured, but it can be challenging at times. Observation of a child is an equally if not more important part. Watching them walk, talk, and interact gives a lot of information. Even before the start of formal examination these observations are very useful. Formal neurological examination in a child is exactly the same as an adult but a child's cognitive ability and cooperation needs to be factored in. By age 7, most children can be fully examined as an adult; equally, it can be at times completed in a 4-year-old.

All children should have weight, height, and OFC measured and plotted on age-appropriate charts.

Gait and posture
- The way a child walks into the clinic should never be missed. Watching the child's standing, sitting, and lying down postures often can give clues to localize the site of underlying problem to a central (brain/spinal cord) or peripheral (muscle/peripheral nerve) source.
- Formal MRC grading of muscle power is often not possible in young children. Observing the child walk, run, jump, hop, and get up from sitting or lying down will clearly indicate the degree and pattern of weakness.

- Hemiplegic, dystonic, and ataxic gaits can be noticed.
- Subtle asymmetries and motor weakness can be uncovered by performing a Fogs' test.

Facial features
- Facial asymmetry when talking or smiling.
- Expressionless, open, tented myopathic facies.
- Ptosis: bilateral in myotonic dystrophy, myopathies, mitochondrial disorders, and myasthenia (can be asymmetric in juvenile myasthenia gravis). Unilateral is Horner's syndrome, third nerve palsy.
- Syndromic: some are easily recognizable such as DS, Angelman syndrome, Turners syndrome, fragile X.
- In others it is important to see both parents before a definitive diagnosis of dysmorphology.

Neurocutaneous markers
Should be looked for, e.g. port wine stains (Sturge–Weber syndrome), ash leaf macules (tuberous sclerosis—may need Wood lamp exam), café au lait (neurofibromatosis).

Other suggestive signs
- Few examples.
- Spinal muscular atrophy (SMA) type 1: hypotonia, tongue fasciculation.
- Peroxisomal disorders: hypotonia, hepatosplenomegaly.
- Ataxia telangiectasia: ataxia, eye or skin telangiectasia.
- Menkes disease: developmental delay, stiff wiry hair.
- MPS: hirsutism, coarse facial features.
- Rett's syndrome: hyperventilation, hand stereotypes.

Other additional pointers
- Note the child's behaviour/interaction for any features of hyperactivity, social communication difficulties, etc.
- Don't forget to examine the parents, e.g. maternal myotonia in a weak hypotonic infant (congenital myotonic dystrophy), parents for cutaneous lesions in infant with infantile spasms (tuberous sclerosis), parental feet in Charcot–Marie–Tooth disease.

Additional examination points in newborn and infant neurological examination
- Neonatal reflexes should be examined and their persistence beyond a certain age documented as abnormal. These include Moro (noting the persistence and asymmetry if any), asymmetric tonic neck reflex, palmar and plantar grasp reflexes, stepping and placing reflexes, and parachute reflex.
- A weak, floppy neonate or infant lying in a frog leg posture with poor antigravity movements and weak cry is suggestive of a neuromuscular disorder.
- An exaggerated startle to a nose tap especially in a stiff neonate with or without cyanotic spells suggests hyperekplexia.
- Neonatal seizures can be subtle especially in preterm babies and may be easily missed. Jitteriness can be seen in hypoglycaemia and hypocalcaemia. Persistent hiccups are sometimes seen in non-ketotic hyperglycinaemia.

- Nerve root injuries (Erb and Klumpke) as well as more traumatic cervical cord injuries may occur during the process of delivery. They can present as focal limb weakness of more generalized weakness in cord injury with areflexia and swallowing and breathing difficulties.
- Hip dysplasias and joint contractures should be noted.

Signs and symptoms

Abnormal head size

- It is important to accurately measure the OFC at its widest point, accounting for gestational age.
- A sequential plot is more valuable than a single measurement.
- Parental head circumference must be measured, and mid-parental head circumference centile worked out.
- Age-appropriate charts must be used.
- OFC has to be interpreted in the context of the child's neurodevelopmental assessment, intracranial pressure, and concerns of regression, if any.

Causes of large head (>2 SD above mean for age)

- Familial large head (most likely).
- Hydrocephalus (true obstructive as in aqueduct stenosis, tumours, Chiari malformation, or poor absorption as in post meningitis or post haemorrhagic).
- Increased extra-axial fluid spaces: this has to be excessive and progressive. It is a common finding on imaging in achondroplasia, Menkes, glutaric aciduria type 1.
- Hydranencephaly: very rare, may be part of holoprosencephaly sequence.
- Megalencephaly: genetic or associated with neurocutaneous syndromes such as neurofibromatosis, tuberous sclerosis, gigantism as in Soto syndrome.
- Metabolic disorders: Alexander and Canavan diseases, galactosemia, glutaric aciduria type 1, MPS, gangliosidoses.
- Subdural effusions/haemorrhages.
- Thickened skull causing large head: rickets, osteogenesis imperfecta, cleidocranial dysostosis, epiphyseal dysplasia, osteopetrosis, etc.

Causes of microcephaly (OFC <2 SD below normal for age)
Primary microcephaly

- Genetic.
- Chromosomal abnormality.
- Anencephaly and encephalocoeles.
- Cortical malformations like lissencephaly or pachygyria.
- Holoprosencephaly.

Secondary microcephaly

- Intrauterine infection/toxin exposure.
- Hypoxic ischaemic injury.
- Intracranial haemorrhage or perinatal stroke.
- Post meningitis/encephalitis.
- Chronic malnutrition.

Abnormal head shape

Postural plagiocephaly is the most common. In the absence of developmental concerns or abnormal examination findings, no further investigation is required.

Causes of abnormal head shape

- Intracranial causes, e.g. hydrocephalus, chronic subdural effusions.
- Extracranial causes, e.g. plagiocephaly, craniosynostosis which may be syndromal, genetic, or associated with other conditions such as MPS, polycythemia, hyperthyroidism, hypercalcaemia, and rickets.
- Well-recognized craniosynostosis syndromes with characteristic head shapes are clover leaf skull of Pfeiffer syndrome, brachycephaly and synostosis of Apert syndrome, and generalized synostosis of Crouzon or Carpenter syndrome. Crouzon has associated facial malformations and Carpenter syndrome could have obesity and hypogonadism.

Floppy infant

- In a floppy infant, the first challenge is to differentiate if floppiness is due to hypotonia, weakness, or ligamentous laxity. In many cases, all three may coexist.
- Ligamentous laxity is very common and often familial and can cause significant motor developmental delay but there is no muscle weakness.
- GDD is unlikely in a pure neuromuscular disorder although there are exceptions with autism and learning difficulty in association with Duchenne muscular dystrophy (DMD)/Becker muscular dystrophy (BMD) and seizures and learning difficulties in congenital muscular dystrophies.
- Hypothyroidism (Semelaigne syndrome) can present with weakness, calf hypertrophy, and raised muscle creatine kinase enzyme levels akin to muscular dystrophies and must always be actively excluded.

As a general approach, one needs to determine if a child is 'floppy but strong' or 'floppy and weak'.

If child is floppy but strong, predominant causes are more likely to be central

For example:
- Hypoxic ischaemic injury.
- Cerebral dysgenesis.
- Metabolic disorders, e.g. Menkes, glutaric aciduria type 1, MPS, gangliosidoses, glycosylation defects, etc.
- Hypothyroidism, rickets, hypocalcaemia, hypophosphataemia.
- Recognizable syndromes, e.g. Prader–Willi syndrome, DS, Angelman syndrome, Rett syndrome, etc.
- Chromosomal abnormality, e.g. 22q11 deletion, trisomies, fragile X, etc.

Examination
Will usually reveal axial weakness, normal limb strength, normal to brisk deep tendon reflexes, global developmental concerns, and dysmorphism.

Investigations
Most likely to help are neuroimaging, chromosome analysis, genetic opinion, and metabolic investigations.

If child is floppy and weak, predominant cause is likely to be a peripheral neuromuscular problem

For example:
- SMA: characterized by normal cognition but profound weakness, flopped/frog leg posture in infants, lower limb weakness in older children, tongue fasciculation, hand tremor (polyminimyoclonus), and absent deep tendon reflexes.
- Myasthenia: if presenting in infancy it is more likely to be a congenital myasthenia and early history is very important. Autoimmune myasthenia can sometimes present as early as second year of life. Transient neonatal myasthenia can carry on into the first few months of life in infants born to mothers with myasthenia gravis. Eliciting a history of or demonstrating fatigue is critical.

- Congenital myopathies.
- Congenital myotonic dystrophy. This is very important to consider and the examination repertoire should include a parental examination to exclude myotonia.
- Congenital muscular dystrophies.
- Other muscular dystrophies that rarely present in infancy: DMD, facioscapulohumeral muscular dystrophy.
- Metabolic myopathies: in particular, Pompe disease can present with early cardiomyopathy, hepatomegaly.
- Mitochondrial myopathies.
- Peripheral neuropathies. Rarely present in infancy.

Examination

Will usually reveal significant axial and limb weakness, depressed or absent deep tendon reflexes, and normal cognitive development in most.

Investigations

Most likely to be useful are thyroid function, creatine kinase, lactate, EMG/nerve conduction studies, and muscle biopsy. DNA analysis can give rapid diagnosis in SMA, DMD, and myotonic dystrophy.

Headache

Headache is very common in school-age children and may be present from infancy in some cases. Distinction must be made between acute and chronic headache, causes of which differ. Further distinction is between symptomatic and idiopathic headaches. Chronic idiopathic headaches are the ones most likely to be encountered in the outpatient setting.

Causes of symptomatic headaches

- Raised intracranial pressure: secondary to acute hydrocephalus, cerebral oedema, idiopathic intracranial hypertension, venous sinus thrombosis, etc. The characteristics symptoms of early morning headache with or without nausea/vomiting, worsening of headache with Valsalva manoeuvres. Cranial nerve palsies and papilloedema are seen as established cases.
- ENT and sinus disease.
- Dental disease.
- Visual acuity problems.
- Vascular—subarachnoid or intracranial haemorrhage from aneurysms, arteriovenous malformations (rare and usually catastrophic).
- Post traumatic, e.g. concussion acutely and chronic headaches.
- Acute infections, e.g. meningitis, encephalitis.
- Metabolic causes, e.g. hypothyroidism.
- Toxins, e.g. analgesic overuse, carbon monoxide poisoning.
- Miscellaneous, e.g. obstructive sleep apnoea, hypoventilation (neuromuscular disorders), hypertension (rare).

Common causes of chronic and paroxysmal idiopathic headaches

- Migraine (with and without aura).
- Variants of migraine, e.g. abdominal migraine and cyclical vomiting.
- Complicated migraines, e.g. hemiplegic migraine, basilar migraine, ophthalmoplegic migraines, confusional migraine.
- Chronic daily headaches (episodic and chronic tension type).
- Cluster headaches (rare).
- Mental health issues like anxiety/low mood (often under-recognized in children).

Migraine

- The common characteristics are as follows:
  - Unilateral (or bilateral especially in young children).
  - Throbbing character.
  - Lasts 3–72 hours.
  - Associated photo and/or phono phobia.
  - Associated nausea and/or vomiting.
  - Often positive family history.
  - Relieved by rest/sleep.
  - Can be precipitated by stress, dehydration, sleep deprivation, long periods of starvation, and menstruation.
  - Aggravated by movement and continued activity.

- The disabling nature of migraine is an important feature to recognize in the history.
- Auras are uncommon in younger children. They take the form of visual auras (positive—scintillation, wavy or crisscross lines, dots, spectral, distortion of imagery, macropsia. Negative—scotomas, micropsia, hemianopias, etc.), auditory, gustatory, olfactory, etc.
- In children with stereotypic episodes with consistent features, no further investigations are indicated.
- EEG will show slowing of background during an attack and is unhelpful. Neuroimaging is normal or may pick up incidental abnormalities which can cause unnecessary anxiety. Both these are not recommended in children with migraines.
- Very rarely an atrial septal defect or patent foramen ovale is present and closure of these can lead to a resolution of migraines.
- Treatment is symptomatic in the form of simple analgesia often in combination with an antiemetic, plenty of fluids (once vomiting has resolved), oral or intranasal triptans. Prophylaxis in frequent attacks is in the form of avoidance of triggers where identifiable; various other drugs such as pizotifen, propranolol, topiramate and sodium valproate.

Tension-type headaches

- Commonly experienced due to life stresses, fatigue, and exertion.
- Headache is dull, constricting in character, and lasts up to a day, sometimes a little longer.
- Chronicity should raise the suspicion of chronic anxiety and depression. The usual history is of a constant headache without typical migraine characteristics and is not disabling in the same way as an acute migraine attack.
- Amitriptyline may be helpful.
- Psychology input is probably most beneficial.

Unsteadiness and falls

There are many reasons for being unsteady and its presence does not equate to a diagnosis of ataxia. Careful history and examination are key.

Important questions in the history

- Onset, duration, and time course: is it a new symptom or has it been since the child started walking and is just more noticeable?
- Is it episodic, paroxysmal, persistent, or progressive?
- Are there any associated concerns, e.g. weakness, speech and articulation problems, vision or hearing difficulties, feeding and swallowing difficulties?
- Are the problems restricted to gait alone or are there upper limb difficulties as well?
- Is there associated nausea, vomiting, vertiginous sensation, etc.?
- Ask questions about all aspects of praxis, e.g. articulation of words, dressing, fine motor skills, sequencing tasks.

Examination

When examining, one needs to focus on certain points such as:

- Presence of true ataxia: is there gait, trunk, and limb ataxia? Are there cerebellar signs, e.g. nystagmus, difficulty with tandem walking, dysmetria?
- Is there any weakness and is it fatigable?
- Is the proprioception intact? Romberg test and finger–nose test with eyes closed, drift of outstretched arm (may be due to weakness).
- Is the coordination appropriate? Sequential finger–thumb opposition, copying a sentence in sequence, performing sequential tasks.
- How is the fine motor coordination, e.g. stringing beads, cutting or folding paper, handwriting?
- Are there any vestibular features, e.g. nystagmus, tinnitus, vertigo?
- Is there any evidence of a neuropathy? Check for weakness and deep tendon reflexes.
- Are there any neurocutaneous markers, e.g. telangiectasia?
- Any other unusual examination findings, e.g. opsoclonus, altered conscious state (non-convulsive status), pupillary abnormalities (toxins), papilloedema (raised intracranial pressure), pyramidal tract signs, tendo Achilles or hamstring contractures, movement disorders, e.g. tremors, dystonia, chorea?

Unsteadiness thus can result from various causes

- Vestibular.
- Peripheral neuromuscular problems, e.g. neuropathies.
- Weakness (often weakness in Guillain–Barré syndrome is interpreted as ataxia).
- Ataxia (see pp. 256–8).
- Developmental coordination disorder (definitions vary between therapists and clinicians). This is essentially 'clumsiness' in the absence of any weakness, ataxia, or other neurological dysfunction. Degrees of functional impairment vary. It affects fine and gross motor function and most markedly sequencing. There are no alarming examination findings and no cerebellar signs. It is static but may become more obvious as more demands on coordinated functioning are placed on a growing school-age child.

Abnormal movements

Abnormal movements

Common movement abnormalities seen are:

Tremor
- Rhythmic oscillation of a part of or whole body.
- Amplitudes can vary.
- It can be postural when trying to maintain a posture or action, or intentional when precipitated by voluntary action (usually cerebellar pathology), and extrapyramidal which is high-amplitude tremor present at rest that gets worse with posture and movement (pathology in superior cerebellar peduncle or substantia nigra).

Chorea and ballismus
- A sudden jerky trunk or limb movement which is purposeless.
- Ballismus is a more severe form with violent, high-amplitude proximal limb movements.
- Typically seen in rheumatic fever when acute and in cerebral palsy alongside athetosis and dystonia. May also be seen in metabolic conditions such as Wilson disease.

Athetosis and dystonia
- Sustained abnormal contractions of agonist and antagonist muscles with cramp-like pain and postures.
- Slow, writhing distal movements that accompany dystonia are termed athetosis. Often coexists with chorea.
- Dystonias may be generalized due to basal ganglia injury from kernicterus, hypoxic ischaemic encephalopathy, genetic/metabolic conditions such as PKAN, Wilson disease, DYT1 dystonia, and focal such as in blepharospasm, torticollis, writer's cramp.

Myoclonus
- Sudden involuntary muscle contraction lasting <250 milliseconds.
- May be focal, multifocal, or generalized.
- May be spinal or cortical.
- May be spontaneous as in epilepsy or triggered by noise or touch.

Rigidity and bradykinesia
- These are features of parkinsonism and are rare in children.
- There is paucity of spontaneous movement and initiation of action.
- There is a persistent abnormal increased tone with increased resistance to passive movement (lead pipe rigidity). There is often superimposed tremor causing the 'cog wheeling' phenomenon.

Tics and other stereotypes
- Various behavioural stereotypes like arm flinging, hand wringing, head nodding, and body rocking are seen in children with learning difficulties but sometimes in developmentally normal children as well.
- Tics are the commonest movement stereotypes.
- They often involve face and limbs and can change from one body part to another over time.

- There are quiescent periods with exacerbations at times of stress.
- They may take the form of simple or complex motor phenomena. Ocular tics may be mistaken for opsoclonus or nystagmus.
- If they persist without remission over >6 months in a 12-month period and are accompanied by vocal tics, a diagnosis of Tourette syndrome needs to be considered. ASD, ADHD, anxiety, and/or obsessive–compulsive disorder can be associated in Tourette syndrome.
- They can be voluntarily suppressed and extinguish in sleep.
- Simple motor tics do not need treatment other than reassurance.
- Psychological input and medication such as clonidine may be needed in more intrusive tics and Tourette syndrome.

Other rare paroxysmal abnormal movements

Include tonic upgaze of infancy, torticollis of infancy, cataplexy, and paroxysmal kinesogenic and non-kinesogenic choreoathetosis.

Epilepsy and non-epileptic paroxysmal events

- When considering paroxysmal events and diagnosing epilepsy, a meticulous history is crucial.
- A comprehensive history including eyewitness accounts, school accounts, and, where possible, video footage even from phone camera can be valuable in making an accurate diagnosis.
- In case of uncertainty, it would be prudent to keep an open mind than to hastily commit to a diagnosis of epilepsy and/or initiate treatment.

A systematic approach to assessment of seizures is important and helpful guide can be using the acronym DESSCRIBE

- Description—describe the observed event in simple terms.
- Epileptic—is it epileptic or non-epileptic or uncertain based on the history?
- Seizure—if epileptic, what is the seizure types(s)?
- Syndrome—is there an identifiable epilepsy syndrome?
- Cause—what is the cause of this epilepsy and which further investigations should be considered?
- RIBE—any relevant impairment of behaviour or educational abilities? These are often ignored but are probably the most relevant in terms of overall management of the child.

> Epilepsy is by definition recurrent, stereotypic unprovoked seizures.

Non-epileptic paroxysmal events

Syncope

- Could be secondary to cardiac arrhythmias such as prolonged QT, breath holding, or reflex asystolic syncope.
- Every child being investigated for epilepsy must have an ECG.
- Reflex asystolic syncope typically presents with episodes of pallor and loss of consciousness precipitated by a painful stimulus. ECG shows a brief asystole.
- Breath holding is a voluntary apnoea induced by holding one breath against a closed glottis causing cyanosis. In both, the secondary hypoxia can induce a seizure but it is not epileptic as it is not unprovoked.

Febrile seizures

- Occurs in 6-month to 6-year age group.
- Associated with fever but not necessarily high pyrexia.
- Developmentally normal child.
- Family history may be present.
- Frequency tails off beyond 2 years.
- If recurrent prolonged febrile seizures, followed by afebrile seizures, myoclonus, and developmental concerns, consider Dravet syndrome.

Gastro-oesophageal reflux (Sandifer syndrome)
- Typically feed related.
- Very painful dystonic posturing with head/neck deviation and back arching.

Shuddering attacks
Looks like shivering, usually in the context of excitement.

Sleep myoclonus
- Occurs at a few weeks of age.
- Only in sleep.
- Synchronous or asynchronous limb jerks which may be quite violent and may occur in clusters.
- Does not involve the face and does not wake the child.
- Normal development.

Self-gratification
- Leg adduction and rubbing, flushed, vacant expression, irritable if disturbed.
- Commonly seen in highchair/car seat.
- Self-limiting.

Behavioural stereotypes
Common in children with learning difficulty but sometimes in developmentally normal children.

Preoccupation (daydreaming)
- Common especially where child is academically struggling at school.
- Commonly mistaken as 'absences'.
- May not respond to voice but will respond to touch (compared to epileptic absences which do not respond to touch as well).

Parasomnias
- Night terrors often confused with frontal lobe seizures.
- Night terrors usually occur in the early part of sleep, are single events/day, and quite long.
- Child has no recollection of the event.
- Frontal seizures are usually numerous/night at any time of sleep cycle and brief.

Benign myoclonus of infancy
- Normal EEG.
- Often difficult to distinguish from epileptic myoclonus.
- Normal development.

Hyperekplexia
- This is caused by a mutation in the gene encoding strychnine responsive glycine receptors.
- Can be dominantly inherited.
- Causes stiffness and exaggerated startle diagnosed by nose tapping to induce opisthotonic posture.
- Can be severe enough to cause cyanosis.
- Treated with benzodiazepines.

Non-epileptic attack disorder (pseudoseizures)
- Seizures are asynchronous limb jerks with pelvic thrusting movements with quick offset and no postictal phase.
- Can coexist with genuine epilepsy and may require video telemetry to untangle epileptic from non-epileptic events.

Paroxysmal kinesogenic dyskinesias
- Precipitated by movement, several times a day, can take form of dystonia or choreoathetoid movements.
- Mutation in *PRRT2* gene.
- Can also be seen in patients with GLUT1 protein deficiency.
- Treated with carbamazepine/phenytoin in case of *PRRT2* mutation and ketogenic diet for GLUT1 deficiency.

Cataplexy
- Can occur in isolation, as part of narcolepsy complex or in some storage disorders like Niemann–Pick type C.
- Sudden loss of posture induced by surprise, laughter, or loud noise.

Paroxysmal torticollis of infancy
- Presents in infancy and resolves by 4–5 years.
- Episodes of torticollis with alternating sides associated with pallor, vomiting, ataxia, and behavioural change.
- Episodes last hours to days.
- Child is entirely normal in between episodes with no neurological signs/symptoms.
- Considered as a migraine variant by some.

Tonic upgaze of infancy
- Early onset.
- Episodic tonic conjugate upward deviation of the eyes. Associated down-beating saccades in attempted downgaze. Can be associated with mild ataxia.
- Normal horizontal eye movements.
- Frequent relief by sleep.
- Normal development and neurological examination.
- Improves with age and no treatment required.
- Some consider it to be a type of paroxysmal dystonia.

Early-onset epilepsies

Some common epilepsy syndromes are briefly covered here.

Benign neonatal convulsions (non-familial)
- Day 1–7.
- Focal clonic or subtle seizures.
- Ictal spikes or slow waves, interictal asynchronous theta rhythm.
- Treatment phenobarbitone/levetiracetam.
- Excellent prognosis. Seizures remission after short-term treatment.

Benign neonatal convulsions (familial)
- AD (ask grandparents for a careful history).
- Can start at day 3 and occur up to 3 months.

- Generalized clonic seizures, occasionally tonic with cyanosis.
- No specific EEG features.
- Treatment carbamazepine/phenytoin.
- Good prognosis—in most cases seizure remission by 6–12 months. In 10–15% seizures can recur later.
- *KCNQ2* and *KCNQ3* commonest genes.

Pyridoxine-dependent seizures
- Neonatal to 18 months (some may present with later-onset epilepsy).
- Multifocal or generalized seizures/infantile spasms.
- Suppression burst or hypsarrhythmic EEG.
- Raised serum pipecolic acid and urine alpha amino adipic semi-aldehyde (AASA).
- Treatment with high-dose pyridoxine 50 -100 mg.
- AR inheritance, *ALDH7A1* or antiquitin gene.
- Trial of pyridoxine should be considered in any intractable infantile epilepsy without a clear aetiology.
- Pyridoxal 5-phosphate dependent epilepsy can present similarly but will only respond to pyridoxal-5-phosphate. *PNPO* (pyridoxamine 5-phosphate oxidase) is the gene and also has AR inheritance.

Early infantile epileptic encephalopathy (Ohtahara syndrome)
- Neonatal to first 6 months of life.
- Tonic seizures.
- Suppression burst EEG.
- Brain malformations common.
- Intractable seizures.
- Poor prognosis for epilepsy and neurodevelopment—may evolve to West syndrome.

West syndrome
- 3–12 months (peak 3–7 months) as opposed to infantile colic which is very rare after 3 months of age.
- Infantile spasms in clusters at sleep–wake interface.
- Developmental plateau or regression (may occur before or after onset of spasms). Loss of previously acquired visual behaviour is commonly noted.
- Hypsarrhythmic EEG with attenuation following spasm (initially wake EEG may be normal, always ask for sleep EEG).
- Idiopathic (better outcome) or symptomatic, e.g. hypoxic ischaemic encephalopathy, tuberous sclerosis, DS.
- Treatment: vigabatrin for tuberous sclerosis; steroids (prednisolone/ adrenocorticotrophic hormone or combined steroid and vigabatrin) for other aetiology.
- Early recognition and initiation of treatment crucial to improve outcome.
- Outcome better if spasms controlled quickly with normalization of EEG but in most cases is also influenced by underlying aetiology.
- Outcome is poor generally. About 70% will have learning difficulties and may evolve to Lennox–Gastaut syndrome.

Lennox–Gastaut syndrome
- 1–8 years.
- Tonic, atonic, myoclonic seizures, atypical absences.
- Slow spike waves in wake and fast spike bursts in sleep.
- Poor prognosis for developmental outcome. Seizures initially intractable but can improve with age though seizure freedom is rarely achieved.
- Treatment options include most broad-spectrum antiepileptics like levetiracetam, sodium valproate, and lamotrigine, and some specific Lennox–Gastaut syndrome options like rufinamide and cannabidiol.
- Ketogenic diet and vagal nerve stimulator can also be considered.

Dravet syndrome
- Prolonged febrile seizures or recurrent febrile status epilepticus with onset not infrequently <6 months. Typically, hemiclonic seizures which change sides. Then afebrile hemiclonic or generalized seizures.
- Developmental plateau or regression usually in the second year.
- Myoclonus appears later.
- Spike waves, polyspike waves on EEG, early photosensitivity can be seen.
- Seizures often intractable.
- Ataxia develops with age, developmental outcome poor.
- 85% have mutation in *SCN1A* gene, usually *de novo*.
- Treatment: sodium valproate, clobazam, topiramate, stiripentol, ketogenic diet, and cannabidiol.

Childhood absence epilepsy
- 3–12 years.
- Typical absences (can be induced by hyperventilating for 3 minutes).
- 3 Hz spike wave discharges on EEG.
- Treatment: ethosuximide, lamotrigine, levetiracetam, sodium valproate.
- Seizures remit in 75%.
- May show subtle cognitive impairment especially if intractable.
- Consider GLUT1 (glucose transporter defect) if intractable absences and early-onset absences.
- Ketogenic diet may be useful.

Benign epilepsy of childhood with centrotemporal spikes (BCECT)
- 3–13 years.
- Focal or generalized motor seizures—orofacial muscles often involved.
- Centrotemporal spikes.
- Treatment—none or carbamazepine.
- Consider MRI brain for any structural abnormality if poor response to carbamazepine (first line).
- Outcome excellent with seizure remission by puberty.

Landau Kleffner syndrome (acquired epileptic aphasia)
- 2–10 years.
- Infrequent generalized tonic clonic or focal clonic seizures (may precede or follow language regression in 60–80% of cases).
- Language regression with normal hearing and audiometry.
- Multifocal spike waves in temporal or parieto-occipital regions. Continuous slow spike waves in slow sleep.

- Treatment with steroids (may need long-term pulse steroids).
- Outcome good for seizure control but guarded for language recovery.

Juvenile myoclonic epilepsy (JME)
- 10–18 years.
- Bilateral symmetrical myoclonus predominantly in arms (typically in the morning); generalized tonic–clonic seizures, absences.
- Generalized spike or polyspike waves (>3 Hz).
- Photosensitivity common.
- Treatment: sodium valproate (males), levetiracetam, lamotrigine.
- Needs treatment to continue into adult life.
- Good response to treatment.

Progressive myoclonic epilepsies
- Generalized or fragmentary myoclonus, generalized seizures, atonic seizures.
- Associated cognitive decline, regression, ataxia.
- Conditions to consider include neuronal ceroid lipofuscinosis, lysosomal storage disorders like sialidosis, Gaucher disease, Unverricht–Lundborg disease, Lafora body disease, mitochondrial disorders like MERRF, Huntington disease, Wilson disease, neurodegeneration with brain iron accumulation including pantothenate kinase (PKAN).
- These need specialist opinions and extensive neurometabolic and neurophysiological investigations.

Investigating epilepsies
- Once a clinical diagnosis of epilepsy has been made, the investigations are an attempt to identify an underlying cause, and classify them into epilepsy syndromes where possible. They also help guide treatment options and prognosis.
- First as an aid to classification of the epilepsies into syndromes an EEG is required. If a wake EEG is normal, it is important to request a sleep EEG. This may be a natural sleep or sleep-deprived EEG or induced sleep with sedation or melatonin.
- If there is doubt about the paroxysmal events being described, it is then important to get more information. There are various methods that can be employed to get additional information, such as:
  - More meticulous history taking.
  - Asking for description from carers, friends, school, etc.
  - Parental video recording with a mobile phone camera, digital camera, or video camera.
  - Arranging an inpatient stay to observe and document seizures.
  - An ambulatory EEG recording over 48–72 hours. This can be complemented by parental records or video footage.
  - Video telemetry (simultaneous video and EEG recording).

It is not possible to have a standard set of investigations to fit all patients.

Nevertheless, some important investigations to consider include:
- Chromosome analysis: including fragile X, ring chromosome 14, 20.
- DNA analysis: single gene analysis, e.g. *SCN1A* mutations in Dravet syndrome, *SLC2A1* in GLUT1 deficiency, etc. or epilepsy panels, whole-exome/genome sequencing when several genes need to be covered.
- Neuroimaging: this should be a good-quality MRI scan. This should include thin sections and volume sequences (epilepsy protocol) especially when epilepsy surgery is being considered.
- Specialized neurophysiology: this includes visual evoked potentials, video telemetry, ambulatory EEG recording, ictal SPECT scanning, magnetoencephalography, or functional MRI scans for functional localization of ictal focus; intracranial grid mats. Most of these investigations are only available in centres that perform epilepsy surgery procedures.
- Metabolic investigations: including urine alpha amino adipic succinyl aldehyde and serum pipecolic acid (pyridoxine-dependant seizures), cerebrospinal fluid (CSF) glucose paired with blood glucose (GLUT1), biotinidase, CSF and serum amino acids, lactate, copper, long chain fatty acids, white cell enzymes, etc.
- Other investigations: e.g. retinal examination, muscle biopsy, etc. may add further information in specific clinical scenarios.

Management of epilepsy

The mainstay of management is with antiepileptic drugs. There are very few data on use of drugs specific to certain syndromes.

NICE guidelines are available on choice of medication in seizure types.

Consider discussion with patient and family at diagnosis
- Safety issues related to epilepsy.
- Sharing diagnosis of epilepsy with educational and childcare settings.
- Risk of sudden unexpected death in epilepsy.

Antiepileptic drugs
The following is only a suggested guide:
- Generalized seizures: sodium valproate, lamotrigine, levetiracetam, topiramate, clobazam.
- Focal seizures: carbamazepine, topiramate, lamotrigine.
- Myoclonic seizures: sodium valproate, levetiracetam, clonazepam, topiramate.
- Atonic seizures: sodium valproate, topiramate, levetiracetam.
- Absences: ethosuximide, lamotrigine, valproate.

Sodium valproate should not where possible be used in girls of childbearing age due to teratogenicity. If no alternative option is suitable, patients should be made fully aware of the risks and the need to avoid becoming pregnant (⌖ https://www.gov.uk/guidance/valproate-use-by-women-and-girls).

It is not essential but prudent to check blood count and liver functions prior to starting antiepileptic drugs. Routine blood tests subsequently are not recommended.

Drug levels are indicated only for toxicity or compliance monitoring.

Non-drug treatments
- Vagal nerve stimulation:
  - Implantable device which sends regular electrical stimuli to vagus nerve in the neck. Swiping a magnet over the device can deliver immediate impulse in acute situation.
  - Mechanism of action unknown.
- Ketogenic diet:
  - A high-fat, low-carbohydrate diet to induce ketosis.
  - Can be considered in most refractory epilepsies.
  - Treatment of choice in GLUT1 deficiency.
- Epilepsy surgery: hemispherectomy, lesional and focal resections, corpus callosotomy, multiple subpial transection.

Further resources

Epilepsy Action: ☎ 0808 800 5050; 🖰 https://www.epilepsy.org.uk/

Ataxia

- Ataxia is the inability to coordinate muscle activity causing inefficiency of voluntary movement. It may involve limbs, head, or trunk.
- Acute to subacute ataxias result from:
  - Post-infectious cerebellitis (particularly 7–14 days post varicella).
  - Acute disseminated encephalomyelitis (ADEM).
  - Toxins.
  - Posterior fossa tumours.
  - Pseudo ataxia from weakness in Guillain–Barré syndrome.
  - Posterior circulation vascular events etc.
  - Opsoclonus myoclonus syndrome.
- Chronic ataxia may be:
  - Cerebellar.
  - Spinocerebellar.
  - Neuropathic.
  - Mixed.

Some causes of ataxia

Opsoclonus—myoclonus syndrome
- Presumed parainfectious or paraneoplastic (neuroblastoma) condition.
- Often presents with altered behaviour and irritability, rapid chaotic synchronous eye movements in all directions of gaze (opsoclonus), and later myoclonus. Ataxia can be an important early component.
- Treatment is with steroids and other immunomodulating agents may be required in some cases.
- Neuroblastoma/sympathetic chain tumour should be probed for.

Mitochondrial cytopathy
- Ataxia is just one component of the myriad symptoms that result from mitochondrial mutations.
- Retinopathy may accompany especially in the condition NARP (neuropathy, ataxia, retinitis pigmentosa with the typical 8993 mtDNA mutation).

Metabolic and degenerative disorders
Several metabolic disorders present with chronic ataxia. Some examples are:
- HARP (hypobetalipoproteinaemia, ataxia, retinitis pigmentosa).
- Hartnup disease.
- Maple syrup urine disease.
- Pyruvate dehydrogenase deficiency.
- Vitamin E deficiency.
- Refsum disease.
- Adrenoleukodystrophy.
- GM2 gangliosidoses (hexosaminidase deficiency).

Genetic ataxias

Some examples are:

Episodic ataxias
Several different types of episodic ataxia recognized. Types 1 and 2 are the commonest.

Type 1
- Potassium channelopathy (*KCN1A* mutation).
- Attacks begin at 5–7 years of age.
- Sensation of spreading weakness and stiffness accompanies the ataxia which lasts for about 10 minutes but can last a few hours.
- Myokymia is seen and an EMG shows continuous spontaneous activity at rest.
- Treatment is with phenytoin or carbamazepine.

Type 2
- Calcium channelopathy (*CACNA1A* mutation).
- Onset in school-aged children with accompanying vertigo and vomiting as well as a migraine.
- Attacks last from 1 hour to 1 day.
- Treatment is with acetazolamide or flunarizine.

Spinocerebellar ataxias (SCA)
- There are an ever-increasing number of progressive dominantly inherited ataxias (SCA 1, 2, 3, 6, and 7 have onset in childhood as also dentatorubral-pallidolysian atrophy—DRPLA).
- They show a mixture of pyramidal, extrapyramidal, and cerebellar features as well as sensory neuropathies.
- The genetic defect is often a trinucleotide repeat.
- Diagnosis is largely based on DNA testing and no specific treatments are available.

Ataxia telangiectasia (AT)
See ➜ p. 263.

Ataxia and oculomotor apraxia
- Ataxia precedes the characteristic feature of oculomotor apraxia. Eventually a motor neuropathy develops.
- Also AR Inherited.

Friedrich ataxia
- Most common recessively inherited ataxia.
- Triplet repeats of Frataxin gene.
- Onset between 2 and 16 years.
- Associated features include scoliosis, dysarthria, diabetes mellitus, and hypertrophic cardiomyopathy. Typically, tendon reflexes are absent in the lower limbs with extensor plantar response.
- Life limiting due to cardiomyopathy.

Investigations in ataxia
- Are based on the clinical picture.
- MRI brain is first line in most cases.
- DNA analysis is the mainstay in genetic ataxias.
- Metabolic investigations should include:
  - Vitamin E levels.
  - Alpha-fetoprotein.
  - Immunoglobulins.
  - Cholesterol and triglycerides.
  - Transferrins.

- Phytanic acid.
- White cell enzymes.
- Plasma amino acids.
- Urine organic acids.
- Carnitine profile.
- Lactate (blood and CSF).
- Muscle biopsy/bone marrow.
- Nerve conduction studies and EMG.
- Eye examination.

Further resources

Ataxia UK: ☎ 0845 644 0606; ⌖ https://www.ataxia.org.uk/

Neurocutaneous disorders

- The skin and nervous system have common embryonic origins as explained on ➲ pp. 218–20.
- Skin malformations and markers are a useful clue in the diagnosis of neurocutaneous malformation sequences.
- One or two café au lait patches occur in 10% of the general population.

Well-recognized neurocutaneous syndromes include:

Neurofibromatosis types 1 and 2

- Both syndromes are dominantly inherited.
- Incidence is about 1:4000 live births.
- More than 50% are new mutations. Incidence 1:3000 live births.
- *NF1* gene lies on chromosome 17q11.2.
- It is a progressive condition with onset in infancy.
- Cutaneous features increase through the first decade of life.

Clinical criteria for diagnosis are at least two of the following
- Six or more café au lait spots (>5 mm prepubertal/>15 mm post-pubertal).
- More than two neurofibromas or one plexiform neurofibromas.
- Axillary or inguinal freckling.
- Optic gliomas.
- More than two iris hamartomas.
- Characteristic bone lesions such as sphenoid wing dysplasia or bone cortex thinning with or without pseudoarthrosis.
- First-degree relative with NF1 diagnosed by the above-listed criteria.

Minor features
- Include microcephaly, short stature, learning difficulties in 60% of cases, epilepsy, hypertension resulting from aortic coarctation, renal artery stenosis, or phaeochromocytoma.
- Scoliosis is present in 10–40% of cases.
- Optic gliomas occur in 20% of cases.
- Other neoplasms associated are brainstem gliomas, malignant transformation of neurofibromas, ependymomas, meningiomas, and medulloblastomas. There is an increased risk of Wilm's tumour, rhabdomyosarcomas, medullary thyroid carcinoma, melanomas, leukaemia, and phaeochromocytoma.
- Children with three to five café au lait patches but no other signs of NF1 should be referred to a specialist with interest in NF1 as they might have mosaic NF1 or NF2.

Main principles of management are monitoring for disease manifestations with regular surveillance and patient education
- Monitoring of visual symptoms, visual fields, and fundoscopy (optic pathway glioma).
- Monitor head circumference (tumour/hydrocephalus).
- Monitoring growth.
- Monitoring blood pressure (renal artery stenosis or pheochromocytoma).
- Monitoring puberty (delayed or precocious due to pituitary/ hypothalamic lesion).
- Monitor spine (scoliosis, compressive plexiform neurofibroma).
- Monitor skin (cutaneous, subcutaneous, and plexiform neurofibromas).

Neurofibromatosis 2

- AD.
- The gene for NF2 lies on chromosome 22q12.2.
- Is less common than NF1 with an incidence of 1:40,000 live births.

Diagnostic criteria

Diagnostic criteria are covered in Box 5.1.

- Presentation in children is different to adults who have bilateral schwannomas as the commonest presentation.
- Children present with subtle skin tumours, small posterior capsular or cortical-edge cataracts, HL, neurological signs due to brainstem or spinal cord compression from tumours, non-eighth cranial nerve mononeuropathy like facial or third nerve palsy or peripheral nerve (wrist or foot drop).
- The main principle of management is tumour surveillance. As children with NF2 develop multiple cranial, spinal, and peripheral nerve tumours, the goal is to preserve function and maximize quality of life as much as possible. This is achieved by close monitoring and timing surgery based on a child's neurological symptoms/signs rather than only imaging findings.
- Genetic counselling for family members is important in both conditions.

Box 5.1 Diagnostic criteria for neurofibromatosis 2

Bilateral vestibular schwannomas (affecting both ears).

Or a first-degree relative with NF2, plus any two of the following:
- Meningioma.
- Glioma (e.g. spinal ependymoma).
- Neurofibroma.
- Schwannoma.
- Juvenile cataracts.

Or unilateral vestibular schwannoma plus any two of the following:

- Meningioma.
- Glioma.
- Neurofibroma.
- Schwannoma.
- Juvenile cataracts.

Or multiple meningiomas (two or more) plus:

- Unilateral vestibular schwannoma, or any two of the following:
  - Glioma.
  - Neurofibroma.
  - Schwannoma.
  - Juvenile cataracts.

Further resources

Nerve Tumours UK (formerly the Neurofibromatosis Association): ☎ 0845 602 4173; 🔗 https://nervetumours.org.uk/

Tuberous sclerosis

- Incidence 1:20,000 live births.
- Dominantly inherited.
- Genes responsible for the syndrome are *TSC1* (chromosome 9q) and *TSC2* (chromosome 16p).
- Two-thirds of cases are de novo mutations.
- Infantile spasm is the commonest presentation.
- Skin associations are ash leaf macules (may need Wood lamp examination to detect), shagreen patch, periungual fibromas, and adenoma sebaceum.
- Multiple cardiac rhabdomyoma in fetus, spontaneous regression is universal.
- Tuberous sclerosis results in multiple hamartomas (tubers) in the brain.
- Subependymal nodules usually occur at the foramina of Munro and can develop into subependymal giant cell astrocytomas (SEGAs) which may cause obstructive hydrocephalus typically in or before the second decade of life.
- Epilepsy can be refractory in two-thirds of cases. If a prominent tuber is epileptogenic, removal of this area may be considered in intractable cases with good outcome.
- Other associations are retinal phakomas, renal angiomyolipomas or hamartomas, polycystic kidneys, bone and lung cysts, and cardiac rhabdomyomas.
- Children usually have severe learning difficulties especially children with early-onset epilepsy.
- Behavioural issues are common—sleep difficulties, aggression, as is ASD (40–50%), ADHD (30–50%), and anxiety issues.

Surveillance

- Renal ultrasound scan at diagnosis for polycystic kidney disease.
- Subependymal nodules needs neuroimaging every 1–3 years through childhood and if concerns of enlarging SEGAs or symptoms of hydrocephalus then more closer interval scans.
- Renal angiomyolipoma: start surveillance from 5 years as risk of bleeding of >3 cm seen in 20% of cases.
- Pulmonary lymphangioleiomyomatosis—exclusively occurs in females and appears at end of teenager years so all tuberous sclerosis female patients should have a CT chest imaging prior to transition to adult care.
- Vigabatrin is the drug of choice for infantile spasms and can be used as long-term antiepileptic as well. Most seizures are focal onset but can secondarily generalize so broad spectrum.
- Newer treatment—mammalian target of rapamycin (mTOR). Inhibitors like rapamycin and everolimus. Everolimus reduces size of SEGAs and renal angiomyolipoma (but they regrow on discontinuation). Emerging evidence of seizure reduction with everolimus but side effect profile risk is high.

Further resources

Tuberous Sclerosis Association UK: ☎ 05602 420809; ⌀ https://tuberous-sclerosis.org/

Sturge–Weber syndrome

- An association of an ipsilateral port wine stain in the first division of the trigeminal nerve dermatomal distribution and leptomeningeal angiomatous malformation causing focal epilepsy, progressive hemiatrophy of the brain, and contralateral hemiparesis.
- It is important to bear in mind that only about 15% of children with port wine stain will have Sturge–Weber syndrome.
- Other associations are learning difficulties (90% of cases), glaucoma (30% of cases), and homonymous hemianopia.
- Seizures may be difficult to control. Intractable seizures may warrant a hemispherectomy.
- Low-dose aspirin prophylaxis aiming to reduce stroke-like episodes is recommended.
- Laser therapy is used to treat the cutaneous angioma.
- Regular ophthalmology follow-up for glaucoma is needed.

Further resources

Sturge Weber UK: ☎ 01392 464675; ℘ https://www.sturgeweber.org.uk/

Ataxia telangiectasia

- Rare disorder with incidence of 1:40,000.
- AR inheritance or *de novo* mutation in *ATM* gene on chromosome 11q22.3.
- Clinical features consist of:
  - Slowly progressive cerebellar ataxia, and dysarthria.
  - Nystagmus and oculomotor apraxia.
  - Telangiectasia of skin and conjunctiva.
  - Increased susceptibility to bronchopulmonary infections (70% of cases) due to IgA and IgE deficiency.
  - Lymphoid tissues (tonsils, adenoids, thymus) may develop abnormally or fail to develop.
  - Raised alpha-fetoprotein and carcinoembryonic antigen.
  - Chromosome fragility.
  - Cognition is not affected.
  - Diabetes.
  - Short stature and progeric changes.
- Life limiting due to increased risk of leukaemia, lymphoma, and skin malignancy.
- Heterozygotes also have increased risk of malignancy especially breast cancer.

Further resources

Ataxia UK: ☎ 0845 644 0606; ℘ https://www.ataxia.org.uk/

Incontinentia pigmenti

- Affects skin, hair, teeth, and CNS.
- Four typical stages:
  - Stage 1: at birth or early infancy redness or inflammation of skin lasting few weeks to several months.
  - Stage 2: blisters develop into a raised, wart-like appearance involving extremities lasting for several months.

- Stage 3: skin darkens with a swirled pattern (marble cake).
- Stage 4: atrophic stage presenting with pale and hairless patches in adolescents and adults.
- Seizures and developmental delay can be associated.

Hypomelanosis of Ito

- Distinctive hypopigmentation as patches, streaks, or whorled/spirals.
- Seizures and developmental delay can be associated.
- Females more affected.

Neurodegenerative disorders

- This is a rare group of conditions presenting with progressive loss of skills (progressive intellectual and neurological degeneration).
- Progressive nature of a new-onset neurodegenerative disease in a developmentally normal child is usually clear but in children with previous developmental issues, there may be difficulty in establishing whether signs and symptoms are truly progressive in the initial phase.
- Pseudo-regression should be considered in the presence of only cognitive impairment without any other progressive neurological signs. For example, a child with pre-existing mild learning difficulties who begins to fail as academic demands increase through adolescence; non-convulsive status epilepticus in a child with epilepsy.

The list is not exhaustive, but the most common neurodegenerative disorders are as follows:

Rett syndrome
- X-linked.
- Presents with language regression and loss of purposeful hand function after a period of normal development, but also with GDD.
- Epilepsy, motor disorder, unusual breathing patterns are associated.
- Methyl-CpG-binding protein 2 (*MECP2*) gene testing is diagnostic.

Krabbe's disease
- AR.
- Presents in infancy with developmental delay or regression, extreme irritability, and stiffness.
- Optic atrophy, sensorineural deafness, spasticity, and epilepsy develop.
- Late-onset milder phenotype in childhood presents with ataxia, fine motor difficulties, and cognitive decline.
- Diagnosis is by white cell enzyme analysis for galactocerebrosidase and genetic testing for *GALC* gene mutations.
- Treatment is symptomatic.
- Death usually by 2 years in the infantile onset.

Adrenoleukodystrophy
- X-linked peroxisomal disorder.
- Two distinct presentations: cerebral presentation with cognitive features (commonest in children) and a myelopathic form with slowly progressive spastic paraparesis and dorsal column sensory disturbance (adult phenotype).
- Presents at 4–10 years.
- New-onset cognitive disturbance, behavioural change, and hyperactivity which progress with evolving visual impairment, HL, and possible hemiparesis.
- Biochemical adrenal insufficiency is universally present but is rarely the presenting feature.
- Typical MRI appearance includes widespread increased T2 signal particularly in the occipital white matter, often involving the splenium of the corpus callosum, with involvement of the descending corticospinal tracts.

- Diagnosis is confirmed by measurement of high levels of saturated very long-chain fatty acids.
- Bone marrow transplant may be beneficial in selected cases.

Metachromatic leukodystrophy (MLD)

- Recessive disorder.
- Two types in childhood: late-infantile MLD and juvenile MLD.
- Late infantile MLD presents in most children before the age of 3 years with difficulty walking, leg weakness with absent reflexes which rapidly progress to flaccid paralysis/decerebrate posturing and optic atrophy.
- Death by 8–10 years.
- MRI shows a tigroid appearance of the white matter.
- Urine exam shows the typical metachromatic granules and nerve conductions show a neuropathy.
- White cell enzymes and genetics confirm diagnosis.
- No treatment currently available.

Niemann–Pick type C

- Recessive disorder.
- Perinatal/neonatal onset with hepatosplenomegaly and liver disease with high early mortality.
- Infantile onset with developmental delay or regression, hypotonia, hepatomegaly.
- Childhood onset with ataxia, fine motor difficulties, cognitive decline. Adolescent onset with behavioural problems, expressive language difficulties, ADHD, psychiatric symptoms (mania or psychosis), and cognitive decline.
- Characteristic early finding is impairment of the ability to look upward and downward (vertical supranuclear gaze palsy). Children lose the ability to rapidly look up and down and compensate by head movement.
- Epilepsy, cataplexy, dystonia, and HL can develop.
- Diagnosis is by analysis of serum oxysterol, skin fibroblasts for filipin staining, or genetic testing for Niemann–Pick type C 1 and 2.
- Miglustat may slow the progression of neurological symptoms associated with Niemann–Pick type C and should be considered.

Neuronal ceroid lipofuscinosis

- Recessive disorder with several genes involved.
- Several types with age of onset from infancy to adolescence.
- Presenting symptoms include visual difficulties, loss of developmental skills/cognitive impairment, and/or seizures.
- Children develop progressive visual failure, refractory epilepsy, and severe neurodisability.
- Depending on the type, age at death can vary from mid-childhood to adolescence to early adulthood.
- Visual evoked potentials are abnormally enlarged in the face of an extinguished electroretinogram.
- Diagnosis is via blood analysis for enzyme activity, and/or vacuolated lymphocytes, inclusion bodies may be seen on skin and conjunctival biopsy and genetic testing.

- No curative treatment available but cerliponase alfa is an enzyme replacement therapy for only neuronal ceroid lipofuscinosis type 2 (TPPT1 deficiency) which shown to slow or halt the progression of the symptoms.

Alpers disease or polymerase gamma (POLG)-related disorder

- Mitochondrial recessive disorder.
- Presents with hypotonia, developmental delay, failure to thrive, seizures, and hepatic dysfunction.
- Can present with developmental regression during intercurrent illness.
- Status epilepticus and hepatic failure results in death.
- Sodium valproate is contradicted as it can precipitate hepatic failure.
- Visual evoked potentials are abnormal with normal electroretinograms.
- Diagnosis is via genetic testing for POLG mutation.
- No treatment currently available.

Wilson disease

- Recessively inherited disorder of copper transport resulting in deposition of copper in brain, liver, and cornea.
- Can present from childhood to adult life, commonly in teenage years.
- Presents with liver dysfunction in the younger child but clumsiness, tremors, difficulty walking, speech problems, cognitive difficulties, and psychiatric manifestation (anxiety, depression, rage) in older children.
- Slit lamp exam shows a Kayser–Fleischer ring.
- Low plasma caeruloplasmin and serum copper is seen, and MRI shows low signal in lentiform nuclei and brainstem. Confirmation by genetic testing for *ATP7B* mutations.
- Chelation with penicillamine or zinc slows disease progression.

Neurodegeneration with brain iron accumulation

- Heterogeneous group of disorders characterized clinically by progressive extrapyramidal syndrome and excessive iron deposition in brain, primarily affecting the basal ganglia.
- Most are AR inheritance.
- Can present from infancy to adulthood.
- Presentation includes GDD in infancy/childhood, developmental regression/cognitive decline, dystonia-parkinsonism, and isolated parkinsonism.
- Optic atrophy and retinitis pigmentosa can develop in some types.
- MRI shows characteristic 'eye of the tiger' appearance but may not be seen in early childhood. Cerebellar atrophy in *PLA2G6* mutation.
- Genetic testing is confirmatory.
- Treatment is symptomatic.

Juvenile Huntington disease

- AD inherited.
- Triplet repeat disorder showing anticipation.
- Presents with rigidity, dystonia. Myoclonic seizures can develop. Adults present more with tremor, chorea, and dementia.

- MRI may show caudate atrophy.
- Diagnosis is via genetics testing for triple repeats in the *HTT* gene.

Progressive myoclonic epilepsy

- Heterogeneous group of epilepsies with onset in childhood or adulthood.
- Developmental regression/progressive cognitive decline with myoclonic seizures as the predominant seizure type.
- Causes include Unverricht–Lundborg disease, Lafora body disease, MERRF, and neuronal ceroid lipofuscinosis.

Mucopolysaccharidoses (type 3 Sanfilippo in particular)

- Initial normal or developmental delay, then behavioural problems and cognitive deterioration followed by progressive motor disorder.
- HL can be associated.
- Diagnosis is by excess urinary heparan sulphate excretion, white cell enzymes assay, and genetic testing.
- Treatment is symptomatic.

Subacute sclerosing panencephalitis (SSPE)

- Late presentation due to measles virus reactivation in nervous tissue.
- Increasing incidence due to drop in measles vaccine uptake.
- Presents between 5 and 15 years with gradual deterioration in behaviour and school performance and myoclonus, tremor, and seizures eventually appearing.
- A retinopathy is associated, and EEG shows suppression burst pattern.
- Rapid motor and cognitive deterioration leading to a coma and death.

Stroke

- A focal neurological deficit lasting >24 hours due to a vascular event.
- A transient ischaemic attack lasts <24 hours.
- A stroke-like event is a stroke of non-vascular aetiology.
- Stroke in children presents as an acute onset of focal neurological deficit and the symptoms depend on the site of the infarct.
- Symptoms include cranial nerve deficits, focal limb deficit (motor or sensory), and ataxia.
- Associated symptoms include seizures particularly in neonatal strokes, headache, vomiting, and depressed level of consciousness in haemorrhagic strokes and neck pain particularly where arterial dissection is aetiology.
- Fever, preceding neck trauma, pre-existing cardiac disease, sickle cell disease, and family history of strokes or stroke-like episodes should be sought.

Causes

- Arterial.
- Venous.
- Haemorrhagic.

Arterial stroke

May result from:

Embolic event

- Paradoxical embolus from the heart in a child with congenital heart disease (right-to-left shunt) or proximal vessels.
- An arterial dissection following a trivial trauma can cause a thrombus to form which later embolizes.

Thrombotic event

- These are rare in children but include prothrombotic deficiencies such as:
  - Protein C.
  - Protein S.
  - Antithrombin 3 deficiency.
  - Homozygous mutations in methyltetrahydrofolate gene (*MTHFR*).
  - Factor V Leiden.
  - Antiphospholipid syndrome.

Vasculopathy

- This is seen in small vessels in post-varicella vasculopathy and large vessels in Moya Moya syndrome, fibromuscular dysplasia, Lyme disease, and *Mycoplasma* arteritis.
- It is also seen in neurofibromatosis, DS, and sickle cell disease.
- Post cranial radiotherapy.

Venous infarction

Polycythaemia

True or as a result of dehydration especially in newborn babies, congenital heart disease, sickle cell disease, etc.

Venous sinus thrombosis
- From infection or hypercoagulable states in particular homocystinuria needs to be considered.
- It may be precipitated by oral contraceptive use.

Haemorrhagic stroke
- *Cerebral aneurysm rupture*: catastrophic with headache, seizures and altered conscious level.
- *Arteriovenous malformation*.
- *Cavernomas*: dominantly inherited, usually causes slow bleeds and seizures.

Investigations
For a stroke include:
- Thrombophilia screen.
- Transthoracic echocardiogram.
- MRI and magnetic resonance angiogram from aortic arch to vertex.
- Plasma homocysteine, sickle cell screen, lactate, lipid profile, lupus anticoagulant, lipoprotein (a), anticardiolipin antibody, and beta-2 glycoprotein-1.
- Transcranial Doppler in sickle cell disease.

Acute management
- Maintain airway, breathing, and circulation.
- Adequate oxygenation and hydration.
- Monitoring blood pressure.
- Treat seizures.
- Neurosurgical intervention—evacuation of haematoma, intracranial pressure monitoring, and craniectomy in the event of raised intracranial pressure.
- Time-critical thrombolysis with tissue plasminogen activator can be considered in some cases of arterial ischaemic stroke. In most cases, management is initial treatment with high-dose aspirin and is followed by low-dose aspirin for secondary prevention.
- Heparinization followed by anticoagulant/antiplatelet treatment needs to be considered in case of underlying congenital heart defect, procoagulant defect, or a definite arterial dissection and in sinovenous thrombosis.
- For ischaemic strokes due to sickle cell disease, initial management includes exchange transfusion followed by regular transfusion for secondary presentation. Sickle cell disease is also associated with silent infarcts. Transcarotid dopplers are used for monitoring and early initiation of regular blood transfusion.

Further resources
Royal College of Paediatrics and Child Health ('Stroke in childhood – clinical guideline for diagnosis, management and rehabilitation'): ℳ https://www.rcpch.ac.uk/resources/stroke-childhood-clinical-guideline-diagnosis-management-rehabilitation

Neuromuscular disorders

These can have a range of symptoms:
- Hypotonia with weakness (hypotonia without weakness usually has a central cause for the hypotonia).
- Delayed motor milestones.
- GDD (DMD/BMD and congenital muscular dystrophy, congenital myotonic dystrophy).
- Absent deep tendon reflexes (SMA, Charcot–Marie–Tooth disease).
- Recurrent chest infections, respiratory failure.
- Cardiomyopathy.

Diagnosis

An anatomical approach to neuromuscular disorders is helpful in achieving a diagnosis.
- Anterior horn cell: SMA types 1, 2, and 3.
- Peripheral neuropathies: inherited (Charcot–Marie–Tooth disease) and acquired (Guillain–Barré syndrome/chronic inflammatory demyelinating polyneuropathy).
- Neuromuscular transmission defects: congenital and autoimmune myasthenia.
- Muscle disease:
  - Congenital myopathies.
  - Muscular dystrophies: DMD, BMD, congenital muscular dystrophies, limb girdle, facioscapulohumeral, Emery–Dreifuss, etc.
  - Congenital myotonic dystrophy.
  - Myotonia and paramyotonia congenita.
- Connective tissue disorders: Ehlers–Danlos syndrome.
- Metabolic myopathies: acid maltase deficiency, muscle phosphorylase deficiency.
- Mitochondrial myopathy.
- Inflammatory myopathies: dermatomyositis.

Congenital hypothyroidism can cause a severe myopathy with raised creatine kinase levels and must always be excluded.

Salient features of the common neuromuscular problems

Duchenne and Becker muscular dystrophy
- XLR inheritance.
- About 30% *de novo* mutations.
- Present with delayed motor milestones, speech delay or GDD, calf hypertrophy, sometimes calf pain and cramps, hip girdle weakness.
- Progressive weakness causes loss of independent ambulation usually between 12 and 14 years in steroid-treated DMD boys. BMD are usually ambulant into adult life and the loss of ambulation can be variable.
- Diagnosis is by raised creatine kinase, DNA analysis identifying a deletion/duplication or point mutation in the *DMD* gene. With advances in the genetic testing, muscle biopsy is rarely performed.
- 40% have associated moderate to severe learning difficulties.
- ASD is also higher.
- Joint contractures and scoliosis are commonly seen.
- Cardiomyopathy and respiratory failure are late complications.

- Long-term steroids are the main treatment to delay motor decline/preserve cardiac and respiratory function but are associated with side effects which need to be monitored for.
- Newer drugs include ataluren for patients with nonsense mutations, eteplirsen (exon 51 skippable), and golodirsen (exon 53 skippable). Access to these drugs is limited.
- Angiotensin-converting enzyme inhibitors are prophylactically initiated around the age of 8 years.
- Non-invasive ventilation for management of respiratory failure.

Congenital myotonic dystrophy

- AD inheritance.
- Trinucleotide CTG repeat. Severity depends on length of repeats.
- Anticipation down generations.
- Maternal grip myotonia and expressionless facies may offer diagnostic clues.
- Polyhydramnios, reduced fetal movements, facial weakness, weakness and hypotonia, arthrogryposis/talipes at birth. Even those neonates who require ventilator support in neonatal period successfully wean off in time so should be supported.
- Most achieve independent ambulation and then can develop adult pattern of weakness.
- Cardiac rhythm defects should be monitored.
- Other issues include recurrent chest infections, bowel issues including constipation, pseudo-obstruction.
- Moderate to severe learning difficulties and higher association with ASD.
- Diagnosis is by DNA analysis of trinucleotide repeats in DM1 gene.

Spinal muscular atrophy

- AR disorder due to deletion of exons 7 and 8 of the SMN gene.
- Classified clinically into:
  - Type 1 (never able to sit independently).
  - Type 2 (never able to stand independently).
  - Type 3 (achieve independent ambulation but get progressively weaker).
- Life expectancy in SMA1 is under 2 years without respiratory support, SMA2 is childhood to adult depending on severity, and normal in SMA3.
- Recurrent chest infections and respiratory failure are main causes of morbidity and mortality.
- Clinical features include progressive proximal weakness (lower limbs > upper limbs) and absent deep tendon reflexes. Those with SMA1 have tongue fasciculation with paradoxical breathing due to intercostal weakness; those with SMA2 and -3 can have a hand tremor (polyminimyoclonus).
- There are new treatment including nusinersen (antisense oligonucleotide) and onasemnogene abeparvovec (gene therapy), both of which show promising benefit in all three types of SMA.

Spinal muscular atrophy with respiratory distress (SMARD)

- AR disorder due to mutation in the IGHMBP2 gene.
- Clinical presentation is usually in infancy with similar phenotype to SMA1 but with predominant diaphragm weakness.
- The same gene can present with later onset progressive neuropathy with distal weakness.

Congenital myopathies
- Various types such as core myopathy, nemaline myopathy, myotubular myopathy, etc.
- Clinical features are arthrogryposis, myopathic facies (marked facial weakness), occasionally ophthalmoplegia, hypotonia, and axial and limb muscle weakness which is relatively non-progressive or slowly progressive.
- Creatine kinase is normal or mildly raised.
- EMG reveals myopathic features with reduced amplitude of CMAP.
- Diagnosis largely rests on muscle biopsy and immunohistochemistry and genetic confirmation by DNA analysis for specific mutations. Muscle MRI showing patterns of differential muscle group involvement may add a piece to the diagnostic jigsaw.

Congenital muscular dystrophies
- Inherited muscle diseases with or without CNS involvement and eye involvement in varying degree.
- Present with hypotonia, weakness, and developmental delay. Weakness is progressive although not very rapid.
- Creatine kinase is usually elevated.
- Learning difficulties, seizures, and visual impairment may be associated.
- Diagnosis is based on muscle biopsy showing dystrophic features, neuroimaging abnormalities such as white matter abnormalities, structural brain defects and cerebellar cysts, confirmed by DNA analysis.

Congenital peripheral neuropathies (Chariot–Marie–Tooth)
- These are inherited neuropathies all genetically labelled as Charcot–Marie–Tooth diseases.
- Several different types.
- Modes of inheritance include AR, AD, and X-linked.
- Most common form is type 1A (AD).
- This presents with delayed motor development, foot drop, weakness of ankle eversion and dorsiflexion, absent deep tendon reflexes, distal leg weakness and wasting, clawing of feet and hammer toes, as well as pes cavus foot deformity. Distal upper limb weakness can develop over time.
- Usually slowly progressive.
- Diagnosis is by nerve conduction studies showing a demyelinating or axonal neuropathy.
- Diagnosis is confirmed by DNA analysis.

Childhood myasthenia syndromes
- Include congenital myasthenia syndrome, transient neonatal myasthenia, and juvenile myasthenia gravis.
- The main clinical presentation is fatiguable muscle weakness.
- Congenital myasthenia gravis is due to a genetic defect affecting proteins involved in neuromuscular transmission. Congenital myasthenia gravis can present with hypotonia, gross motor delay, weakness, ptosis, ophthalmoparesis, bulbar difficulties, and recurrent respiratory crisis. Treatment depends on the underlying genetic mutation and includes

pyridostigmine and salbutamol. Some congenital myasthenia gravis types can deteriorate on pyridostigmine so await genetic result prior to treatment initiation.

- Transient neonatal myasthenia is seen in infants born to mothers with myasthenia gravis due to transfer of maternal antibodies. Clinical features include hypotonia, feeding difficulties, ptosis, and respiratory difficulties. Treatment is supportive care and pyridostigmine, as symptoms resolve in 3–4 months.
- Myasthenia gravis is due to antibody-mediated impaired neuromuscular transmission. It can present with isolated eye involvement (ptosis, ophthalmoparesis) or generalized (eye, bulbar, limb weakness and respiratory involvement). Antibodies include anti-acetylcholine receptor, anti-muscle specific kinase (MuSK), and anti-low-density lipoprotein receptor-related protein (LRP4). First-line treatment is pyridostigmine, most patients require immunosuppression with steroids or steroid-sparing agents. Thymectomy should considered in acetylcholine receptor-positive patients.

Investigations of neuromuscular disorders

- EMG and nerve conduction studies (myopathy and neuropathy).
- Repetitive nerve stimulation and single-fibre EMG (myasthenia).
- Raised creatine kinase (muscular dystrophies) and lactate (mitochondrial myopathies).
- Tensilon test (myasthenia—rarely performed).
- Muscle biopsy.
- Muscle MRI scan.
- Brain MRI scan (congenital muscular dystrophy).
- DNA analysis.

Management

This is largely supportive though specific treatments available in some conditions as previously discussed.

Three main areas of management are:

Managing orthopaedic complications

- Tendon release and lengthening for contractures.
- Use of orthotic appliances.

Scoliosis managed by using body braces and spinal jackets and eventually insertion of metal rods to stabilize the spine.

Managing respiratory complications

- Advocating immunization including seasonal influenza vaccination.
- Aggressively managing respiratory infections with a low threshold for using antibiotics, chest physiotherapy, and use of assisted cough devices and non-invasive ventilation.
- Regular lung function monitoring is important as well as seeking early symptoms of hypoventilation (early morning headaches, nausea, excessive daytime lethargy).

Managing cardiac complications
- Prophylactic use of angiotensin-converting enzyme inhibitors to delay the onset of cardiomyopathy.
- Regular monitoring of cardiac function is very important as well as monitoring for cardiac rhythm disturbances.

Further resources

Duchene UK: ♒ http://www.duchenneuk.org
Muscular Dystrophy Campaign: ♒ http://www.muscular-dystrophy.org
Myaware: ♒ http://www.myaware.org
Myotonic Dystrophy Support Group: ♒ http://www.myotonicdystrophysupportgroup.org
Spinal Muscular Atrophy UK: ♒ http://www.smauk.org.uk

Neural tube defects

- Birth defects of the CNS originate during embryogenesis and result from failure of complete neural tube closure.
- Commonest are spina bifida and anencephaly.
- Spina bifida can take various forms depending on which part of the neuraxis is involved such as:
  - Meningocoele (meninges only).
  - Myelomeningocoele (spinal cord and meninges).
  - Lipomyelomeningocoele (intra/extradural fat, meninges, and spinal cord).
- This is often associated with other developmental anomalies such as lipomas, dermoid cysts, neurenteric cysts, and diastematomyelia (cord split by bony or fibrocartilaginous spur).
- There are other anatomical anomalies like a low-lying spinal cord or a tethered spinal cord, a syrinx, or low-placed cerebellar tonsils (Chiari malformation).
- Hydrocephalus is seen in 80% of children with myelomeningocoele.

Aetiology

- Complex with both genetic (polygenic) and environmental factors.
- Environmental factors include maternal folic acid deficiency, poorly controlled diabetes mellitus, and sodium valproate use.
- Incidence of neural tube defects is about 0.5–2 per 10000 live births with a larger proportion being fetal losses.
- There is about a 2–5% recurrence risk of non-syndromic neural tube defects in siblings of affected cases which significantly reduces with pre-conceptional folate supplementation.
- Antenatal diagnosis is by anomaly scanning at about 20 weeks' gestation showing ventriculomegaly and vertebral arch defects, fetal MRI scans, and raised maternal serum alpha-fetoprotein levels.

Management

- Multisystem and multidisciplinary.
- Prenatal surgery has emerged as an option though this at present remains contentious due to the risks of preterm birth versus the benefits of surgery.
- At birth, the defect is assessed as to whether there is skin cover. This determines time of repair with open defects needing to be closed earlier.
  - Open defects: a mixed upper and lower motor neuron picture is seen on examination. Bladder and bowel involvement needs urological input and investigations. There is often associated scoliosis and talipes.
  - Occult defects: are often heralded by skin pigmentation, dermal sinuses, or hair over the spine.
- An MRI scan determines the anatomical level of the lesion. The neurological level is often higher than the anatomical level and is a prognostic indicator of future disability.
- It is important to assess antigravity movement, spinal reflexes, and sacral sensations as well as sphincter tone.

- Associated Chiari malformations, syrinx, and hydrocephalus need attention.
- Syndromes such as VACTERL (vertebral anomalies, anal atresia, cardiac anomalies, tracheo-oesophageal fistula, (o)esophageal atresia, renal anomalies, and limb defects) associations warrant investigations to look for other system involvement.
- Talipes and scoliosis need orthopaedic intervention and monitoring or surgical correction.
- Neurogenic bladder and constipation often exist and needs appropriate treatment. Bladder dysfunction results in incomplete emptying against sphincter resistance leading to vesicoureteric reflux and nephropathy.
- Other associated problems to monitor:
  - Hydrocephalus.
  - Tethering of the spinal cord.
  - Growth and nutrition.
  - Psychosocial issues.

Prognosis

- The neurological level of lesion is the main predictor of future needs.
- Ankle dorsiflexion predicts walking outdoors and independent transfers. Presence of knee extension predicts household ambulation and standing for transfers. Trunk stability and hip flexion predicts non-functional ambulation and wheelchair use.
- There is usually no overt LD.
- Hydrocephalus, shunt infections, renal failure, and surgical interventions determine mortality and morbidity.

Further resources

Shine (formerly the Association for Spina Bifida and Hydrocephalus): ☎ 01733 555988; 🖰 https://www.shinecharity.org.uk/

Chiari malformation

- A downward displacement of posterior fossa contents through the foramen magnum.
- There are different types of Chiari malformation based on degree of involvement of the posterior fossa structures.

Chiari 1 malformation

- Cerebellar tonsils descend below the foramen magnum.
- There may be a secondary syrinx in the spinal cord.
- A large displacement is often symptomatic with occipital headaches (worsened by cough, straining, or bending down), cerebellar signs, limb paraesthesia, and reduced pain sensation due to the syrinx.

Chiari II malformation

- There is additional malformation of the pons and the pons and fourth ventricle are abnormally low.
- This is often associated with spina bifida.

Chiari III malformation

- There is herniation of posterior fossa contents through a posterior meningocoele.
- Management is by decompression of the foramen magnum with other additional surgery depending on associated conditions.

Hydrocephalus

- Increased volume of CSF spaces in the brain eventually causing raised intracranial pressure.
- This may be non-communicating or communicating.
- Incidence is 5–8 per 10,000 births.

Obstructive hydrocephalus

Can be due to various causes such as:
- Aqueduct stenosis: genetic (X-linked *L1CAM* mutations), acquired from intrauterine infections.
- Dandy–Walker malformation: cystic dilatation of fourth ventricle with vermis hypoplasia.
- Tumours and cysts, e.g. medulloblastomas, giant cell astrocytomas, colloid cyst of third ventricle, ependymomas.
- Vascular malformations: arteriovenous malformations, aneurysm of vein of Galen.
- Intraventricular haemorrhage: premature babies with grade 3 and 4 intraventricular haemorrhage develop progressive ventricular dilatation.

Communicating hydrocephalus

- Post infectious, e.g. meningitis.
- Post haemorrhagic, e.g. intraventricular haemorrhage, post traumatic, subdural, and subarachnoid haemorrhage.
- Venous sinus thrombosis.
- Craniosynostosis and achondroplasia.
- Neural tube defects, e.g. myelomeningocoele, encephalocoele, and Chiari malformations.
- Other conditions associated with hydrocephalus are DS, myotonic dystrophy, NF1, Hurler syndrome, etc.

Symptoms and signs of hydrocephalus

- Increasing head circumference crossing centile lines.
- Infants: irritability, poor feeding, drowsiness, sun setting eyes.
- Older children: headache, vomiting, new-onset squint/visual difficulties.
- Signs: sun setting eyes, prominent scalp veins, papilloedema is a late and unreliable sign.

Investigations

- Congenital hydrocephalus can be diagnosed antenatally by ultrasound scan or fetal MRI scan.
- Ultrasound scan if fontanelle is open.
- CT scan.
- MRI scan.

Treatment

- In neonates: serial ventricular taps and lumbar puncture.
- Shunt: ventriculoperitoneal (mostly), ventriculoatrial, ventriculopleural, and lumboperitoneal shunts (rarely).
- Endoscopic third ventriculostomy: for obstructive hydrocephalus mainly due to aqueduct stenosis.

Shunt complications

Infection

- 10% overall incidence of infection.
- Present with fever, drowsiness, irritability, vomiting, and seizures.
- Infection screen and shunt tap by neurosurgical team often required for diagnosis.
- Requires long courses up to 6 weeks of intrathecal and IV antibiotics.
- Externalization of shunt for the duration of antibiotic therapy followed by shunt replacement is often required.

Shunt block or disconnection

- 60–80% of shunts inserted in infancy require revision within 10 years.
- Symptoms are similar to infections but can be less acute.
- They include lethargy, headache, visual disturbance, behaviour change, intermittent vomiting, and occasionally seizures.

Over-drainage

- Symptoms are lethargy, headache worse on sitting up and improved by lying down.
- CT or MRI show slit ventricles and at times tonsillar descent.
- Intracranial pressure monitoring is required for diagnosis.
- Treatment is by inserting shunts with programmable high resistance valves.

Shunt migration, colonic perforation, and peritonitis

Common sites of migration are perforation of the bowel, migration to the genitourinary region, abdominal wall, chest/thorax, intracranial, cardiac/intravascular system.

Associated problems in children with hydrocephalus

- Learning difficulties.
- Fine motor impairment and tremor.
- Epilepsy.
- Visual impairment.
- Endocrine disturbances.

Idiopathic intracranial hypertension

- Also known as benign intracranial hypertension or pseudotumour cerebri.
- It causes raised intracranial pressure in the absence of any intracranial pathology.
- Symptoms include headache (worse after lying down), pulsatile tinnitus, double vision, and visual difficulties.
- Signs include papilloedema and sixth nerve palsy. Asymptomatic visual field impairment with enlargement of the blind spot and inferonasal visual field loss are early signs.
- Neuroimaging (CT brain/CT venography or ideally MRI brain with magnetic resonance venography) is mandatory to rule out alternative cause for raised intracranial pressure and must be performed prior to lumbar puncture.
- MRI findings suggestive of idiopathic intracranial hypertension include empty sella, enlarged perioptic subarachnoid space with or without a tortuous optic nerve, flattened posterior globe/sclera, and intraocular protrusion of optic nerve head. Magnetic resonance/CT venography is required to rule out venous sinuses thrombosis.
- An appropriately performed lumbar puncture reveals opening pressure of >28 cmH$_2$O.
- Risk factors include obesity, cerebral venous abnormalities, medications including oral contraceptives, tetracyclines, retinoids, steroids, vitamins D and A, Addison disease, hypoparathyroidism/hyperparathyroidism, hypothyroidism/hyperthyroidism, and obstructive sleep apnoea.
- Treatment is by lumbar puncture to reduce closing pressure to <20 cmH$_2$O. In severe cases, serial lumbar punctures may be required.
- Acetazolamide is usually used for medical management post lumbar puncture.
- Lumboperitoneal and ventriculoperitoneal shunting as well as optic nerve sheath fenestration may be needed in refractory cases.
- Visual fields and function need close monitoring.

Mental health and behaviour

The moon moves slowly, but it crosses the town.

African proverb

Introduction

Community paediatric teams and primary care professionals play a vital role in recognizing, evaluating, and improving the mental well-being of young people.

Mental disorders are common in children and adolescents, with a mean overall prevalence of 15.8%. Rates in general paediatric clinics have been reported to be as high as 28%. Most mental health problems are long-standing, often lasting >1 year, yet it is estimated that half of these children receive no professional help. Professionals need to be able to recognize mental illness, understand the nature and severity of the disorder, and know when to refer to specialist services.

The assessment of mental health in children can be challenging due to several factors:

• Multiple environmental and psychosocial factors contribute to the child's presentation and parents, family, friends, and school may need to be involved in the assessment and treatment plan.

• The child's symptoms and response to stress must be interpreted in the context of the child's age and development level to avoid the risk of mislabelling normal behaviour as pathological.

• Children's symptoms can be transient, appear to lack the severity necessary for a diagnosis, and they frequently present with a range of symptoms which may either meet the diagnostic criteria for several conditions or not fit neatly into any categorical diagnostic system. Comorbidity is common.

Despite these challenges, the early recognition of problems and timely intervention can prevent and relieve a significant amount of distress for children and carers.

Working with child and adolescent mental health services

Child and adolescent mental health services (CAMHS) structure

In the UK, service delivery is arranged in a tiered approach and/or a pathway model. Both arrangements are predominantly outpatient based with few adolescent inpatient units.

Tiered model

Increasing complexity of mental illness is associated with a higher tier. Professionals are 'gatekeepers' for higher tiers. Higher tiers provide consultation to lower tiers.

- Tier 1: GP, HVs, social services, school nurses, voluntary agencies.
- Tier 2: professional groups working as individuals—community paediatricians, clinical and educational psychologists, social workers, psychotherapists.
- Tier 3: CAMHS—multidisciplinary team, often includes psychiatrist, psychologist, family therapist, and mental health practitioners (nurse, OT, child psychotherapist, social worker, dietician).
- Tier 4: CAMHS specialized services—inpatient units, day services, intensive outreach, and other specialist services such as forensic, neuropsychiatry, and LD.

Pathway model

All referrals are directed to a central single point of access, which covers a larger geographical area. These are processed and directed towards other services or CAMHS teams. The CAMHS teams are organized based on diagnosis/need and can include getting help team (emotional/mood disorders), eating disorders (EDs), neurodevelopmental team (ASD/ADHD), forensic, early intervention in psychosis, crisis team, and assertive outreach service (wrap-around service, challenging to engage young people, chronic conditions).

Depending on local service requirements and commissioning, there may be access to other teams: dialectical behaviour therapy service, dialectic behaviour therapy (mindfulness and CBT techniques to manage self-harm); school in-reach teams (shorter-term interventions), hospital/liaison team.

Local CAMHS teams can refer to nationally based services if a second opinion is required or the work is highly specialized, e.g. gender identity disorder services.

Referrals to CAMHS

- Ideally there should be a local policy document regarding the nature and the severity of conditions seen by specialist CAMHS.
- Discuss the case with CAMHS if uncertain whether to refer.
- Parents can feel that they have 'failed' if a mental health referral is required, so 'framing' the referral is important.
- Ensure the family understands the reasons for the referral and obtain assent where possible.
- Consider the motivation of the family—poorly motivated parents may not engage with an assessment or treatment.

- Include what the child and parents want/expect from CAMHS in the referral information.
- Community CAMHS timescale for assessments varies considerably based on local team structure and demand. Generally, 'emergency' assessments should be within 24 hours, 'urgent' within 7 days, and 'routine' within 4 weeks (often longer). Neurodevelopmental (ASD/ADHD) assessments may have a considerably longer wait.

Assessment, diagnosis, and management

Prior to the assessment, information is often gathered by sending questionnaires to school, GP, and the family. Initial assessments may be telephone/internet based or face to face. They usually involve one or two team members. As well as seeing the family as a group, the assessment should also include some separate time with both the carers and the child.

Two manuals are used to diagnose:
- *International Classification of Diseases*, 11th revision (ICD-11), produced by the WHO, released 2018, with implementation from 2022. Most commonly used in the UK.
- *Diagnostic and Statistical Manual of Mental Disorders*, fifth edition (DSM-5), produced by the American Psychiatric Association, released 2013.

The family may need to be seen more than once before a formulation, diagnosis, and management plan can be concluded.

A written plan and letter should be shared with the family and professional network regarding the outcome of the assessment.

UK mental health services use a 'Care Programme Approach' to assess health/social needs, and formulate a care and risk management plan. A team member takes responsibility as 'care coordinator', providing the principal source of contact/liaison with the family and other agencies. Regular reviews occur (usually 3–6 months) and professionals involved in the child's and the family's care may be invited to attend or copied into Care Programme Approach review documentation.

Working with CAMHS

- Meet the local psychiatry consultants, team manager, and team members at least once!
- Consider regular contact: review cases that have physical and mental health needs, feed back on consultations for each other, agree referral pathways (particularly for emergency/urgent cases), review areas of good practice/need for improvement, and review overlap/division of labour, e.g. ASD/ADHD assessment and management.
- Regular communication prevents 'splitting' by parents.
- Consider joint paediatrician and psychiatrist clinics.
- Encourage paediatric and psychiatric trainees to sit in on clinics.
- Joint research, audit, and teaching.
- Shared virtual/physical library of resources, e.g. patient information leaflets, commonest websites, and local support groups.

Further resources

Diagnostic and Statistical Manual of Mental Disorders, fifth edition (DSM-5): https://www.psychiatry.org/psychiatrists/practice/dsm
International Classification of Diseases, 11th revision (ICD-11): https://icd.who.int/browse11/l-m/en

The psychiatric evaluation

The psychiatric assessment in children involves:
- An initial warm-up period.
- Defining the reason for referral and current difficulties.
- Assessing for comorbidities.
- Assessing family and school functioning.
- Conducting a mental state examination.
- Risk assessment and formulation.
- Generating a treatment plan.

▶ History taking should be a cathartic and therapeutic intervention.

General approach
- Ask the family to introduce themselves.
- Use an initial period of 'unstructured' conversation as a 'warm up' focusing on engagement and observing the child, family, and their interaction. Begin with neutral topics (hobbies, friends, school, pets).
- Family members may want you to 'side' with their opinion—adopt a neutral stance.
- Use active listening (brief summaries and paraphrasing to check understanding, use body language to convey attention, reduce interruptions).
- Divide time: all together, parent alone, child alone, back together at conclusion of session.
- Outline the limits of confidentiality with older children and adolescents.
- Use single questions and language appropriate for the developmental level of the child.
- Age of child will influence approach with greater emphasis on drawing and play for children aged <6 years.
- Use drawings or pictures of emotional faces in books for children struggling to express themselves.
- Reference to a third party ('I knew a boy who ...') when children are struggling to express their worries.

Presenting complaint

What are the child's and family's understanding of the reasons for the referral? What would they like to get out of the session?
Problem: antecedents, onset, duration, and severity.
- Circumstances: pervasive/specific situations? Explore 'exceptions': what is different about those times when the problem is less prominent?
- Consequences: degree of emotional distress, social/academic functioning, family relationships, impact on development.
- Explore any global statements by obtaining specific examples of behaviour—when did that happen last? Tell me about that?
- What strategies have the child and family utilized to tackle the problem? What has been helpful?
- Review current support: friends, school counsellor, teacher, youth worker, extended family.

Review of other symptoms

Emotions

- Family may be unaware of the extent of the child's distress.
- Worries, fears, anxiety, depression, and somatization (abdominal pain, headaches).
- Suicidal ideation ('Have you ever felt so bad that you wanted to run away/end it all?').

Conduct

- Oppositional/defiant behaviour, lying, empathy, destructiveness, aggression (threats, verbal, physical, bullying).
- 'Do you ever get into fights at school?'

Screen/review other problems

- Current level of functioning not covered in the presenting complaint.
- School: academic level and progress, motivation, special educational needs, bullying, relationship difficulties, school refusal/truancy, behavioural problems.
- Cognitive: memory, attention, concentration.
- Activity level, self-care, diet, exercise, sleep, play.
- Sensory processing issues (hypo- or hypersensitivity to touch, taste, sound, position).

Past psychiatric, medical, and developmental history

(See ➜ pp. 234–7.)

Previous diagnosis, duration, and impact of interventions. Traumatic events and maltreatment.

Family history

Genogram, quality of relationships, family stresses and life events, family history of mental illness, and current treatment.

Social history

Housing, recent geographical moves, employment, and social services input.

Alcohol, substance use, and forensic history

Pattern of drug use and how is it funded; assaults, damage to property, theft, fire setting, cruelty to animals, police involvement, and youth offending service support.

Premorbid behaviour/personality

What has changed? How would friends/significant others describe them before illness?

Future

- Hopes and aspirations in the short and long term.
- Assess motivation to change: 'How much would like … [e.g. mood] to improve/change?' 'How confident are you that you can change?' Rate both out of 10.
- Hypothetical questions: 'If the problem went away what would you be doing?' 'How would you know things had improved?' 'What would other people see?'
- In younger children, use three wishes/magic wand question to explore how things would look if your worries were gone.

▶ Always review the child's strengths: what strengths can the child and the family identify? How does the child react to their parent's comments?

Observing the child

The Mental Status Examination (MSE) provides a systematic and structured approach for recording observations of the child.

Mental status examination

Appearance and behaviour

- Physical appearance, dysmorphic features, nutritional status, bruises, injuries, clothes (clean, unusual).
- Social responsiveness: shy, withdrawn, disinhibition, friendliness, reciprocity, rapport, can you 'connect' with the child?
- Interaction with carers: warmth, affection, ease of separation and reaction on reunion.
- Aggression, non-compliance, impulsivity.
- Nature of play: concrete, imaginary, main themes (e.g. loss, sexualized, violent, death), age appropriate.
- Non-verbal communication: eye contact, gestures, posture.
- Motor: hyper/hypo-activity, fidgeting, mannerisms, tics, stereotypies, gait, fine and gross motor difficulties.

Speech

Rate, rhythm, volume, prosody, immediate and delayed echolalia (repetition of phrases), neologisms (made up words). Appropriate for developmental level? Ability to 'chit-chat'/maintain reciprocal conversation.

Mood and affect

Subjective and objective mood, symptoms of depression (decreased energy, sleep, appetite, concentration, self-esteem, and loss of interest in hobbies), range and appropriateness of affect.

Thoughts

- Content: view of self, world, and future; preoccupations, fears, phobias, obsessions, compulsions and delusions (fixed, firmly held belief out of keeping with person's culture, content, e.g. persecutory, grandiose), fantasies, suicidal ideation, and hopelessness.
- Form: poverty, flight of ideas (racing thoughts).

Perceptions

Abnormalities in auditory, visual, and other sensory modalities. Types: altered perceptions—external object present, e.g. illusions and false perceptions; no external object present, e.g. hallucinations (occur in external space); and pseudo-hallucinations (inside head).

Cognition

Concentration, orientation in time/place/person, short and long-term memory, age-appropriate vocabulary/drawings.

Insight

Recognition of current difficulties and need for treatment, willingness to accept treatment.

Observing the family

- Parent–child interaction: overly close, distant, warm, punitive.
- Parental response to their child's distress. Emotional availability.
- Do the parents set effective limits/boundaries? How does the child respond?
- Problem-solving skills during the session.
- Discrepancy between how the parents treat the child and siblings?
- Parental relationship: supportive, conflictual.
- Signs of mental illness in family members.
- Could the family interactions be maintaining the problem?

Other sources of information

- Questionnaires to explore generalized psychiatric symptoms or specific areas.
- Consider using specialist investigations: ADOS assessment in ASD, computerized assessment of attention in ADHD, cognitive assessment.
- School observation/questionnaires/reports.

Summary

- Key findings, including relevant 'negatives' that would make a diagnosis less likely.
- Risk: to self and others including self-injury, self-harm, aggression, vulnerability, child protection issues.
- Strengths: personal, environment, school, family.

Further resources

International Association for Child and Adolescent Psychiatry and Allied Professions (IACAPAP), free to download e-textbook with chapters covering a range of mental health topics including assessment. Available at: ℘ https://iacapap.org/english/

Strengths and Difficulties Questionnaire (brief screening questionnaire, 3–16 years, free download). Available at: ℘ http://www.sdqinfo.org/a0.html

Psychological aspects of learning disability

One-third of children with a mild LD and 50–70% of children with a moderate/severe LD (see ➋ pp. 136–41) meet diagnostic criteria for a coexisting mental illness.

- Any psychiatric disorder may occur; anxiety (17%), ADHD (see ➋ pp. 126–34), ASD (see ➋ pp. 114–25), stereotyped movement, e.g. rocking, self-harm (SH) (head banging, biting) (see ➋ pp. 334–6), and depression are especially common.
- Full diagnostic criteria may not be met and with increasing severity of LD more emphasis is placed on observed behaviour.
- Medical comorbidity is often unrecognized despite being common: epilepsy (22%), CP (20%), and sensory processing issues.
- Children with LD (see ➋ pp. 136–41) are more likely to experience poverty, social exclusion, and bereavement.

Comorbid LD and psychiatric illness increases care-giver/placement strain considerably. Consider a coexisting psychiatric disorder before rationalizing behavioural symptoms as an integral part of the LD.

Factors predisposing to behavioural problems

- Communication difficulties: speech and hearing impairments (5–10%) hinder understanding and communication of needs, can contribute to social exclusion (see ➋ Chapter 4).
- Non-verbal behaviours, e.g. hitting, self-harm used to attract attention (see ➋ 334–6).
- Limited coping strategies: receiving adult attention for shouting or aggression potentially reinforces the use of such behaviour when faced with a problem perceived as unsolvable.
- Undetected physical illness: e.g. infection, pain, or constipation can lead to behaviours such as rocking or hitting painful body part.
- Boredom: self-injury may serve to reduce boredom in severe LD.
- Epilepsy: both seizures and antiepileptic medication can worsen behaviour (see ➋ pp. 248–55).
- Brain damage (moderate/severe LD).
- Psychosocial factors (particularly mild LD): bullying (see ➋ pp. 318–19), abuse, increasing self-awareness of limitations with age, all increase risk of low self-esteem, anxiety, and depression (see ➋ p. 286).
- Behavioural phenotypes: Prader–Willi (hunger with overeating, inattention; see ➋ p. 518), Lesch–Nyhan (self-injury), fragile X (social anxiety, gaze avoidance, associated with ASD; see ➋ pp. 516–17).

Medication for behavioural problems

- Consider other psychosocial management strategies before medication.
- Aim to use medication in combination with other interventions.
- Very limited evidence base and most used off licence.
- Document target symptoms, doses: 'start low, go slow', and review regularly.
- Short-term use of antipsychotics (aripiprazole, risperidone) can reduce challenging behaviours and are anxiolytic.

- Children with LD may be more likely to experience medication side effects: extrapyramidal side effects, neuroleptic malignant syndrome, anticholinergic, worsening cognition with sedative medication, or paradoxical disinhibition with benzodiazepines.

Sleep problems
(See ➲ pp. 466–8.)
Common, often present since infancy. Key factor in family breakdown. Both decreased need for sleep and difficulty falling asleep can occur. Improving sleep can improve behavioural problems. Sleep hygiene is mainstay of treatment. If inadequate, especially in autism, melatonin can be helpful.

Eating disorders
(See ➲ pp. 342–4.)
Pica (ingestion of inedible substances), regurgitation, under- and over-eating common. Anorexia rare.

ADHD
(See ➲ pp. 126–34.)
Hyperactive subtype particularly common. Consider child's developmental level when deciding if hyperactivity and decreased attention present. Symptoms should be present across several situations. Children with LD are more prone to medication side effects particularly decreased appetite.

Autism spectrum disorder
(See ➲ pp. 114–25.)
Seen in 7.8–19.8% of LD; 66–80% ASD have LD. Behavioural problems are largely mediated through anxiety, often situational and worse at home.

Depression
(See ➲ pp. 330–2.)
Consider depression if new or increasing challenging behaviours (irritability/aggressive, social withdrawal), particularly in adolescence or in absence of change in environmental factors.
Less likely to express hopelessness, low mood. Appetite and sleep often affected (can increase or decrease) as are concentration (decreased) and pleasure.
SSRIs helpful. Adapted CBT may have a role depending on degree of LD.

Anxiety
(See ➲ pp. 338–40.)
In non-verbal children, avoidance and agitation may suggest the diagnosis.

Psychosis
- Not to be confused with 'self-talk', which is common in children, especially if LD. Talking to self includes thinking out loud, directing behaviour, processing emotions, and stimulation.
- True psychosis rare. In LD, visual and tactile hallucinations more common than complex delusions. Usually associated with decreased functioning and altered personality. If suspected, need EEG and brain imaging.

OCD

(See ➔ p. 340.)

Repetitive actions, e.g. washing, tidying that reduce anxiety. Differentiate from stereotypies (repetitive, non-goal directed, e.g. rocking, hand-wringing). Consider ASD in differential diagnosis.

Further resources

Mencap (UK charity): ⅏ https://www.mencap.org.uk/learning-disability-explained/what-learning-disability

LD Online (US website on LD and ADHD): ⅏ http://www.ldonline.org/

Autistic spectrum disorders: CAMHS aspects

(Also see ⮞ pp. 114–25–p. 125.)

Children with ASD have higher rates of mental illness and behavioural problems. 70% of children with ASD have one co-occurring mental health condition and 41% have two or more conditions.

ADHD (see ⮞ pp. 126–34), anxiety disorders (see ⮞ pp. 338–40), oppositional defiant disorder (ODD), and depression (see ⮞ pp. 330–2) are common. If symptoms of mental illness are significant enough to warrant a comorbid diagnosis, then management should follow the standard treatment protocols for the relevant disorder.

Children with ASD often present with clusters of symptoms that do not fit into diagnostic criteria and we will focus on their management in this section. Common difficulties include aggression, agitation, anxiety, self-injury, repetitive behaviours, behavioural rigidity, sleep difficulties, and 'ADHD-like' symptoms.

▶ There are no curative treatments for ASD and many of the interventions aimed at addressing the core symptoms of autism have insufficient evidence to recommend routine use.

Non-pharmacological interventions

Many of the 'generic' behavioural management techniques (behaviour therapy (see ⮞ p. 366) and challenging behaviour strategies (see ⮞ p. 363)) will be appropriate. However, the core symptoms of ASD and common coexisting LDs should be considered when adapting these techniques.

- Systematically review possible precipitants for the behaviour, including routine changes, transition from an activity of interest, anxiety, sensory overload, and physical discomfort.
- Gather collateral information: have there been changes that parents are unaware of (contact school, carers)?
- Exclude physical causes or exacerbating factors (pain, fatigue, sleep disorders, seizures, menstrual cycle).
- Reduce frustration by enhancing communication: use visual augmentation (pictures) (see ⮞ p. 408).
- Encourage the use of structured environments, predictable daily routines, and consistent responses to behaviour at home and at school.
- Support from special educational services, including opportunities for social skills training at school (see ⮞ pp. 656–8 and pp. 122–3).
- Parent support: training (see ⮞ pp. 122–3) and support groups for parents and siblings.

Pharmacological interventions

- Use to target specific behaviours that cause significant distress or impairments in functioning and education.
- Increased risk of side effects and paradoxical effects so 'start low, go slow' and monitor closely.
- Symptoms often return upon discontinuation.
- Evidence supports the use of risperidone and aripiprazole for challenging and repetitive behaviours. Limited evidence to support the use of other medications, although they are frequently used.

Risperidone and aripiprazole
- Use: commonly used to treat irritability (aggression, tantrums). Possible benefit: repetitive behaviours, self-injury, stereotypies, behavioural rigidity, obsessional symptoms.
- Short-term treatment at low doses.
- High likelihood of side effects: weight gain, sedation.

Methylphenidate
- Use: hyperactivity, inattention, impulsivity.
- May increase risk of agitation, irritability, emotional outbursts, and stereotypic behaviour.

SSRIs (fluoxetine and sertraline)
- Use: repetitive behaviours, anxiety, obsessions. May help depressive phenotype (social withdrawal, crying, reduced energy). Need to assess impact over weeks to months.
- Side effects: nausea, restlessness, insomnia, transient increase in suicidal ideation and agitation.

Melatonin
- Use: sleep difficulties unresponsive to behavioural interventions.

Benzodiazepines
- Try to avoid as decreased evidence to support use, potential paradoxical effect (disinhibition), and they are only suitable for short-term use.

Clonidine and guanfacine
- Decreased evidence to recommend routine use but may help hyperactivity, aggression, self-injury, and sleep dysfunction.

Refer to CAMHS if there is a high likelihood of comorbid mental illness, or if family therapy or highly structured individual work for older/higher functioning individuals is required.

Further resources

American Academy of Child and Adolescent Psychiatry (2014). Practice parameter for the assessment and treatment of children and adolescents with ASD. Available at: ℘ http://www.aacap.org/AACAP/Resources_for_Primary_Care/Practice_Parameters_and_Resource_Centers/Practice_Parameters.aspx

Autism Society of America: ℘ https://www.autism-society.org/

National Autistic Society: ℘ https://www.autism.org.uk/

National Institute for Health and Care Excellence (2013, updated 2021). Autism spectrum disorder in under 19s: support and management. Clinical guideline 170. Available at: ℘ https://www.nice.org.uk/Guidance/CG170

High-functioning autism spectrum disorder

High-functioning autism spectrum disorders were previously commonly described as Asperger syndrome, or pervasive developmental disorder-not otherwise specified. DSM-5 and ICD-11 have merged these, along with autism, into a single umbrella category called 'autism spectrum disorder' (ASD).

Autism spectrum disorder clinical features (adapted from DSM-5)

Persistent deficits in social communication and interaction across multiple contexts

- Deficits in social–emotional reciprocity (abnormal social approach, reduced normal back and forth conversation, reduced sharing interests/emotions/affect, reduced initiate/respond to social interactions).
- Deficits in non-verbal communicative behaviours (poorly integrated verbal and non-verbal communication, eye contact, facial expression, posture, gesture).
- Deficits in developing, maintaining, and understanding relationships (adjust behaviour to social situation, sharing imaginative play, making friends, reduced interest in peers).

Restricted, repetitive patterns of behaviour, interests, or activities

At least two of:

- Stereotyped and repetitive motor mannerisms (hand/finger flapping or twisting, complex whole-body movements), use of objects (lining up toys > imaginative play), or speech (echolalia, set phrases).
- Insistence on sameness, inflexible adherence to routines or ritualized patterns of verbal or non-verbal behaviour (distress at small changes, transitions, rigid thinking, greeting rituals, same school route, and foods).
- Restricted, fixated interest/preoccupation that are abnormal intensity or focus (excessively circumscribed or perseverative interests, preoccupation with unusual objects).
- Hyper- or hypo-reactivity to sensory input or unusual sensory aspects of environment (indifference to pain/temperature, sensitive to sounds/textures, excessive smelling or touching of objects, fascination with lights or movement).

Other

- Severity: mild, moderate, severe.
- Onset in 'early developmental period' but may present later.
- Symptoms cause clinically significant impairment in social, occupational, or other important areas of current functioning.
- Disturbances are not better explained by ID or GDD.

- Prevalence: wide variation in estimates due to historically differing diagnosis criteria, ♂ > ♀.
- Aetiology (see ➔ pp. 117–18).
- Family members—higher risk of ASD phenotype, 2–18% risk in siblings.

Assessment

- Individuals with higher functioning ASD tend to present to medical services later than children with more severe forms of autism. This may reflect better learned or innate coping strategies, so symptoms only become manifest when demands exceed a child's capacity to cope.
- Referrals are common around school transitions (home/junior school/ high school) when social interaction difficulties become more noticeable and children must cope with greater change.
- No pathognomonic sign or definitive medical test.
- Development history as for ASD (see ➔ pp. 119–20).

Enquire about

- Increased or decreased interest/desire for friendship and inability to initiate or maintain friendships, social isolation; better relationships with younger children and adults.
- May be content in their own company, or very small group of friends, or desperately want to fit in with peers but struggle to do so.
- Play with others: insist on taking the lead or overly passive, desire for 'sameness' in play, precisely follow rules.
- Enquire about behaviour at parties and when children visit the home— more interested in toys and food than peers? Could they cope with not being the centre of attention? Excessively shy? Follow rules of party games—ignore them, rigid adherence, cope with others response?
- Decreased recognition of emotions and viewpoints of others.
- Sensory processing issues with hypo- or hypersensitivities to sound, texture, odours, and taste.
- Motor clumsiness.
- Struggles to understand and follow social rules, e.g. need to always tell the truth, behaviour considered odd by peers.
- Hobbies/interests—can include excessive computer use/addiction, collecting all toys/objects of a set.
- Different symptoms vary in intensity and over time.

Look for

- Subtle speech and pragmatic language impairments—abnormal prosody/ inflection voice, formal pedantic language, literal/concrete use of language with decreased understanding of sarcasm, proverbs, and implied intent.
- Content to discuss their topics of special interest.
- Tendency to talk 'at' you rather than 'with' you.
- Impaired 'chit-chat'. Initial conversation may be appropriate as it tends to follow a more fixed pattern. Deficits may become more apparent as the conversation builds or strays away from usual topics. You may be told the same anecdote more than once.

▶ Eye contact, smiling, and displays of affection/secure attachment to family members do not exclude a diagnosis of ASD.

▶ Features in girls compared to boys: better social skills, areas of interest are less concrete/object orientated and more 'social', e.g. soap operas, celebrities, friends, makeovers, animals, psychology. May struggle to share a best friend with peers. Physical changes of puberty may be particularly distressing.

Investigations
- Screening and diagnostic tools (see ➲ p. 117).
- Developmental and/or psychometric evaluation for overall level of functioning and discrepancy between verbal and non-verbal performance.
- Physical examination (see ➲ pp. 119–20).

Differential diagnosis
(See Table 6.1.)

Significant risk of comorbidity, 20–70% develop concurrent mental illness: depression, anxiety, ADHD, tic disorders, dyspraxia, aggression, oppositional behaviour, or self-injury.

Management
- Psychoeducation for child and family.
- Inform school—appropriate educational support and educational psychology assessment if appropriate.
- Support with accepting diagnosis—increased awareness of difference from peers, bullying.
- Managing social situations—social stories groups at schools, help at home, practice social scripts.
- Treat common comorbidity including ADHD, anxiety, and tics.
- Refer to occupational therapy for assessment if hypo/hypersensitivity or difficulties in motor development.
- Behavioural interventions (see ➲ pp. 412–13).
- Refer to CAMHS if comorbid mental illness.

Table 6.1 Differential diagnosis

Disorder	Differentiating features
ADHD	Able to form, but not necessarily sustain, friendships. Appropriate non-verbal communication. Less rigidity/structure in play compared to ASD
Attachment disorder	History of adverse caregiving, improvement in social deficits in response to a more appropriate environment. Imaginative play preserved and lack unusual interests
Selective mutism	Able to converse appropriately with family, normal non-verbal communication, and imaginative play
OCD	Obsessions and compulsions are often accompanied by distress, social skills preserved, onset >4 years
Social anxiety/phobia	Better social interaction with family and as a younger child, no restricted interests. ↓ anxiety with people they know

Prognosis

- Lifelong condition: some improvement with increasing age, particularly once they can commence more specialist education/work.
- More likely to live independently, establish a family, and to be employed compared to people with moderate/severe ASD.
- Higher IQ improves prognosis.

Further resources

Anxiety scale for children—autism spectrum disorder (ASC-ASD), 24 item child and parent versions, derived from RCADS, free to download at: ℘ https://research.ncl.ac.uk/neurodisability/leafletsandmeasures/anxietyscaleforchildren-asd/

Attwood T (1998). Asperger's Syndrome: A Guide for Parents and Professionals. London: Jessica Kingsley.

Gray C (2015). The New Social Story Book. Arlington, TX: Future Horizons.

Healthtalk.org (several videos of people discussing their experiences of autism): ℘ https://healthtalk.org/life-autism-spectrum/overview

National Autistic Society: ℘ http://www.autism.org.uk

National Institute for Health and Care Excellence (2011, updated 2017). Autism spectrum disorder in under 19s: recognition, referral and diagnosis. Clinical guideline 128. Available at: ℘ https://www.nice.org.uk/guidance/cg128

Tic disorders

Description of tics

- Rapid, recurrent, non-rhythmic motor movement, or utterance (verbal tic).
- Involuntary, may be suppressed for short periods of time and may be preceded by premonitory sensation.
- Often occur in bouts, wax and wane in frequency, and type of tic can vary.
- Precipitants include excitement, anxiety, fatigue, and heat.

Classification

- *Simple*: single muscle group—eye blinking, head and shoulder jerks, facial grimacing, grunting, sniffing, throat clearing, coughing.
- *Complex*: multiple muscle groups—repetitive touching, tapping, squatting, echopraxia (copying actions), copropraxia (obscene gestures), self-injury, coprolalia (profane verbal tic, 10% Tourette syndrome), echolalia (copying heard phrases), palilalia (repeating own sounds).

ICD-11 classification

- Transient tic disorders: <12 months' duration, 6–20% of children.
- Chronic motor or vocal tic disorder: >12 months' duration, single type of tic, 4% of children.
- Tourette syndrome: multiple motor tics and at least one vocal tic, >12 months' duration, 1% of children.

Epidemiology

- Onset 4–8 years, 3:1 ♂:♀.
- Simple tics more common and develop earlier than complex tics. Motor tics more common and develop earlier than vocal tics.

Aetiology

- Tics occur in 10–15% of first-degree relatives.
- Neurodevelopmental condition with imbalance in dopaminergic system, basal ganglia implicated.
- Possible association with post-streptococcal infection autoimmune response (PANDAS).

Assessment

Observe child during discussion of tics (discussion can often precipitate tics). Is there a video recording of the tics?

Explore

- Onset, triggers, relieving factors, possible tic suppression, and tic-induced pain.
- Impact on emotional, social, academic, and family functioning, especially interference with daily tasks, isolation, stigmatization, bullying, and self-harm.
- Tic severity may not correlate with subjective distress.
- Yale Global Tic Severity Scale—assess and monitor response to treatment.

- Comorbidity ADHD (60%), OCD (30%), depression (see ➨ pp. 330–2), anxiety (see ➨ pp. 338–40), learning difficulty (see ➨ pp. 136–41), sleep disorders (see ➨ pp. 466–8), conduct disorder (CD), ASD (see ➨ pp. 114–25).
- Physical examination. Myoclonus (see ➨ p. 246), dystonias (see ➨ p. 536), choreas, dysmorphic features, self-injury (see ➨ p. 363).

Differential diagnosis

OCD (see ➨ p. 340), ADHD (see ➨ pp. 126–34), dystonia (see ➨ p. 536), stereotypies (earlier onset, fixed pattern, rhythmic, no premonitory urge), absence seizures (see ➨ p. 252).

Management

- Assess and treat comorbidities: ADHD—methylphenidate hydrochloride; OCD—CBT; mood/anxiety—monitor, ask about suicidal thoughts and refer to CAMHS.
- Management is determined by impact of tics on psychosocial functioning.
- Psychoeducation regarding prognosis and consider watchful waiting.
- Support groups/charities.
- Avoid caffeine (may exacerbate tics).
- Try regular exercise, relaxation techniques, provide safe place in which to tic.
- Practising tics, e.g. before school: deliberate tic repetition for several minutes resulting in tic free period of >1 hour.
- First-line treatment: behavioural intervention training which includes relaxation practice and habit reversal training—psychologist led, increase tic awareness and generate alternative behaviours.
- Second-line treatment is medication: has limited impact with 35–50% tic reduction. Aim to reduce psychosocial impairment. Assess response to medication over several months as tics naturally wax and wane.
  - Alpha agonists—clonidine, guanfacine. Reduce motor tics > vocal tics. Monitor pulse, blood pressure, sedation.
  - Risperidone or aripiprazole (atypical antipsychotics). Greater evidence base but more side effects than clonidine.
  - Alternatives: haloperidol, topiramate, botulinum toxin injections—for adolescents with severe localized tics.
  - Note: alpha agonists and antipsychotics can cause QT prolongation.

Prognosis

Severity peaks 8–12 years, average duration 4–6 years, usually improves during adolescence with 80% significant reduction in tics by age 18. Poor prognosis associated with comorbidity. Increased risk of mood and anxiety disorders with severe tics.

Further resources

Tourettes Action (UK charity): ℔ http://www.tourettes-action.org.uk/
Yale Global Tic Severity Scale: ℔ https://dcf.psychiatry.ufl.edu/files/2011/06/TIC-YGTSS-Clinician.pdf

Conduct disorder and oppositional defiant disorder

Definitions

Conduct disorder (DSM-5)/conduct-dissocial disorder (ICD-11)
- Repetitive, persistent behaviour where basic rights of others or age-appropriate societal norms are violated. Includes aggression (towards people/animals), destruction property, deceitfulness, theft, serious violation rules.
- Causes significant impairment—personal, family, social, or educational.
- Behaviour pattern >12 months.

Oppositional defiant disorder
- Defiant, disobedient, provocative, or spiteful behaviour, more frequent than peers.
- Prevailing, persistent angry or irritable mood; frequent severe temper outburst; headstrong, argumentative, and defiant behaviour.
- Severity causes significant impairment in personal, family, social, or education.
- Lasts >6 months.

Epidemiology

- CD: 4–9%, ♂:♀ 3:1, increased prevalence in lower socioeconomic groups.
- ODD: 1–16%, ♂ > ♀ in young children, ♂ = ♀ older children/adolescents. Onset usually by 8 years.

Aetiology

Complex interaction of multiple risk factors especially inherited vulnerability, negative parenting, and environmental factors.
- *Biological*: temperament (lack guilt, empathy), dyslexia, LD, low IQ, ADHD, CNS disorders, autonomic under-arousal, abnormal prefrontal cortex, prenatal toxin exposure, neurotransmitter abnormalities (serotonin, noradrenaline, dopamine), low cortisol, high testosterone, family history of CD/substance abuse/ADHD.
- *Psychosocial*: parenting style (harsh, inconsistent, ineffective, rejection of child), insecure/disorganized attachment, parental mental illness and substance misuse, family dysfunction, socioeconomic disadvantage, poor social information processing.

Differential diagnosis and comorbidity

ADHD, substance abuse, adjustment disorder, anxiety, depression, developmental disorder, LD, psychosis, chronic paediatric illness. ASD (two-thirds of children excluded from primary school have social and communication problems).

Assessment

- Multiple informants to assess behaviour in different settings (family, school, community, legal system—often low rate of agreement between informants).
- Empathic non-judgemental engagement of the young person to elicit their views and motivation for change.
- Description of current behaviour problems: nature, onset, duration, frequency, context, functional impact. Children may be reluctant to discuss their externalizing behaviour.
- Children with ODD are more likely to be oppositional/defiant around people they know.
- Comprehensive history to identify aetiological factors (particularly family history, social history, and parenting style and parents' response to the behaviours).
- Identify comorbid conditions especially ADHD, substance misuse (very common and can improve symptoms and prognosis if treated).
- Physical examination with attention to neurological factors.
- Psychological assessment and/or review of school reports to assess IQ, language, reading, and arithmetic skills.

Risk assessment

- Historical: violence/non-violent offending, exposure violence at home, maltreatment, parental criminality, self-harm.
- Individual: impulsivity, anger problems, low empathy, negative attitudes.
- Social: peer delinquency/rejection, coping strategies, personal support, parental management.
- Protective factors: social support, attitude regarding intervention and authority, commitment to school, personality.

(Adapted from Structured Assessment of Violence Risk in Youth (SAVRY), 2003.)

Management

- Multimodal and multilevel interventions required (child, family, school, community). One-off, short-term, fear-inducing treatments ineffective and can be harmful.
- Provide behavioural management advice (see ➜ p. 366 and p. 363).
- Parent management training: group-based training. Most effective intervention for children < 12 years. *NICE recommends*:
  - Curriculum informed by social learning theory (decreased positive reinforcement of unwanted behaviour, e.g. giving child attention when misbehaving, increased positive reinforcement of desired behaviour, selective use of punishment, e.g. time-out, loss of privileges). Reinforcement and punishment should be consistent, contingent, and immediate.
  - Individual treatment for families with especially complex needs.
  - Role play in session and homework (apply techniques to home situation between sessions).

- School: focus on positive behaviour, support parents, individual classroom support, assess learning difficulties/social and communication difficulties with educational psychologist input, social skills groups, and if mainstream education not possible then consider special educational placements.
- CAMHS input will depend upon local service arrangements and the presence of any comorbid mental illness.
- Child-focused individual interventions are only modestly effective, may not generalize and are less likely to be effective in older children (>10 years). Include CBT problem-solving skills, anger management, emotional recognition.
- Family therapy: little evidence.
- Pharmacological: no first-line medications recommended. Only use if psychological interventions inadequate to control severe behaviour, or to treat comorbidity, e.g. stimulants for ADHD, antipsychotics (risperidone, aripiprazole) for aggression.
- School-based intervention: support for language, cognitive, and social deficits. Specialist schools and residential treatments.
- Specialist foster placements for adolescents with chronic CD.

Prognosis

- Of those with ODD, 30–50% develop CD. CD persists (40%) into adulthood manifesting as antisocial personality disorder, substance abuse, mood disorders, criminality, interpersonal difficulties, incomplete schooling, and unemployment.
- Poor prognosis: early onset (<10 years), number and severity of behaviours, late treatment intervention, comorbidity (especially ADHD).

Further resources

National Institute for Health and Care Excellence. Antisocial behaviour and conduct disorders in children and young people overview. Available at: ℘ https://pathways.nice.org.uk/pathways/antisocial-behaviour-and-conduct-disorders-in-children-and-young-people

Encopresis and faecal soiling

Definition

The passage of normal stool in an inappropriate place (clothing, floor), ≥1 events/month for ≥3 months' duration. Can be involuntary or intentional. Occurs in a child at least 4 years old. Behaviour not caused by substance (e.g. laxative) or medical condition, except through a mechanism involving constipation (adapted from DSM-5).

Classification

- *Primary*: bowel control never established.
- *Secondary*: independent bowel control achieved for at least 6 months.
- *Retentive*: leads to constipation and overflow incontinence. Some consider this subtype more appropriately termed faecal soiling than encopresis.
- *Non-retentive*: deliberate soiling in inappropriate places. 'True' encopresis and the minority of cases.

Epidemiology

- 3:1 ♂:♀.
- 5% of 4-year-olds, 1–2% of 7-year-olds, and 1% of 11-year-olds.

Aetiology

- *Primary*: LD, dyspraxia, poor toilet training.
- *Retentive*: toilet fears/phobia in anxious children especially in public places, poor toilet training, multiple causes of constipation and painful defecation.
- *Non-retentive*: regression secondary to psychosocial stressors, psychological distress that the child is unable to communicate directly, sexual abuse, conduct issues. There can be inappropriate deposition of faeces and smearing.

Assessment

▶ Very important to exclude maltreatment and possible organic cause (anorectal malformations, Hirschsprung disease, neurological disorders, nutritional problem, thyroid disorders, inflammatory bowel disease, medication side effects) by history, physical examination, and investigations.

Enquire about

- When are bowels open, consistency of stools, discomfort, drinks/day, and fibre intake. Nature and pattern of soiling, antecedents, family reactions, and impact of attempted treatments.
- Environmental influence, e.g. bullying or anxiety about passing stool at school can lead to encopresis only occurring at home.
- Child's attitudes and access to toilets and reasons for avoidance, e.g. fear of monsters in the toilet.
- Developmental age of child.
- Stress or negative life events, e.g. parental separation, birth of sibling, starting school.

- Presence of emotional or psychiatric disorders, e.g. anxiety, phobia, ADHD, ODD, or CD.
- Presence of regressive behaviour including separation difficulties, clinging.
- Family dysfunction and parent–child conflict (can be cause and effect).
- Secondary low self-esteem, guilt, and shame.

Management

- Psychoeducation: explain it is a common condition, aim for bowels to be open at least 3 times/week and ideally 1–3 bowel movements/day. Family to keep record of stool frequency and consistency (use the Bristol Stool Form Chart).
- Address specific stressors and social difficulties: both causative and consequences, e.g. to reduce shame child should be able to leave class without asking to and have access to a private toilet.
- Treat constipation with fluids (6–8 drinks/day), dietary fibre (≥5 portions of vegetables/fruit), exercise, and stimulant and softening laxatives (see ➜ p. 440).
- Behavioural intervention: cooperation of both parent and child essential. Reduce punitive measures (they often increase soiling). If accident occurs, parents should reassure and help. Praise and reward charts (star chart) for appropriate passage of stool. Regular post-prandial toileting for 10 minutes without pressure to produce stool. Reading book or special toy just for use on toilet. Ensure toilet is comfortable and use a step to support feet.
- Family may require additional support from HVs or social services to manage behavioural programme.
- Graded exposure and rewards for toilet phobia.
- Family therapy techniques: externalization of the problem as 'Sneaky Poo'. The child and family describe how 'Sneaky Poo' causes them both difficulties, helping to reduce scapegoating, and work together to 'out sneak Sneaky Poo'. Humour is used in this approach. Useful if there is an aggressive (smearing) component to encopresis. See website in 'Further resources'.

Prognosis

The majority of uncomplicated cases resolve by adolescence. Poorer prognosis associated with non-retentive subtype, and significant family or social dysfunction.

Further resources

ERIC (The Children's Bowel & Bladder Charity; UK children's charity dealing with bedwetting, daytime wetting, constipation, soiling, and potty training): ℘ http://www.eric.org.uk/
Heins T, Ritchie K (1988). Beating Sneaky Poo: Ideas for Faecal Soiling, 2nd ed. Leaflet free to download at: ℘ http://www.dulwichcentre.com.au/beating-sneaky-poo-2.pdf

Enuresis

Definition

The DSM-5 criteria for enuresis is as follows:
- Repeated voiding of urine into bed or clothes (whether involuntary or intentional)
- Manifested by either a frequency of twice a week for at least 3 consecutive months or the presence of clinically significant distress or impairment in social, academic or occupational functioning
- Chronological/developmental age is at least 5 years
- The behaviour is not due to medications (e.g. diuretic, antipsychotic or SSRI) or a medical condition (e.g. polyuria, loss of consciousness, diabetes, etc.)

Classification

- Primary enuresis (85%) (never acquired bladder control).
- Secondary enuresis (15%) (achieved bladder control for at least 6 months).
- Nocturnal, diurnal, or both.

Epidemiology

- 4-year-olds: 12–25%; 8-year-olds: 7–10%; 12-year-olds: 2–3%.
- <12 years old: ♂:♀ 1.5:1.
- >12 years old: ♂ = ♀.
- Nocturnal enuresis more common than daytime enuresis.

Aetiology/associations

- Genetic (70% have first-degree relative with functional enuresis), learning difficulties, behavioural and emotional difficulties, lower socioeconomic status, institutionalized care, abuse, psychosocial stressors, and/or psychiatric disorder, e.g. ADHD.
- Secondary enuresis is most commonly associated with psychosocial factors.

Assessment

- Essential to exclude organic cause of urinary symptoms (urinary tract infection, diabetes, constipation, structural abnormality, neurological problem, medication) by history, physical examination, and urinalysis.
- Consider how much urine is being produced, bladder capacity, and child's ability to respond/wake to full bladder.

Enquire about
- Toileting patterns (including bowel habit) and fluid intake.
- Onset, frequency, and timing of wetting.
- Anxiety and level of access to school toilet.
- Keep diary—to monitor progress and record degree of wetting, e.g. '+' pants/PJ, '++' clothes/bottom sheet, and '+++' puddle/top sheet.
- Sleep and sleeping arrangements.
- Previous interventions, including duration, consistency of approach, and degree of success.
- Impact on the child (guilt, bullied, loss confidence) and family (disturbed sleep, frustration, blame child). Consider motivation for change.
- Aetiological factors as previously listed.

Management

- Psychoeducation and support groups.
- Practical measures: hygiene, mattress protectors, disposable products, and changes of clothes. Praise for even small improvements.
- See NICE guidelines on bedwetting in children and young adults.

Nocturnal enuresis

- Behavioural management: avoid punishment and criticism; reward charts and praise for appropriate fluid intake and toileting during daytime, utilizing toilet prior to sleep, taking medication, or utilizing an enuresis alarm.
- Enuresis alarm: 'bell and pad' sounds an alarm when damp. Slow response but reduced rate of relapse compared to medication. Assess response after 4 weeks. Terminate use after 2 weeks without wetting.
- Medication:
  - Desmopressin (synthetic antidiuretic hormone): first-line medication from 5 years old. Low risk of side effects. Nasal spray, tablet, and melt. Rapid onset of action. Review after 1–2 weeks and consider dose increase. Consider 1-week medication holiday after 3 months to review response. Recommence if wetting returns.
- Second-line medication:
  - Oxybutynin (anticholinergic): short-acting. Elixir or tablet. Can be combined with desmopressin.
  - Imipramine (tricyclic antidepressant with anticholinergic effects): low dose 3 hours before bedtime. Toxic in overdose so avoid in DSH and depression. Review after 3 months.

Diurnal enuresis

- Psychoeducation, behavioural programme with regular toilet times, and bladder retraining.
- Oxybutynin (anticholinergic)—relaxes bladder and delays initial desire to void.
- Bladder scan, urine flow test if persists.
- A MDT approach may be required.

Prognosis

Improves with age. Prevalence in 16-year-olds 1–3%. Small proportion will continue into adulthood.

Further resources

Bladder and Bowel UK: ✆ https://www.bbuk.org.uk/
ERIC (The Children's Bowel & Bladder Charity; UK children's charity dealing with bedwetting, daytime wetting, constipation, soiling, and potty training): ✆ http://www.eric.org.uk/
National Institute for Health and Care Excellence. Bedwetting in children and young people overview. Available at: ✆ https://pathways.nice.org.uk/pathways/bedwetting-in-children-and-young-people

Preschool behavioural problems

Although behavioural issues are common in preschool children, the proportion of children with serious difficulties is low. It can be challenging to categorize the difficulties as they may not meet diagnostic criteria for the conduct, hyperactivity, and emotional disorders seen in older children.

Common issues

- Feeding and sleeping problems are the commonest. Emotional behaviour (fears, worries, disruptive (aggression, tantrums)), relationship issues, concentration and overactivity, wetting and soiling, and comfort habits (rocking, head banging, masturbation).
- Moderate/severe behavioural problems in 7–9%, mild in 13%.
- Comfort habits, sleep, appetite, and toileting problems are usually transient; however, others often persist. Problems identified age 3 persisted to age 8 in 73% of boys and 48% of girls.
- A history of preschool fears and worries, overactivity, and disruptive behaviour is often present in older children with emotional disorders, ADHD, and ODD/CD respectively.

Assessment and management

- Consider aetiology of presentation (biological, psychological, and social). Obtain thorough developmental history, information about family background, life events, and the average day at home.
- Where problems are part of a psychiatric disorder management, proceed as described in the relevant chapters.
- Physical symptoms are often present, e.g. stomach aches with emotional issues. However, do consider if a physical disorder could be causing or exacerbating the behavioural issues.
- Consider who wants change (parents, nursery staff, child). What does the child want? How will you know when enough change has been achieved?
- Establish the parents' view of 'normal behaviour' as this can vary dramatically between families. Is it developmentally appropriate behaviour being pathologized and by whom? Consider the parents' mental health and childhood experiences.
- Consider the severity of the behaviour, pattern (present in different environments with variety adults/children), associations with change, and impact of behaviour on child. Use behaviour diary/questionnaires.
- Is more information or support required from other sources, e.g. social services, nursery staff, or behaviour support services?
- If problems are possibly transient than intervention may be unnecessary. Consider watch and wait, depending on severity.
- If the behaviour does not require intervention at present, consider that it may be an early warning sign of future difficulties, e.g. autism.
- Behavioural modification approach (for management of behavioural problems, see ➜ pp. 412–13) is the mainstay of treatment.

Disruptive behaviour

Includes attentional and oppositional problems, ADHD, and ODD.
Common problem in early childhood (8%). ♂ > ♀ in >3-year-olds.

- Aetiological factors: individual factors, e.g. child temperament, ineffective parenting strategies (low-quality parent–child interactions, inconsistent/harsh/unresponsive parenting), low-quality and high-volume day care, other factors as for CD (see ➔ pp. 306–8).
- Co-occurrence of ADHD and oppositional problems associated with persistence of problems into adolescence.
- Management: HV support, self-help parent behavioural management books/internet, and parenting programmes.

Sleep difficulties

(Also see ➔ pp. 466–8 for sleep disorders and management.)

Occur in approximately one-third of 0–3-year-olds. Large spread of normal sleep variations depending on parental attitudes and tolerance. Takes >1 hour to settle 6%, frequently wakes 10%, sleeps with parents 10%.

Insufficient sleep

- Circadian rhythm sleep disorders: causes include chaotic bedtime routine, ADHD, and LD.
- Treatment includes behavioural approach to re-establishing appropriate bedtime routine (internet and local support), specialist sleep clinic, and melatonin.
- Upper airway obstruction: causes include tonsillar hypertrophy, obesity, and structural abnormality. Associated with daytime somnolence and decreased attention.
- Consider other physical causes: threadworms, enuresis, or eczema.

Parasomnias

- Night terrors: child wakes a few hours after sleep onset, afraid, inconsolable, partially or unresponsive to attempts to communicate. Child does not recall the disruption next morning. (Different to nightmares, which occur later in night, child is consolable, responsive to parent, and may recall details on waking.) Management: wake child 15 minutes before terror usually occurs. Usually effective within a few nights.
- Somnambulism (sleep walking).

Eating/feeding difficulties

(See ➔ pp. 436–7.)

Feeding problems are the most common behavioural problem in children <5 years.

- Exclude physical causes.
- Consider meal (type of food offered, timing meals, seating, environment), child's behaviour (faddy, sensory processing issues regarding texture and taste), and parents' response to child's behaviour (encouragement, frustration, punitive).
- Children with ASD can often have sensory processing issues and rigidity regarding food.

Food refusal
- Reduced appetite 11%, faddy 12%, and both 14.7%.
- Possible means of child asserting independence.
- Multifactorial aetiology: child temperament, parenting skills, family stress, feeding experiences, parental anxiety over poor intake leading to bribes or increased attention, and child learning to manipulate parents.
- Management: eat as a family to remove focus on the child, consider distractions—turning TV off/on, remove conflict and manage parental anxiety, offer balanced meal and remove without comment if not eaten, aim for a graded approach to increase food intake, praise for eating, and reduce intake between meals.

Pica
- Consumption of non-food items, e.g. plastic, paint, faeces, dirt. Associated with autism (see ➲ pp. 114–25), learning difficulties (see ➲ pp. 136–41), adverse social situations, and poor parental supervision.
- Consider causes and consequences: iron deficiency anaemia, vitamin deficiency, elevated lead levels (paint consumption), toxoplasmosis, bowel obstruction. Complete physical examination.
- Consider developmental stage of child, <2 years eating non-digestible substances more common.
- Treat with a graded feeding plan, review safety of child environment, reduce child boredom, and consider dietician input.

Further resources

Cerebra (sleep advice service): ⅍ https://cerebra.org.uk/get-advice-support/sleep-advice-service/

Bullying

Definition

Intentional use of power and aggression that is repeated against another to cause distress or exert control. The power imbalance between bully and victim can be perceived or actual, physical, psychological, or social. Bullying can be direct or indirect, physical, or verbal.

- *Direct*: hitting, kicking, property destruction, sexual harassment, taunting, name calling.
- *Indirect*: exclusion from a group, manipulation of friendships, spreading rumours, cyberbullying (internet, text/video messaging, social media).

Epidemiology

Bullying typically occurs at school. Prevalence is highest in boys in primary and early secondary school but decreases in both sexes with age. Boys engage more in physical and verbal bullying, and indirect bullying is more prevalent in girls.

Characteristics of children who bully: aggressive, hot temperament, positive attitude to violence, lack empathy, home environment characterized by domestic violence, lack of parental affection and involvement. Antisocial personality disorder or ADHD may contribute to behaviour.

Characteristics of victims of bullying: quiet, anxious, unassertive, low self-esteem, physically weak or disabled, obese, poor social skills, socially isolated (few and poor-quality friendships), over-protective/enmeshed family. Consider victim's sex/gender, race/ethnicity, and sexual orientation.

Note: there is no one clinical type of bully or victim and some children alternate between the two ('bully-victims' or reactive bullies).

Physical and psychosocial health problems associated with bullying

- Symptoms seen in both bullies and victims:
  - Physical signs/symptoms: bruises, headache, stomach ache, symptoms often present on school mornings/Sunday night.
  - Psychosomatic symptoms (difficulty sleeping especially if school is the next day, bed-wetting).
  - Depression, anxiety, suicidal thoughts.
- Children who bully may misuse alcohol or substances and drop out of school. Victims may demonstrate school refusal or absenteeism and a drop in academic performance. 'Bully-victims' may experience the highest level of pathology.
- Belongings becoming lost or damaged, and money/valued objects can be requested or disappear from the family home.
- Can persist into adulthood.

Screening and assessment

Given the high prevalence, substantial health and psychosocial consequences of bullying, and the reluctance of victims to seek help, it is important that professionals are attentive to identifying children involved. Appropriate intervention can minimize short- and long-term consequences.

Consider bullying in any child possessing the characteristics of bully or victim just described or who present with the described physical and psychosocial problems. Follow-up with questioning about peer relationships and school functioning:

- Have you ever been bullied? How are you bullied? What about? Where? How often?
- What do you do when others pick on you? Have you ever told a teacher?
- How do you feel when you are bullied?

Frequent and prolonged bullying associated with greater health risks. Screen for psychiatric comorbidity: depression, anxiety, CD.

Children who admit to being bullied must be believed and reassured they were right to report it. Explain the potentially serious consequences to parents and encourage them to contact the school.

Management

- Multidisciplinary approach: parents, teachers, school counsellor or nurse, and mental health specialists. Essential that all disciplines understand the potentially serious health consequences and need for early intervention.
- Hate crime (crime due to disability, identity, race, religion/belief, sexual orientation) can be reported to school staff and the police.
- School should follow an anti-bullying policy.
- Online abuse: report abusive posts/videos to the social media companies as soon as possible and request removal. Online gaming bullying—ensure games are age appropriate; use closed virtual groups.
- Block calls/texts from specified numbers rather than removing child's mobile.
- Address relationship difficulties, e.g. social and cognitive skills training, anger management, assertiveness training, and treating psychiatric comorbidity.

Further resources

Anti-Bullying Network (not-for-profit company): http://www.antibullying.net/
NSPCC (UK charity providing information and support for children and carers): https://www.nspcc.org.uk/what-is-child-abuse/types-of-abuse/bullying-and-cyberbullying/
Parentline Plus (advice to parents regarding bullying): http://www.familyandparenting.org/ or helpline ☎ 0808 800 2222.
Thinkuknow (UK organization to protect children on- and offline with age-appropriate information): https://www.thinkuknow.co.uk/
Young Minds (UK charity): https://youngminds.org.uk/find-help/feelings-and-symptoms/bullying/

School refusal

Emotionally based school avoidance.

Definition and clinical features

- Severe difficulty in attending school associated with emotional distress.
- Presentation varies with age. Children: somatic symptoms (GI, muscular, autonomic), tantrums, self-harm. Adolescents: anxiety and mood disorders (see → pp. 338–40).
- Onset can be acute or gradual. Refusal can be complete or partial.
- Explicit desire to not attend school, no attempt to conceal non-attendance.
- Willing to complete homework.

► Note contrast with truancy: lack school-related anxiety, conceal non-attendance from parents, intermittent absence, avoid going home, disinterested in schoolwork (see → pp. 650–1).

Epidemiology

- Incidence 1–2%. ♂ = ♀, mean age 11 years.
- No association with intelligence or socioeconomic level.
- Peaks rates at school transitions (5/6 years and 11/12 years).

Aetiology

- *Predisposing*: separation anxiety, social phobia.
- *Precipitating*: starting new school or following breaks from school (holidays or illness), life events (parental illness or separation, moving home), school fears, bullying (especially cyberbullying), tests, group work, teacher relationship.
- *Maintaining*: fear of explaining absence to peers, secondary gain (access to parent, TV, computer at home).

Assessment

- Presentation: tears, aggression, refusal to get ready, insomnia, psychosomatic illness.
- Frequency and timing of symptoms—present outside school hours?
- School-related fears and other aetiological factors.
- Family history of dysfunction (conflict, enmeshment, ineffectual discipline), school absence in siblings, family's response to school refusal.
- Parental anxiety and illness.
- School information: academic and attendance reports, peer and teacher relationships, educational psychologist reports.
- Exclude physical cause of somatic symptoms.
- Look for early warning signs—arriving late for school, conceal absence from parents, drop off in behaviour and academic performance.
- Tools: School Refusal Assessment Scale—Revised, Strengths and Difficulties Questionnaire.

Comorbidity: anxiety disorders (separation anxiety disorder, simple phobia, generalized), CD, mood disorders, ADHD, learning difficulties, social interaction difficulties, ASD.

Differential diagnosis: truancy (affects 6% of children), mixed group (0.5% truancy + emotionally based school refusal), child caring for ill parent.

Management

- Take a medical history and conduct a physical examination. If appropriate, reassure parents that there is no physical illness.
- Emphasize the benefit of early reintegration to school. A coordinated, consistent approach involving the child, both parents, and school is essential.
- Identify a teacher to assist with liaison who can meet the child and parent at home.

Behavioural approaches

- Work collaboratively with the family and school. Acknowledge that the family may have been struggling with attendance for some time, leading to numerous disagreements and parental guilt. Parents may be worn out and feeling hopeless. Let them know you and the school have been through this before, and you will work together.
- Aim for a graded return for chronic school non-attendance. School will need to flex normal school rules; consider later arrival time, earlier leaving, and part-time attendance. Everyone should know what to expect and when with the school.
- The child should be welcomed to school with identified staff member, consider separate room away from classroom, allow warm-up period, don't push work when initially at school. Identify a safe place at school.
- Regular, brief, time-out sessions during day.
- Develop a system to communicate to teacher that anxiety is increasing, e.g. use of cards, hand sign such as touching over heart with fingers, thumbs up/middle/down, exit cards, traffic light colours.
- Develop a plan for break times—prefer quiet areas, company of one or two friends, or in a noisy playground?
- Start on Sunday nights—plan for Monday morning at home, relaxing activities, and appropriate sleep.
- Consider the incentives to remain at home (computer, TV, no homework, parental attention). Reward (child and parents) with any successes no matter how small.
- Rapid return (flooding): only appropriate for short absence and can be very stressful for children and parents.

Anxiety management

- Use in conjunction with a behavioural approach. Exploring the child's fears and recommending relaxation techniques.
- 'Self-help' literature for parents.
- Social skills training.
- Refer to specialist CAMHS if mental illness, severe anxiety, or protracted school refusal.

Education

- Schools can contact educational psychologists for consultation.
- Schools can refer to welfare/school attendance officers if parental condoned absence is suspected.

- Home tuition at home, at neutral site (library), or online tuition.
- Consider off-site pupil referral unit/learning centre in prolonged school refusal with comorbid mental illness. Note: risk of encouraging school non-attendance or worsening anxiety.

Prognosis

- Short-term difficulties: peer and family relationships, reduced academic performance, isolation, impaired self-esteem.
- 70% return to school. One in three experience emotional or social difficulties as adults. Increased risk of unemployment as adult.
- Poor prognosis associated with adolescent onset, duration >2 years, lower IQ, comorbid depression.

Attachment disorders

John Bowlby researched the importance of the relationship between a child and their caregiver in the early years of life. The quality of the relationship (attachment) impacted the child's functioning and was a blueprint for the child's future relationships.

Definitions

Secure attachment: primary caregiver provides safe base for exploration. Child readily comforted if distressed. Child seeks and maintains contact with mother after period of separation.

Attachment disorder: significant abnormalities in social relationships, evident before age 5, associated with emotional disturbance, reactive to changes in patterns of rearing. Two clinical syndromes: reactive (inhibited) type and disinhibited type.

Clinical features

Reactive type
- Fearfulness and hypervigilance, non-responsive to comforting.
- Look miserable, lack emotional responsiveness.
- Limited initiation of/response to social interaction.
- Ambivalent or contradictory social responses especially on parting or reunion.
- Growth failure.
- Associated with severe parental abuse/neglect (caution in making the diagnosis in the absence of abuse/neglect).

Disinhibited type
- Clingy infants, attention seeking and indiscriminately friendly children.
- Inappropriate approaches to unfamiliar adults, willingness to 'go-off' with stranger without checking back with primary caregiver, may seek physical interaction with stranger.
- Difficulty in forming close, confiding relationships with peers.
- Unconcerned by changes in caregivers.
- Associated with institutional rearing from birth, extremely frequent changes in caregivers, absence of primary caregiver.

Both types: overactivity, reduced concentration, learning difficulties, aggression to self and others, low self-esteem.

Epidemiology

Prevalence low in general population but disinhibited attachment is significantly increased if institutional care from birth.

Risk factors

- *Caregiver*: young, isolated, inexperienced, depressed, substance addiction, family dysfunction, poverty.
- *Child*: difficult temperament (e.g. anxious), sensory impairment, ID.

Assessment

- Quality (appropriate, indiscriminate, inappropriate), level, frequency, and pervasiveness of social interactions.
- Quality of care by current caregivers.
- Combination of caregiver interview and observed interactions including a degree of distress to activate child's need for caregiver (e.g. novel/ scary toy).
  - Does s/he relate preferentially to parents rather than strangers?
  - Does s/he refer back to parents in play?
  - Does s/he move away and play independently?
  - Evidence of stranger anxiety?
  - Disinhibited behaviour, e.g. attempting to sit on clinician's lap.
- Manchester child attachment story task (MAST)—uses puppets to assess quality of attachment.
- Note: important to distinguish attachment disorder from ASD. Latter associated with lack/reduced capacity for social relationships, difficulties do not remit in normal rearing environment, coexisting language disorder, circumscribed interests.

Differential diagnosis

ASD, ADHD, anxiety disorders, PTSD, ODD, or selective mutism.

Interventions

- Social services input is often required due to the association with inadequate parental care.
- Provide a safe and emotionally secure care setting for the child, with consistent, positive emotional responses and appropriate behavioural management from caregivers. Young children can improve in enhanced caregiving environment.
- Enhance caregiver's understanding of child's behaviour, emotional sensitivity, and responses to child.
- Severely affected children may require residential placement.
- CAMHS referral to assess and treat comorbidity (anxiety, PTSD, ADHD).

Prognosis

- Enhanced caregiving improves reactive type; however, interpersonal difficulties often persist.
- Disinhibited type persists in a significant proportion despite enhanced caregiver environment.
- Increased risk of mental illness in adolescence and adulthood.
- Enhances to caregiving before age 2 years improves prognosis.

Consequences of child maltreatment

The consequences of child maltreatment are multiple, varied, and often persist into adulthood despite cessation of the abuse. It can be difficult to clearly distinguish between cause, effect, and confounding factors. Maltreatment and its consequences share common risk factors. Which consequences are a direct result of maltreatment and which may have resulted from the disordered family environment?

The outcomes of different types of maltreatment (see ➔ pp. 560–1)—physical, emotional, sexual, and neglect—are very similar (possibly due to the overlap between different types of abuse):

Physical

- Non-organic failure to thrive, psychosocial short stature.
- Impaired brain development:
  - Impaired physical, mental, emotional development.
  - Chronic stress → hyperarousal → vulnerability to sleep disturbance, psychiatric disorder.
- Sexually transmitted diseases.

Cognitive

- Decreased verbal and non-verbal ability and decreased academic achievement.
- Consequence of neglect > abuse.
- Combination of prenatal and postnatal (e.g. decreased nutrition) factors and decreased stimulation (decreased exposure to language and fewer opportunities for cognitive development).

Interpersonal difficulties

- Insecure and disorganized attachment often persist into adulthood.
- Decreased empathy.
- Decreased trust and more likely to attribute hostile intent in others.
- Decreased peer relationships and decreased ability to initiate and maintain relationships.
- Increased negative and conflictual behaviour even with close friends.
- Increased aggression (secondary to hyperarousal, paranoia, and decreased empathy).

Behavioural problems

- Delinquency, teen pregnancy, juvenile and adult criminality, and violence.
- Risk of juvenile arrest increased by 59%, adult arrest by 28%.
- Hoarding food. Overeating.
- Self-soothing when stressed: rocking, head banging, self-injury, masturbation.

Emotional dysregulation

- Withdrawal, emotional blunting, emotional lability.
- Anger.
- Low self-worth.

Psychiatric disorder

- Depression, anxiety, EDs ($♀ > ♂$), PTSD, dissociative disorder, borderline personality disorder, alcohol and substance misuse, ADHD, CD ($♂ > ♀$).
- Self harm($♀ > ♂$), suicidal behaviour.
- 80% have at least one psychiatric diagnosis by 21 years.

Intergenerational transmission of maltreatment

About 30% of abused children become abusive parents.

Additional consequences of sexual maltreatment

- Guilt, feeling responsible for abuse or family break-up.
- Anxiety, nightmares, and PTSD (21–48%).
- Helplessness and hopelessness.
- Inappropriate sexualized behaviour (sexualized play, seductive behaviour to strangers, public masturbation) → prostitution.
- Anxiety regarding sexual orientation ($♂ > ♀$) difficulty with adult sexual relationships.

Factors increasing the impact of maltreatment

- Prolonged, frequent, coercive, violence, penetrative.
- Close relationship with abuser, denial of abuse by abuser.
- Response of non-abusive carer (believe/reject).

Factors diminishing the consequences of maltreatment

- *Individual factors*: 'resilience' (self-esteem, optimism, intelligence, creativity, independence).
- *Community factors*: access to caring adult, neighbourhood and family stability, positive social relationships, access to healthcare.

Management

- Range of consequences which require a range of services and interventions. Social services, school, and CAMHS support.
- Assess, document, and manage risk of the child and other children.
- Ensure safety of child and treat child in context of family.
- Use age-appropriate information for the child and maximize child's control and participation in treatment decisions.
- Psychological debriefing should not routinely be used to reduce the risk of developing anxiety, depression, or PTSD.
- Parental/carer interventions: aim to promote carer/child relationships by enhancing carer communication skills, empathy, and emotional availability. Parent–child interaction therapy, for physical abuse/neglect, with direct coaching of carers while interacting with child.
- Trauma-focused CBT or interpersonal therapy for PTSD (see → pp. 358–9).
- Manage and treat emotional, behavioural, and psychiatric disorders.
- Consider pharmacological interventions only in specialist (mental health) settings.
- Neuropsychology testing to identify cognitive strengths, weaknesses, and assist with enhancing school performance.

Further resources

MOSAC (UK charity supporting non-abusing parents and carers of sexually abused children): ℜ http://www.mosac.org.uk/

WHO guidelines for the health sector response to child maltreatment: ℜ https://www.who.int/publications/i/item/who-guidelines-for-the-health-sector-response-to-child-maltreatment

Depression

ICD-11 diagnostic criteria

- Symptoms present almost daily for >2 weeks.
- Core symptoms: low mood or diminished pleasure and interest (anhedonia).
- Additional symptoms: decreased concentration, feelings of worthlessness or guilt, hopelessness, recurrent thoughts of death or suicide, changed appetite or sleep, psychomotor agitation or retardation, decreased energy.
- Severity determined by nature of symptoms and impact on daily functioning (school, home, social):
  - *Mild*: functioning with some, but not considerable, difficulty in some areas.
  - *Moderate*: considerable difficulty in several areas of functioning. Possible psychotic symptoms.
  - *Severe*: very limited functioning in all domains. Psychotic symptoms may occur.
- Presentation in younger children: describe low mood or guilt less frequently than adolescents. Presentation may be 'atypical' with irritability, anger, somatic complaints (abdominal pain), eating difficulties, and school difficulties. Death and suicide themes may be present in play and drawings.

Epidemiology

- Children: prevalence <3% ♀:♂ 1:1. Adolescents: prevalence 2–8%, ♀:♂ 2:1.
- Risk factors: genetic (heritability 40%), low female birth weight, early-onset female puberty, late-onset male puberty, physical illness, illicit substance use, family dysfunction, traumatic life events.

Assessment

Interview child with parents and then alone. Enquire about:
- Impact of mood on academic and social functioning.
- Decreased self-esteem, guilt; negative views of oneself, future, and the world.
- Important: explore self-harm, suicide plans, and attempts (for suicide and SH see ➔ pp. 334–6). Social media use including support, cyber-bullying, pro-self-harm/suicide websites.
- Preparation for death: written will, given away possessions, 'signed off' to online friends.
- Mood swings and hypomania (increased energy, reduced sleep, impulsiveness, rapid speech).
- Recent life events and relationship difficulties.
- Family history of mental illness.
- Family capacity to cope.
- Illicit substance and alcohol use.

Instruments: Mood and Feelings Questionnaire, Birleson Depression Self-Rating Scale, Child Depression Inventory, Beck Depression Inventory.

Physical examination: chronic physical illnesses can cause or exacerbate depression. Consider anaemia, hypothyroidism, diabetes, medication side effects. Look for evidence of self-harm. Consider the impact of weight and acne on self-esteem.

Comorbidity: CD, anxiety disorders, illicit substance use, ADHD, attachment disorders.

Differential diagnosis: anxiety disorders, acute stress reaction, bipolar affective disorder, organic conditions.

Management

- The management and the urgency of a referral to specialist services will be dependent upon the degree of risk and the severity of depression.
- Early consultation with mental health services for advice.
- A multimodal approach is required with support for child and family.
- Psychoeducation regarding nature of depression and advice on keeping child safe (removing sharps, medication, and ensure family has emergency contact details for GP).
- Clear plan for family and child on how they can seek out-of-hours help or escalate a referral to mental health team if there is a deterioration in mood or increase in risk.
- Use self-help websites and books.
- Schedule in daily activities that promote sense of achievement and pleasure. 'Keep busy' (activity scheduling: TV, drawing, favourite music, walks, exercise), 'look after yourself' (regular healthy eating and sleep hygiene), and talk to someone (family, school counsellor/nurse, youth worker).
- Consider safety of child in different environments; consider risks at school, communicate these with teachers, and explore additional support from staff.
- Mild episode:
  - Self-help websites/books and/or counselling.
  - Consultation with a probable referral to mental health team.
- Moderate or severe episode:
  - Refer to mental health team as soon as possible for treatment.
  - Psychological therapies (CBT, interpersonal psychotherapy, family therapy).
  - Use fluoxetine in combination with therapy for rapid response or if insufficient improvement with therapy.
  - Alternative SSRIs with/without antipsychotics if no response to fluoxetine.
  - Note: commencing SSRIs may initially increase suicidal ideation and agitation.

Prognosis

- Approximately 10% of adolescent depression follows a protracted course.
- Relapse rate of 40–60% necessitates follow-up for 12 months after symptom remission or 2 years if one or more previous depressive episodes.
- Recurrence in adulthood seen in 40–70% of depressed adolescents.

Further resources

Childline: ☎ 0800 1111; ℅ http://www.childline.org.uk

Get Connected (UK confidential helpline signposting to sources of help): ☎ 0808 808 4994; ℅ http://www.getconnected.org.uk

Young Minds (UK charity to improve mental health of children and young people. Downloadable publications on depression): ℅ http://www.youngminds.org.uk/

Suicide and self-harm

Definitions

- Suicide: intentional taking of own life.
- Suicide attempt: non-fatal act undertaken with the intent of taking own life.
- Self-harm: act intending to cause harm to self but with a non-fatal outcome. Includes cutting, overdose, biting, burning skin, head banging, hair pulling, piercing, jumping from heights, dangerous driving, and other risk-taking behaviours.

Epidemiology

- SH: ♀ > ♂ 4:1. Other risk factors: looked after children, comorbid mental illness, substance use, young offenders, low socioeconomic groups, homosexual, transgender, prisoners, asylum seekers, veterans of armed forces, history of being neglected, bullied, abused (physical, emotional and sexual). Prevalence increases with age: 1.3% (5–10 years), 2.1% (11–15 years), 3.1% (13–15 years). True prevalence unknown as only minority (10–20%) present to services. One-third of young people who self-harm will go on to self-harm again.
- Suicide: third leading cause of death in 0–19-year-olds (16% of all deaths). ♂ > ♀. Males use more lethal methods (hanging, guns), females (self-poisoning). Suicide is not always preceded by self-harm.
- Suicidal phenomena rarer in <12 years, ♂ > ♀, hanging, suffocation, walking into traffic, throwing self down stairs most common (i.e. easily available, less complex but more lethal acts possibly due to less awareness of the finality of death).

Assessment

- Interview young person alone for part of the session.
- Asking about self-harm/suicide does not increase the risk of these occurring. Be clear that you may need to share information with others in order to keep young person/others safe.
- Self-harm:
  - Review purpose: one-off episode or persistent self-harm, coping strategy to relieve challenging emotions and provide temporary sense control, communicating distress/need for help, self-punishment. Aim to distinguish between self-harm as a coping strategy and self-harm with intent to die.
  - Assess injury, medical risk.
  - Explore risk of further self-harm/suicide plans.
- Suicidal thoughts:
  - Common (experienced by 15–50% of adolescents); become abnormal when associated with intent/plan.
  - Assess intensity, frequency, duration of thoughts and any protective factor preventing acting on thoughts.
- Collateral information from parents/third party essential.

▶ Review current medication. SSRIs and atomoxetine can increase agitation and suicidality, particularly during the initial 1–2 weeks of commencing treatment.

- Physical examination (for depression see ➋ pp. 330–1).
- Investigations: Scale for Suicide Ideation (SSI), Beck Scale for Suicide Ideation (BSI).
- Consider risk to themselves, risk the young person poses to others (e.g. younger siblings, peers), and risk from other people (e.g. vulnerability of young person).

Risk factors for suicidal behaviour

- Past suicide attempts (strongest predictive factor for future suicide attempt).
- Seriousness of past attempts or plans.
- Psychiatric disorder: bipolar, depression, psychosis, anxiety, CD, ODD, substance misuse and chronic physical illness (90% of completed suicides had psychiatric disorder, especially depression).
- Personality: impulsivity, aggression, perfectionism, hopelessness.
- Family: parental mood disorder, suicide attempts, substance misuse, family violence, poor supervision and communication, trauma/abuse.
- Precipitating and maintaining stressors: relationship break-up, peer difficulties, school failure, bullying (especially <12 years), feeling marginalized.
- Exposure to self-harm, e.g. in friends, media, video-sharing websites.
- Lack of coping skills or support.

Assessment of seriousness of self-harm/suicide attempt

- Purpose of attempt: suicide, escape, get attention, manipulate environment?
- Expectations of outcome act: thought act likely/possibly/unlikely to result in death?
- Objective lethality of act (does not always correspond with child's expectations of act).
- Degree of premeditation: impulsive, contemplated, research on social media and pro-self-harm/suicide websites?
- Final acts, e.g. saying good bye, giving away belongings, suicide note, planning for funeral?
- Behaviour at time of act: did they take precautions to avoid discovery? Attempt to get help afterwards?
- Ongoing suicidal ideation, regret act unsuccessful?
- What does the young person want to happen?

PATHOS overdose assessment tool (more features mean increased risk)
- *P*roblems >1 month?
- *A*lone when overdosed?
- Planed overdose for more than *T*hree hours?
- *HO*peless about future?
- *S*ad most of time prior to overdose?

Management

- Any untreated recent overdoses will require admission for physical assessment and treatment.
- Treat physical effects of self-harm, e.g. infection, medication ingestion.

- Restrict access to means of self-harm and ensure adequate parental supervision.
- Provide self-help information and access to mental health crisis lines if appropriate.
- Advise using distraction (music, mindfulness breathing, exercise, phone friend, drawing, stress ball) and talking to manage urges to self-harm. Alternatives: snap elastic bands, hold ice cubes/chilli, punch bag.
- Install hope: recovery from self-harm is possible.
- Referral for psychiatric assessment. Urgent assessment if serious intent, ongoing suicidal ideation, hopelessness, or significant symptoms of mental illness contributing to self-harm.
- CAMHS management of recurrent self-harm: treat underlying mental illness, try to avoid admission to inpatient CAMHS, CBT, dialectic behaviour therapy, improve self-esteem, and develop alternative ways to regulate emotions.

Further resources

Mood and Feelings Questionnaire (screening tool for depression, free to download): ℜ https://www.corc.uk.net/outcome-experience-measures/mood-and-feelings-questionnaire/

National Self Harm Network (UK charity, has downloadable advice leaflets for young people): ℜ http://www.nshn.co.uk

Young Minds (has information on self-harm and suicidal thoughts): ℜ https://youngminds.org.uk/find-help/feelings-and-symptoms/self-harm/

Anxiety disorders

Generalized anxiety disorder

Panic disorder

Agoraphobia

Specific phobias

Social phobia disorder

Separation anxiety disorder

Anxiety disorders

Anxiety disorders differ from normal fear and worry (common in children) in that they cause significant distress and impact the child's functioning. Normative fears change with developmental age from concrete external things (e.g. loud noises, strangers, the dark) to internalized abstract issues (e.g. social and academic performance, health). One in ten young people suffer from one or more anxiety disorders before the age of 16 years.

Generalized anxiety disorder

Excessive and unrealistic concerns about competence, past and future. Anxiety is 'free-floating' and not limited to specific circumstances. Symptoms include restlessness, irritability, poor sleep and concentration, and overactivity. Symptoms must be present most days for several weeks. Sufferers are often perfectionistic and high-reassurance seekers.

Onset in middle childhood/adolescence. Prevalence 2%. High rates of comorbidity (90%) with other anxiety disorders and depression. Poorer prognosis, often persists into adulthood.

Panic disorder

Repeated unprovoked episodes or severe anxiety with rapid onset and not restricted to any particular situation. Intense fear of impending doom, dying, losing control. Physical symptoms of anxiety are interpreted in catastrophic fashion. Onset in adolescence. $♀ > ♂$. Prevalence 3–6%.

Panic attacks are a feature of agoraphobia: fear of a panic attack occurring in a place from which escape would be difficult. Leads to anticipatory anxiety and avoidance.

Agoraphobia

Marked fear or anxiety in multiple situations where escape might be difficult, e.g. public transport, being in open spaces, in a crowd/standing in a line, being outside home alone.

Specific phobias

Marked fear that is out of proportion to the objective threat of a specific object or situation and leads to avoidance. Common phobias: animals, dark, thunderstorms, heights. Onset usually in childhood. Incidence 5%. $♀ > ♂$. Good prognosis if treated.

Social anxiety disorder

Anxiety in social situations (e.g. parties, eating, or speaking in public). Fear of scrutiny, ridicule, embarrassment, and humiliation. Can lead to avoidance of social situations despite desire for social contact. Onset in early adolescence. Prevalence 5–15%. $♀ > ♂$. Comorbidity 30–60% (anxiety disorders, mood disorders, substance misuse).

Separation anxiety disorder

Developmentally inappropriate and excessive anxiety regarding actual or anticipated separation from attachment figures or home that results in impaired functioning. Associated with sleep disturbance, nightmares, somatization, school refusal, and oppositional/defiant behaviours on separation. Occurs in 3.5% of children. ♀ > ♂. Associated with panic disorder and agoraphobia in adulthood.

Selective mutism

Consistent selectivity in speaking in social situations (typically school, public), despite speaking in other situations (typically home) with >1 month duration. May avoid eye contact or appear anxious. May nod/shake head or speak a few words. Occurs in 1/140 young children, ♀ > ♂, usually starts preschool (2–4 years), comorbidity anxiety disorders (social anxiety, separation anxiety). *Differential diagnosis*: ASD, disorder speech/language development, sensory integration dysfunction, mutism secondary to trauma/PTSD (sudden rather than gradual onset). *Management*: speech and language therapist assessment and behavioural treatment, school support (consider self-esteem, loneliness, academic impact) and treat comorbidity.

Risk factors

Inhibited temperament ×7 risk (timid, shy, emotionally restrained, reticent), parental anxiety disorder ×2 risk, genetic (25–50% heritability rates), overprotective and critical parenting styles, insecure attachment, negative life events, cognitive style (overestimate risk, underestimate coping skills).

Differential diagnosis

Adjustment disorder, acute stress reaction, PTSD, depression, ADHD, psychosis, PDD, hypothyroidism, hypoparathyroidism, migraine, asthma, caffeine, iatrogenic, endocrine and CNS disorders.

Assessment

- Differentiate unrealistic anxiety from fear of real threats, e.g. bullying. Use multiple informants and questionnaires (see 'Further resources').
- Review situations in which anxiety experienced, severity of symptoms, impact on functioning, child and family coping skills, school support, positives, and exceptions when the anxiety is not present/managed (what is different about these occasions?).

Management

- Stepped care approach with lower levels anxiety treated with psychoeducation and self-help (bibliotherapy, parent-led CBT if younger and books/computerized CBT if older); otherwise refer to CAMHS.
- CBT: first-line treatment, relaxation techniques, graded exposure to real or imagined anxiety-provoking situations, cognitive restructuring, social skills training, relapse prevention. 10–20 sessions, parents can join depending on age of child.
- Reduced evidence for the use of other psychological therapies.
- Medication: often used in combination with CBT, SSRIs (sertraline) effective in short–medium term.
- Involve parents (especially younger children): encourage consistency, avoid excessive reassurance, manage parents' anxieties/guilt.

Longitudinal course of anxiety disorders

Comorbidity with other anxiety disorders (60%), mood disorders, and substance misuse. Severe child anxiety symptoms with significant impact on functioning are associated with anxiety, mood, and substance disorders in adulthood.

Obsessive–compulsive disorder (OCD)

OCD was previously classified as an anxiety disorder but is now grouped with other obsessive disorders such as body dysmorphic disorder, hypochondriasis, and hoarding disorder.

* *Obsessions*: persistent thoughts, images, impulses (e.g. contamination, sexual thoughts, harm occurring to others) that are intrusive, distressing, time-consuming, and senseless. Recognized as one's own thoughts.
* *Compulsions*: mental or physical behaviours/rituals undertaken in an attempt to reduce the anxiety associated with obsessions (e.g. hand washing, checking, counting).

Symptoms present on most days for 2 weeks and impair functioning.

Prevalence: 0.5%. Onset in adolescence (prepubertal onset more common in boys, family history of OCD).

Aetiology: genetic vulnerability, external stressors (meningitis, head injury, PANDAS, stressful life events). Differential diagnosis: normal developmental rituals, tic disorder, Sydenham's chorea, ASD.

Management: refer to CAMHS, CY-BOCS questionnaire. CBT: exposure to intrusive thoughts coupled with response prevention, anxiety management. SSRI.

Further resources

Creswell C (2007). Overcoming Your Child's Fears and Worries: A Self-help Guide Using Cognitive Behavioural Techniques. London: Constable & Robinson.

Children's Yale–Brown Obsessive Compulsive Scale (CY-BOCS): ꙮ https://iocdf.org/wp-content/uploads/2016/04/05-CYBOCS-complete.pdf

Generalised Anxiety Disorder Assessment (GAD 7) and Revised child anxiety and depression scale (RCADS) (both free to download): ꙮ https://www.corc.uk.net/outcome-experience-measures/

Eating disorders

(See ➌ pp. 314–6 and pp. 532–5.)

It's not unusual for adolescents to consider dieting and/or to have concerns regarding weight. However, if you suspect a possible ED then refer to mental health services as soon as possible. Early intervention = better prognosis.

Anorexia nervosa

- Underweight: body mass index (BMI)-for-age under <5% centile in children and adolescents or < 85% expected for age and height (either lost or never achieved). (Note: in adults BMI <18.5.)
- Self-induced weight loss: excessive exercise, vomiting, misuse of laxatives, appetite suppressants, diuretics.
- Body image distortion: fear of fatness.
- Restricting or binge eating/purging types.

Bulimia nervosa

- Persistent preoccupation and craving for food.
- Recurrent out-of-control binges (≥1/week for ≥1 month) often associated with guilt or disgust.
- Compensatory behaviour: vomiting, laxatives, appetite suppressants, diuretics, enemas, exercise.
- Fear of 'fatness'.
- Normal weight and menses.

Binge eating disorder

Binges like bulimia nervosa but no regular compensatory behaviour.

Other specified feeding and eating disorders (OSFED)

▶ OSFED replaced DSM-5 'Eating Disorders Not Otherwise Specified' (EDNOS). OSFED is a cluster of EDs where a person does not meet all the criteria of anorexia nervosa or bulimia nervosa (up to 50% of children with ED).

▶ 'Atypical' presentation of ED more common <13 years: less binge and purging, more premorbid anxiety, ♀~♂, often move between ED diagnosis.

- Anorexia nervosa: ♀ > ♂ 10:1, onset mid teens, prevalence 0.3%.
- Bulimia nervosa: ♀ > ♂ 30:1, onset mid–late teens, prevalence 0.9%.
- Risk factors: adolescent dieting, family and twin studies support genetic component to aetiology (possible perfectionistic, harm avoidance, and rigidity traits), athletes, performers (ballet, modelling), severe life events.

Assessment

- Presentation: weight loss/growth failure of unknown cause, delayed or arrested puberty, amenorrhoea, symptoms of low weight (dizziness, syncope, fatigue, easy bruising, cold intolerance, shortness of breath, palpitations, headache, GI symptoms, menstrual irregularities), complications of low weight, weight loss associated with chronic disease.

- Obtain information from parents: degree of weight change, lying about food consumption, eating slowly, cutting up food and moving round plate, feeding to pet, eating alone, wearing disguising clothes, internet history regarding pro-eating disorder websites.
- Spend part of the session alone with child.
- The child will have been struggling with the disorder for several months or more, afraid of the consequences of informing others, and be reluctant to relinquish control. Guilt, low mood, poor self-esteem, and comorbid mental illness are common.

▶ Children with EDs are secretive, skilled at hiding signs from family and professionals, and may reassure you that eating is under control. Avoid agreeing and minimizing symptoms.

- Talk through an average day of eating and drinking, calorie-counting, and food avoidance.
- Family: very stressful for family members to manage behaviour, possible dysfunctional family interactions; history of ED, obesity, or OCD.

Physical examination for medical complications
Pale complexion, facial wasting, flat or anxious affect, muscle wasting, decreased blood pressure with postural hypotension, bradycardia, cardiac arrhythmias, murmur (mitral valve prolapse), failure to develop secondary sexual characteristics, dry skin, brittle hair, lanugo hair, cold extremities, swollen parotids, pitted dental enamel, Russell's sign (calluses on knuckles from self-induced vomiting).

Additional medical complications
Decreased: K, Mg, PO_4, Na, Glu, Ca, thyroid function tests; increased: urea, cholesterol, liver function tests. Anaemia, prolonged QT interval, oesophagitis, gastric reflux (see ➔ pp. 438–9), constipation (see ➔ pp. 440–1), cognitive deficits, growth retardation. Long term: infertility, decreased bone density (see ➔ pp. 556–7), osteoporosis.

Investigations

Screening questionnaires
- SCOFF Questionnaire:[1]
  - Do you make yourself Sick because you feel uncomfortably full?
  - Do you worry you have lost Control over how much you eat?
  - Have you recently lost more than One stone in a 3-month period?
  - Do you believe yourself to be Fat when others say you are too thin?
  - Would you say that Food dominates your life?
- 1 point for every 'yes'; >2 indicates a likely case of anorexia nervosa or bulimia, (sensitivity: 100%; specificity: 87.5 % in adults).
- Self-report questionnaires: EAT (>13 years), ChEAT (8–13 years), EDI-2.

Bloods
- FBC, urea and electrolytes, liver function tests, Ca, Mg, glucose, thyroid function tests, Fe, folate, vitamin B_{12}.

---

1 Reprinted with permission from Morgan JF, Reid F, Lacey JH. The SCOFF questionnaire: assessment of a new screening tool for eating disorders. British Medical Journal 1999; 319:1467.

- ECG if cardiovascular system signs/symptoms.
- CAMHS to determine need for pelvic ultrasound and bone densitometry.

Comorbidity

Comorbidity very common with high rates of depression and anxiety (social phobia, generalized anxiety disorder, PTSD and OCD), ASD, DSH, substance misuse (bulimia nervosa > anorexia nervosa, anabolic steroids in boys).

Differential diagnosis

See 'Comorbidity'; inflammatory bowel disease, malabsorption syndrome, hyperthyroidism, Addison disease, diabetes, malignancy, chronic infection.

Management

General

- Water or mouthwash post vomiting (brushing erodes tooth enamel).
- Psychoeducation, check bloods and refer to specialist CAMHS—sooner rather than later if organic causes are unlikely.
- Parents in denial/unaware of the eating behaviours may be reluctant to consider a psychiatric cause/referral to CAMHS. Try to avoid putting off the referral with unnecessary investigations.

Anorexia nervosa

- Family therapy 'Maudsley' approach:
  - Phase 1: parents initially take charge of meals, avoid debates regarding food at mealtimes, supportive approach.
  - Phase 2: increased weight associated with increased child responsibility for own eating.
  - Phase 3: weight restored, child development issues addressed.
- Individual sessions and dietician input.
- Eat (three meals + three snacks)/day, aim for 0.5 kg/week weight gain.
- Psychotropic medication only for comorbid mental illness—low mood and anxiety usually improves as weight increases.
- Intensive outpatient or inpatient treatment (only if failure of outpatient treatment, rapid and ongoing weight loss, medical compromise).

Bulimia nervosa

- More an individual approach due to increased age.
- CBT, fluoxetine, family therapy.

Prognosis

- Anorexia nervosa: 50% recover fully, 30% partial recovery, 20% chronic course, ~2% die by suicide or starvation, good prognostic factors: early intervention, early onset, healthy relationships friends and family.
- Bulimia nervosa: 50% recover, 25% partial recovery, 25% chronic course.

Further resources

BEAT (UK charity): ℘ http://www.b-eat.co.uk/Home

Eating disorder examination questionnaire (free download): ℘ https://www.corc.uk.net/outcome-experience-measures/eating-disorder-examination/

Somatizing disorders

Definition and classification

Psychological distress in children can often present as physical (somatic) symptoms without a demonstrable physical cause. Symptoms are not consciously produced. An identifiable stressor may or may not exist.

Three commonest somatizing disorders (adapted from DSM-5 and ICD-11):

Somatic symptom disorder (DSM-5)/bodily distress disorders (ICD-11)

- One or more distressing bodily symptoms present most days for at least several months.
- Excessive attention on the symptoms (thoughts, feelings, behaviours).
- No diagnosable medication condition can fully account for the symptoms.
- Repetitive health-seeking behaviour and the person is not reassured by appropriate clinical examination/investigations.
- Symptoms are not caused intentionally, are usually multiple, and may vary over time.
- Severity: mild, moderate, severe.

Conversion disorder (DSM-5)/dissociate neurological symptom disorder (ICD-11)

- Motor, sensory, or cognitive symptoms suggest a neurological or other general medical cause.
- The symptoms are not intentionally produced or feigned.
- The symptoms, after investigation, cannot be explained by a medical condition, substance abuse, or culturally sanctioned behaviour.
- Symptoms cause significant distress/impairment.

Chronic fatigue syndrome

(See ➋ pp. 350–2.)

Clinical features

- GI, neurological, and musculoskeletal symptoms most common.
- Young children: functional recurrent abdominal pain—diffuse abdominal pain usually lasting few hours then remitting with normal abdominal examination. Can be accompanied by limb/joint pain. Headaches less common.
- Older children and females: headache, loss of limb function, and neurological symptoms.
- Polysymptomatic presentation increases with age.
- Presentation may mimic symptoms in family members.

Epidemiology

25% of childhood presentations with headache, abdominal or muscle pain attributed to somatizing. Somatization disorders are uncommon, occurring in <10% of children. Recurrent abdominal pain (prevalence 10%), pain disorders, fatigue, and dissociative disorders are most common. Onset: childhood/early adolescence; conversion disorder later at 16 years.

Aetiology

Predisposing: female, low IQ, depression/anxiety, personality (anxious, obsessional, perfectionist), low socioeconomic class, parental ill-health (somatization, chronic disease or disability, depression/anxiety) family dynamics (enmeshed, over-protective, poor conflict resolution, parental mental illness/somatization), abuse.

Precipitating: stressful life events, physical illness, anxiety, depression, academic pressure, family, or social problems.

Maintaining: excess attention on symptoms (medical investigations, parental over-concern), difficulty in recovering without 'losing face', secondary gain (benefits of sick role), secondary physical changes, e.g. muscle wasting.

Differential diagnosis

School phobia/refusal, depression, anxiety, elective mutism, adjustment disorder, factitious disorder (intentional fabrication of symptoms), unidentified physical disorder.

Comorbidity: 30–50%, depression, anxiety disorder, school refusal, ADHD, ODD.

Management

- Exclude physical illness, be aware that somatizing disorders can coexist with physical illness.
- Stop investigations, as over-investigation could reinforce belief of physical cause.
- Therapeutic alliance is crucial.
- Establish family's attitude to and understanding of the symptoms.
- Explain and reassure that no evidence of organic disorder while acknowledging the symptoms are real and not 'put-on'.
- Present model of mind and body not being separate, have a reciprocal relationship on each other, e.g. stress causing physical symptoms with a tension headache, physical symptoms causing stress.
- Explore stressors in child/family.
- Avoid conflict and confrontation. Aim for consensus with family on presentation and management while acknowledging diagnostic uncertainty. Explain that medically unexplained symptoms are common.
- If child/parent convinced about physical aetiology avoid disagreement and focus on need for 'rehabilitative' treatment, e.g. graded return to previous level of functioning.
- Be positive regarding prognosis and outcome.
- Allow child to recover without 'losing face' rather than 'catching them out'.
- School: develop support strategies (mindfulness, environment changes), reduced timetable, graded return.
- Consider referral to or joint working with liaison psychology/CAMHS.
- Use written records: record short/medium/longer-term goals, keep goals realistic/achievable/allow sufficient time, diary to monitor progress; aim for marathon rather than sprint approach, assume setbacks/temporary worsening of symptoms may occur.

- Family-based CBT: problem-solving skills training, encourage well behaviour, positive reinforcement of health improvements, and removal of positive reinforcement of illness behaviour.
- Family work/therapy to improve communication, explore uncommunicated stressors/maintaining factors.
- Medication is not recommended unless treating comorbid conditions, where there could be a role for antidepressants, analgesics.

Prognosis

Most children improve, with good functional recovery. A proportion can persist to adulthood. Openness to psychological factors and engagement with treatment are good prognostic indicators.

Further resources

Child Somatization Inventory (24-item child and parent questionnaire, free to download): ℘ https://www.psychtools.info/csi24/ or ℘ https://www.childrenshospital.vanderbilt.org/uploads/documents/CSI_Manual.pdf

Chronic fatigue syndrome/ myalgic encephalitis

Definition

Generalized fatigue persisting after routine investigations fail to identify an organic underlying cause. Symptoms can fluctuate in severity and change over time.

Definition of chronic fatigue syndrome/myalgic encephalomyelitis
(Adapted from NICE guideline 2007; note: updated guidance due 2021.)
  Fatigue has all of the following features:
- New or had a specific onset (i.e. it is not lifelong).
- Persistent and/or recurrent.
- Unexplained by other conditions.
- Has resulted in a substantial reduction in activity level characterized by post-exertional malaise and/or fatigue (typically delayed, e.g. by at least 24 hours, with slow recovery over several days).
- Persists for at least 3 months.

  And one or more of the following symptoms:
- Sleep difficulties (see ➲ pp. 466–8).
- Muscle and/or joint pain that is multisite and without evidence of inflammation.
- Headaches (see ➲ pp. 242–3).
- Painful lymph nodes without pathological enlargement.
- Sore throat.
- Cognitive dysfunction (e.g. impaired concentration, short-term memory, word-finding, organizing thoughts, and information processing (see ➲ pp. 416–18)).
- Physical or mental exertion exacerbates symptoms.
- General malaise or 'flu-like' symptoms.
- Dizziness and/or nausea.
- Palpitations in the absence of identified cardiac pathology.

Note: chronic fatigue syndrome was previously classified as neurasthenia/post-viral fatigue in the ICD-10. In the ICD-11, it is classified under 'other disorders of the nervous system' as 'post-viral fatigue syndrome'. If the fatigue does not occur with a virus, then consider coding under disorders of bodily distress disorder.

Epidemiology

- Prevalence 0.05% <18 years. Slightly higher in girls, no difference between socioeconomic groups.
- Onset 11–14 years, gradual or sudden, often preceded by acute illness (influenza, gastroenteritis, glandular fever).
- Risk factors: mental illness (anxiety, depression), childhood trauma, sexual abuse (see ➲ pp. 584–5).

Assessment

- Impact on child's functioning, current activity levels (>50% bed-bound at some stage) and possible maintaining factors.
- Psychiatric symptoms, depression (50%) (see ➔ pp. 330–2), anxiety (see ➔ pp. 338–40), suicidal ideation, self harm (see ➔ pp. 334–6), hopelessness.
- Ascertain child's problem-solving skills.
- Impact on family (disruption, emotional, financial), family response to illness (over-involved, conflictual), family history of chronic physical or mental illness.
- Physical examination: lymphatic, liver, spleen, and tonsillar enlargement. Palpation over nasal sinus, lying and standing blood pressure and heart rate. Neurological examination.
- Investigations: no test is diagnostic, FBC and film, urea and electrolytes, creatinine, Ca, liver function tests, glucose, thyroid function tests, ESR or plasma viscosity, C-reactive protein, creatine kinase, gluten sensitivity, ferritin. Viral serology if history of infection (Epstein–Barr virus-IgM, IgG, Epstein–Barr nuclear antigen). Urinalysis.

Differential diagnosis

Infection (Epstein–Barr virus, influenza, tuberculosis, HIV), neuroendocrine (diabetes, Addison's, hyper/hypothyroidism), haematological (anaemia, lymphoma, malignancy), psychiatric (depression, anxiety), neurological. Obstructive sleep syndromes (see ➔ pp. 448–9), iatrogenic, fabricated, or induced illness (see ➔ pp. 580–3).

Management

- Be aware child/family may have seen several medics prior to assessment.
- Establish collaborative relationship, avoid debates regarding cause, and adopt pragmatic approach.
- Education and information provision including local and national support groups.
- Regular paediatric reviews (monitor progress, development of new physical/psychological symptoms, review diagnosis, support needs). Avoid frequent changes of medical practitioner with resultant anxiety and unnecessary investigations.
- Multidisciplinary management: paediatrician, liaison psychology service, OT, school, and CAMHS (see ➔ p. 288).
- Functional management:
  - Activity pacing.
  - Rest periods of 30 minutes maximum with no sleeping, or physical or mental exertion.
  - Sleep: regular bed and wake times, reduce daytime napping.
  - Healthy diet.
  - Relaxation techniques.
- Education: consider home tuition and gradual return to school.
- Referral to specialist service in moderate to severe cases:
  - CBT: 12–16 sessions (establish baseline activity level, use diary, develop problem-solving skills, alter pessimistic beliefs and maintenance cycles, address over-vigilance to symptoms/checking, reduce distress and symptoms (see ➔ p. 366)).

- Graded exercise therapy and activity management (obtain baseline of activity, gradually increase, add in exercise, maintain activity levels at less than full capacity to avoid 'boom and bust').
- Family therapy.
- Medication: no known pharmacological treatment or cure available; manage symptoms as per usual clinical practice, treat comorbid mental illness, melatonin for sleep difficulties.
- Relapse management: relapse part of normal recovery, generate plan before relapse occurs.

Prognosis

Average duration ~37–49 months with 12 months off school; 60–80% full or partial recovery.

Further resources

Chalder Fatigue Scale (adult scale can be adapted for adolescents, free to download): ℬ http://www.goodmedicine.org.uk/files/assessment,%20chalder%20fatigue%20scale.pdf

National Institute for Health and Care Excellence. Chronic fatigue syndrome: guidelines regarding assessment and management. Available at: ℬ https://www.nice.org.uk/guidance/conditions-and-diseases/chronic-fatigue-syndrome

Chronic illness and mental health

Mental illness in the context of a chronic medical condition is common. Psychiatric disturbance occurs in 20–50% of children, with increased rates of anxiety, depression, and CD. The type of chronic medical condition influences the risk of psychiatric disorder: physical illness (increased ×2), physical illness with disability (increased ×3), CNS illness (increased ×5).

- The degree of functional impairment from the chronic medical condition, rather than just severity, is a key moderating factor.
- Mental illness can impair recovery from physical illness, increase the risk of psychosomatic symptoms, and complicate pain management.
- The link between physical and mental illness can be causal or coincidental (mediated via family/psychosocial factors).

Psychiatric disturbance associated with chronic medical conditions include: depression, anxiety, decreased self-esteem, altered self-concept, anger, hyperactivity, CD and other disruptive behaviour, psychosis. Slightly increased risk of self harm, suicidal ideation/attempts.

Factors that hinder adaptation to the illness are risk factors for psychiatric problems. The impact of risk factors is influenced by developmental stage of child and can change with time:

- Age at illness onset: early recurrent hospitalizations disrupting attachment, disruption to family/social/academic life in childhood, impede peer group attachments/intimate relationships in adolescence.
- Diagnosis: delayed, misdiagnosis, emotional issues ignored, uncertain prognosis.
- Illness: chronicity, degree of disability, functional loss, CNS involvement.
- School: bullying and health-related school absenteeism associated with increased risk of mental health problems.
- Stigma (especially school age/adolescence): physical disfigurement, intrusive treatment regimen/adverse effects, distress associated with self-perception of being different from peers.
- Personality: avoidant coping (poor adjustment, decreased self-esteem, anxiety), denial (treatment non-adherence), over-acceptance of illness (increased anxiety, illness takes over life).
- Parental response: inconsistent, overly attentive/controlling (adolescents need to take increasing responsibility for illness/treatment), parental depression/anxiety, family dysfunction, poor communication/emotional expressiveness.

Asthma

- Increased prevalence of emotional disorders. Psychosocial stress (acute and chronic), emotional arousal (anger, depression) can precipitate symptoms and worsen prognosis.
- Asthmatics and their parents are more anxious than controls.
- Moderating factors: lower socioeconomic status, symptom severity, comorbid CD.
- Treatments (e.g. steroids) can precipitate emotional and behavioural disorders.

Diabetes

- Increased rates of emotional disorders in type 1 diabetes.
- Stress and depression associated with poor glycaemic control.
- Treatment non-compliance/recurrent hospitalizations with ketoacidosis associated with family conflict, parent–child conflict, depression.
- Adolescents can struggle with balancing an intrusive monitoring and treatment regimen with the desire for autonomy.

Epilepsy

(See ➜ pp. 248–55.)
- 30% psychiatric comorbidity.
- Multiple causes: direct result of brain pathology/seizure, medication side effect, psychosocial (stigma, academic and social limitations).
- Risk of comorbidity increased by neurological cause for epilepsy, high seizure frequency, cognitive impairments, family difficulties, young, male, low socioeconomic status.

Assessment

- Screen for existence of and risk factors for psychiatric morbidity.
- Cognitive assessment (impairments influence coping and problem-solving). Educational disability can result from school absence, reduced expectations of child.
- Social, academic function, quality of life. Family and child need opportunity to discuss social and psychological concerns in addition to physical ones.
- Non illness-related stresses facing the family (child's chronic illness associated with marital conflict, behavioural disturbance in siblings, financial difficulties).

Management

- Repeated education about illness/treatment including developmentally appropriate written information (aids treatment compliance). Most effective if both parents and child present. Ensure child is included in treatment decisions.
- Recognize difficulties caused by the illness. Focus on and build on strengths (of child, parents, siblings, and wider system) rather than just negatives.
- Encourage child to be as independent as possible.
- Encourage school attendance, prevent bullying, and provide additional school support.
- Communication with other agencies, education, GP, social services, and HVs.
- Contact with self-help organizations, other families with similarly affected children, and internet support.
- Treat psychiatric comorbidity.
- Consult with liaison psychology service or refer to CAMHS for persistent behavioural/emotional problems.
- Individual therapy: counselling, narrative therapy, CBT, role play.

- Family work: enhance communication, facilitate acceptance/adaptation to diagnosis, allow ventilation of feelings. Allow siblings space to talk. They may feel neglected by parents, worried they could develop the same condition, and feel anger/embarrassment towards the illness and missing out on opportunities.

Further resources

Healthtalk.org (website with young people/families discussing their real-life experiences with a wide range of conditions, including long-term health conditions): ℞ https://www.healthtalk.org/long-term-health-conditions/overview

Post-traumatic stress disorder

Definition

Post-traumatic stress disorder

Definition

Psychological distress secondary to a traumatic event, e.g. motor vehicle collision, abuse (see ⊃ pp. 560–1), natural or man-made disasters, exposure to death, serious physical illness (particularly requiring hospitalization or invasive interventions).

PTSD diagnostic criteria (adapted from the ICD-11):

- Symptoms persist for at least several weeks and cause significant impairment in functioning.
- Re-experiencing the traumatic experience in the present: repetitive and intrusive thoughts, dreams, daytime images ('flashbacks'). Associated with strong emotions, usually fear, and physical sensations.
- Avoidance of traumatic reminders (thoughts, memories, activities, places, and people associated with the trauma).
- Heightened sense of current threat including hypervigilance or an enhanced startle reaction.

Complex PTSD, includes the above-listed diagnostic criteria and adds:

- Affect dysregulation.
- Negative self-concept (thoughts worthlessness, guilt, shame, failure).
- Difficulties in sustaining relationships and feeling close to others.
- Often associated with prolonged/repetitive exposure to threat.

Epidemiology

Children and adolescents: lifetime prevalence 3–10%, probably under-reported in children.

Risk factors

- Trauma: life-threatening, 'man made', proximity to trauma, duration of trauma.
- Individual: ♀ > ♂, pre-existing mental illness, history of neglect/ abuse, low socioeconomic class, lack of social support, distressed/ unsupportive adults.

Assessment

- Presentation varies with age and developmental stage. Younger children more frequently present with physical symptoms and repetitive play incorporating aspects of the trauma.
- Consider PTSD in children with new-onset behavioural disorder, anxiety, agitation, aggression, or self-harm (all possible signs of hyperarousal).
- Flashbacks or recalling traumatic memories may be accompanied by dissociative episodes which can be confused with absence seizures.
- Encourage the child to draw or play in the assessment.
- Enquire about:
  - Sleep disturbance, recurrent nightmares.
  - Negative view of themselves/world/future.
  - Excessive blame on self or others for causing the trauma.
  - Did the child think they were going to die?
  - Withdraw from life/normal interests, numbness/flattening affect, outbursts.

- Coping strategies: including self-harm and illicit substance use.
- Were other family members traumatized?
- Is child now in a safe environment?
- Physical examination to assess possible maltreatment or injuries if appropriate.
- Instruments: Children's Revised Impact of Event Scale (CRIES), Post-Traumatic Cognitions Inventory—child version (cPTCI) (🔎 http://www.childrenandwar.org/measures).

Comorbidity

Depression (see ➔ pp. 330–2), behavioural disorder (see ➔ pp. 412–13), sleep disorder (see ➔ pp. 466–8), ADHD (see ➔ pp. 126–34), self-harm (see ➔ pp. 334–6).

Differential diagnosis

Acute stress reaction (negative life event; develop emotion/cognitive/somatic/behavioural symptoms such as anxiety, confusion, despair, in/overactivity, social withdrawal, stupor; usually resolves within few days or following removal from traumatic situation), adjustment disorder (negative life event, e.g. bereavement, symptoms resolve within 6 months), anxiety (see ➔ pp. 338–40), depression (see ➔ pp. 330–2), ADHD (see ➔ pp. 126–34), attachment disorder (see ➔ pp. 324–5), CD (see ➔ pp. 306–8), sleep disorder (see ➔ pp. 466–8).

Management

Early detection and treatment within CAMHS.
- No clear benefit from single session debriefing immediately post trauma.
- Trauma-focused CBT—strongest evidence. Ten to 20 weekly sessions. Consider group CBT if mass trauma.
- Eye movement desensitization and reprocessing (EMDR)—recall traumatic event while moving eyes side to side or tapping.
- Narrative exposure therapy (NET)—construct a 'lifeline', narrative account of individual's story is produced, evidence for use in asylum seekers who have experienced multiple traumas.
- Family therapy. Children and parents may avoid discussing the trauma for fear of distressing each other. Depression, anxiety, or PTSD in family members exposed to the trauma should be considered and treated. Parents may struggle with guilt, particularly if the child has been abused.
- Medication should not be routinely used. Consider SSRIs in severe PTSD or if comorbid depression/anxiety.

Prognosis

Most resolve completely within a year but some cases become chronic. Prognosis negatively influenced by severity of episode, believing they would die during trauma, premorbid adversity, comorbidity, and post-trauma environment (lack of supportive parents, family dysfunction).

Alcohol and substance misuse

Definition

Experimental and recreational use of illicit substances and alcohol often commences in adolescence:

- *Harmful use*: pattern of use causes mental/physical harm to user, is criticized by others, and causes adverse social consequences.
- *Dependence syndrome*: compulsion to take substance, withdrawal, tolerance, neglect of alternative interests, persisting use despite harmful consequences, reinstatement after abstinence. (Note: withdrawal symptoms less common in adolescents than adults.)

Epidemiology

- Those aged 11–15 years have tried alcohol (44%), tobacco (19%), cannabis (8%), nitrous oxide (4%), or novel psychoactive substances (2%).
- Prevalence: alcohol abuse 0.6–4.3% of adolescents, substance abuse 3.3% of 15-year-olds, 9.8% of 17–19-year-olds.
- Inhaled solvents used more frequently by younger teens (6–7% of 11–12-year-olds).
- Polysubstance use is common.
- About 75% of adolescents obtain substances from friends or relatives.
- Parental attitude to alcohol use has a significant influence on an adolescent's alcohol consumption.

Aetiology/risk factors

- Availability of substance.
- Association with antisocial and marginalized groups where there is social acceptance of drug use.
- Male; sibling with drug use; genetic vulnerability.
- Impulsivity, mental illness (CD (see ➔ pp. 306–8), ADHD (see ➔ pp. 126–34)), adversity/trauma.
- Ineffective parenting (see ➔ pp. 364–5), parental substance misuse, childhood sexual abuse (see ➔ pp. 584–5), traumatic life events.
- Unclear role of socioeconomic status.

Clinical features

Common presentations include changes in academic and social functioning, cognition (reduced concentration, psychotic symptoms, flashbacks), mood (agitation, irritability, somnolence, withdrawal, impulsivity, hypervigilance, fatigue), antisocial behaviour, changing friendship groups, change of interests, appetite change, and/or missing money/valuables.

Assessment

- Interview the young person alone for part of the session and explain limits of confidentiality.
- Pattern of alcohol/substance use: current amount, frequency of use, binges, range of substances, used socially or alone, features of harmful use or dependence.
- Risk: self-harm (see ➔ pp. 334–6), suicide, unprotected sex, aggression, criminal behaviour, funding of habit (theft, prostitution).

- From family: premorbid functioning, parental alcohol/substance use, access to alcohol/substances at home. Have the parents raised their concerns with the adolescent?
- Review positives: supportive relationship with adult, link with local community, positive school experiences, clear boundaries at home.
- Physical examination: self-care, weight deficit, accidental injuries, DSH, infection, skin reactions, signs of nicotine and alcohol use, rash around mouth and nose (inhaling solvents from a bag), gynaecomastia (anabolic steroid use).
- Bloods in IV drug use: hepatitis B/C, HIV.
- Urine toxicology not routinely required.

Comorbidity

Comorbidity in 60–75%. CD, ODD (see ➜ pp. 306–8), ADHD (see ➜ pp. 126–34), depression, anxiety disorders, PTSD (see ➜ pp. 358–9), EDs (see ➜ pp. 342–4).

Management

- Non-judgemental approach.
- Treat comorbid physical illness.
- Discuss/provide information about substances and associated risks.
- Encourage engagement with local drugs advisory service or specialist treatment services dependent upon severity of substance use.
  Treatment usually involves:
  - Engagement and analysis of difficulties.
  - Aim to improve life skills, independent thinking, and assertiveness.
  - Address risk including child protection and safe sex.
  - Individual and group work incorporating cognitive and behavioural approaches (see ➜ pp. 412–13).
  - Motivational interviewing: non-confrontational approach designed to lead adolescent to desire change (includes pros and cons of substance misuse, alternative means of achieving 'pros').
  - Relapse prevention: cue avoidance, social pressures, alternative coping strategies.
  - Harm reduction approach if abstinence impossible, advise use of safer drugs, clean needles, and first aid.
- Referral to mental health team to treat mental illness (see ➜ p. 288).

Prognosis

Majority of addictive behaviour terminated by adulthood.

Further resources

Drugscope (independent UK charity): ℘ http://www.drugscope.org.uk
FRANK (independent UK government-funded website offering information and support): ℘ http://www.talktofrank.com/
Healthtalk.org (video for young people): ℘ https://healthtalk.org/drugs-and-alcohol/advice-to-young-people-about-drugs-and-alcohol

Challenging behaviour

Challenging behaviour is an umbrella term. It describes a variety of behaviours which put a child or others at risk and has a negative impact on the quality of their life. The term is more frequently applied to younger children, and children with learning difficulties and autism.

Common types: aggression, tantrums, destruction, sexualized behaviour, self-injury, stereotyped behaviours, running away. There is often a repetitive nature to the behaviours and they can interfere with functioning and development.

In order to accurately interpret behaviour, the developmental age of the child should be considered, e.g. tantrums in a 2-year-old are 'normal' but may be inappropriate for 10-year-olds.

All children will at some point 'challenge' their carers or teachers, so obtaining a detailed history of difficulties is key to distinguishing 'normal' behaviour and the management of 'challenging' behaviour.

Assessment

Who perceives the behaviour as challenging, what is their understanding/explanation of the origin and purpose of the behaviour, and why do they find it challenging/distressing?

Review potential causes of behaviour with SPACE (Sensory, Pain, Access to tangibles/support, Communicate needs, Escape/Avoidance). Consider:

- Long-term triggers: chronic pain, distressing event/thought, anxiety, sleep difficulty, puberty.
- Short-term triggers: communication with others (go away, come here, need help), sensitivities to light/sound, boredom, inability to cope with change in routine, sensory stimulation, self-soothing (sexualized behaviour), acute pain.

Utilize a functional analysis approach (for management of behavioural problems see ➲ pp. 412–13).

- Look for patterns of precipitants and perpetuating factors. Consider keeping a behaviour diary.
- Is the behaviour pervasive or only present in certain environments or company?
- What is the child trying to communicate?
- How have carers, family members, and the school responded to the behaviour?
- Range of interventions tried, duration, and consistency.

What is the child's explanation for the behaviour? They will have been asked this before by other adults and may be understandably wary of discussing the issue, particularly if they feel embarrassed or believe that you may tell them off or judge them. Children may often 'not know', and be unable or unwilling to communicate why they behave in a certain manner, so consider approaching the issue indirectly.

If possible, see the child alone for part of the session. Using drawings or models can help. A non-judgemental approach throughout the session can facilitate discussion.

Management

- Exclude physical cause for behaviour, comorbid mental illness, LD (see ➲ pp. 136–41), and neurodevelopmental disorder (see ➲ pp. 36–8).
- Assess risk to self and others.
- Everybehaviour is a form of communication and has a function. Understanding the behaviour guides the intervention.
- Use behavioural interventions (for management of behavioural problems see ➲ pp. 412–13) and ensure that behavioural interventions involve a coordinated response from school and family.
- Consider the impact of:
  - Changes to physical and social environment.
  - Methods of enhancing communication—visual forms of communication such as pictures, objects, 'emotional' faces, thumbs up/down/middle, traffic light colours.

Anger management: parent management training and individual behavioural training (for CD and ODD see ➲ pp. 306–8).

Sexualized behaviour: feedback regarding where and when the behaviour is appropriate, review causes including possible sexual abuse (see ➲ pp. 584–5).

Self-injury: often used to communicate, behavioural treatments, enhance communication skills (functional communication training) (for suicide and SH see ➲ pp. 334–6; for ASD CAMHS aspects see ➲ pp. 298–9).

Education: SEN support including behavioural support services, and/or educational psychologist input (see ➲ pp. 656–8).

Medication: only consider after behavioural analysis and interventions, identify which symptoms will be targeted, conduct a thorough risk:benefit analysis before commencing, determine how the response will be measured and monitored (child's report, carer/school reports, questionnaires).

Refer to CAMHS if listed interventions inadequate.

Further resources

Challenging Behaviour Foundation (charity for children and adults with severe LDs; has information sheets for managing behaviour): ✆ http://www.thecbf.org.uk/

Greene RW (2021). The Explosive Child: A New Approach for Understanding and Parenting Easily Frustrated, Chronically Inflexible Children, 6th ed. New York: HarperCollins.

Also see 'Further resources' in 'Parenting', ➲ p. 365.

Parenting

Parenting is an immensely rewarding but at times challenging 'job'. A balanced authoritative parenting style that is flexible and meets the child's developmental needs will be most successful. Excessive authoritarian, permissive, or disengaged approaches are more likely to be associated with difficulties.

Supporting parents

- Use attentive listening when reviewing the parents' concerns—it is itself therapeutic, increases the likelihood of parental change/following your advice, and models 'how to listen' to their children.
- Try to avoid judging and blaming the parent—it will not help the child or parent.
- The parents are part of the solution.
- Empathize—all parents get frustrated and parenting can be more challenging and stressful if a child is 'unwell'.
- Address parental guilt—parents may feel as if they have 'failed' or are responsible for their child's illness, particularly if mental illness. Make time to explore parental concerns.
- Are the parents being too hard on themselves? Aim to be a 'good enough' parent rather than a perfect parent.
- Review the parental relationship—impact of illness, degree of cooperation, conflict, triangulation with child.
- Review parental closeness with child and advise as appropriate—too close leading to inhibition (enmeshment) or too distant.

General advice/approach

- Externalize—the behaviour is the issue rather than the child.
- Encourage a consistent approach from both parents that is also consistent over time.
- Encourage parents to 'tune in' to the child—what would it be like to be in their child's shoes? What is the child attempting to communicate? What are they feeling?
- Reward appropriate behaviour—learn to recognize and encourage desirable behaviours. Be generous with praise.
- Learn to ignore minor issues.
- Keep instructions short and focus on what you want the child to do. Speak slowly and check understanding.
- House rules should be few, fair, followed by everyone, reviewed regularly, and on display.
- Enjoy your child—spend time doing things together. Let the child lead the play. When is the parent–child relationship working well and what is different about these times? Look for patterns and schedule more.
- Let the child know they are special—listen to them and express your affection.
- Provide security and stability—routines and order will help reduce child anxiety.
- 'Time out' for parents—anger and frustration will alter a parent's response to a situation. If the situation is emotive, internally count to ten or walk away, before responding to child.

Advice for managing specific behaviours—see individual topics or management of behavioural problems topic (see ➜ pp. 412–13).

Other sources of parental support:
• Self-help.
• Parenting programme: 12 weekly sessions, behaviour-based interventions supporting parenting skills can reduce child behaviour problems and improve parental mental health.
• Local and national support groups (see ➜ p. 23).
• Family, friends.
• HVs (see ➜ pp. 676–7), GP, social services (see ➜ pp. 682–3), school (see ➜ pp. 656–8).
• Mental health service—family therapy (see ➜ p. 367).

Parental mental illness

• Is the 'unwell' child actually bringing their parents/family for treatment?
• Recognition is key, so always ask. Enquire about postnatal depression, affective disorders, past and current input from GP/mental health services, and any other family history of mental illness.
• Consider genetic risk in child.
• Could there be a common aetiology, e.g. parental stress reaction caring for a seriously ill child, shared exposure to traumatic event?
• Review capacity of parent to cope with current situation and child. Parents often try to shield their children from their illness.
• Chronic difficulties such as parental personality disorders are often more damaging for children than acute episodes of illness.
• Individual assessment and treatment for parent—GP/mental health services.
• Family therapy—adult mental health team or CAMHS (see ➜ p. 288).
• Review the impact of the parental illness on the child.
• Review risk to children. Ensure your concerns are explained to the parent and communicated to other professionals (for child protection see ➜ pp. 560–1 and pp. 596–602).

Further resources

Faber A, Mazlish E (2012). How to Talk So Kids Will Listen & Listen So Kids Will Talk. New York: Scribner.

Family and Parenting Institute: ℘ http://www.familyandparenting.org/

MindEd for Families (parenting tips and managing common issues): ℘ https://mindedforfamilies.org.uk/young-people/

The Incredible Years: ℘ http://www.incredibleyears.com

Young Minds Parents Helpline (offers information and professional advice): ☎ 0808 802 5544; ℘ http://www.youngminds.org.uk/

Young Carers Net (UK website for <18-year-olds who look after someone in their family who has an illness, disability, drug/alcohol addiction, or mental illness): ℘ http://www.youngcarers.net

Psychotherapeutic interventions

Psychotherapeutic interventions are one of the commonest treatments for child mental illness. The choice of intervention is determined by the needs of the child and family, evidence base, and local availability.

Behaviour therapy

For management of behavioural problems see ➜ pp. 412–13.

Cognitive behaviour therapy

- Recommended for depression, anxiety disorders, OCD, and EDs. Has a significant supporting evidence base.
- Structured therapy that focuses on the links between thoughts (cognitions), emotions, and behaviour in different situations.
- Changing cognitions will change emotions and behaviour.
- The therapist is a 'coach' working collaboratively with the child to develop a formulation of the problem and maintenance cycles.
- 'Socratic' questioning (encouraging the child to reach their own conclusions to reveal new perspectives) is utilized to identify and alter unhelpful cognitions associated with psychopathology.
- Common cognitive distortions include black and white thinking, jumping to conclusions, mind-reading, magnification, personalizing, and over-generalization.
- 'Homework' is used between sessions and includes 'thought diaries' and behaviour experiments.
- The behavioural therapy component of CBT may be enough to induce change with little cognitive therapy, e.g. activity scheduling for depression.
- Usually individual therapy but group/family CBT possible. Parents can join sessions for younger children.
- Time limited, approximately six to 24 sessions.

Counselling

- A supportive, cathartic, client-led therapy that focuses on the discussion of distressing issues.
- Problem-solving and advice can be incorporated.
- Children and adolescents can value the contact with an 'independent and non-judgemental' adult.
- Used in schools and local youth support organizations.
- Evidence base is limited.
- Commonly used to manage mild depression and anxiety, significant life events, relationships, school difficulties, and substance misuse.

Creative therapies

- These include art, play, music, and drama.
- Most suitable for younger children and those with learning and communication difficulties.

Dialectic behaviour therapy

- Used to manage self-harm and emotional dysregulation.
- Incorporates elements of CBT, mindfulness, and problem-solving.
- Both individual and group work.
- Not widely available but effective.

Family therapy

- Family treated as a whole, rather than just the child.
- Reduces feelings of guilt and 'scapegoating' in children.
- Sometimes only part of family seen.
- Therapist maintains neutrality.
- Use 'reflective team' and a one-way mirror.
- Lower-frequency sessions compared to other therapies, approximately six to 12 sessions over several months.
- Widely utilized, best evidence: EDs, depression, substance use.

Interpersonal psychotherapy

- Focuses on relationship difficulties including conflicts and adapting to life events.
- For those aged >11 years, ~12 sessions.
- Used in depression, grief reactions, and EDs.

Mindfulness

- Involves increasing awareness of thoughts, body sensations, and emotions. Teaches how to accept thoughts rather than challenge or judge them, pay attention to the present, not aim for a set goal, and uses meditation techniques. Encourages individual to take a compassionate approach to themselves. It is flexible and can be practised for short periods of time every day.
- Useful to manage stress, anxiety, and distressing recurrent thoughts.
- Can be used in individual and group settings with a growing evidence base for school-based interventions.

Parenting programmes

Provide group support and teach positive parenting skills (see 'Further resources').

Psychodynamic psychotherapy

- Brief or intensive (one to three sessions/week over 1 year).
- Aim to gain insight into unconscious processes that maintain psychopathology.
- Parents can be seen separately in parallel with the child.
- Use in anxiety and depression.

Further resources

Royal College of Psychiatrists (website has information leaflets regarding a range of therapies and a section on young people's mental health): ℘ https://www.rcpsych.ac.uk/

Treatment non-adherence

Treatment adherence is rarely complete. In children and adolescents with chronic conditions, it is estimated at 58%, with adolescents adhering less than children (WHO data). Non-adherence can result in mortality or chronic morbidity depending on the underlying medical condition.

Factors that may increase non-adherence

Illness and treatment-related factors

- Chronic illness, relapsing–remitting course.
- Demanding, complicated, intrusive, long-term treatments.
- Suboptimal treatment response or delayed onset of action.
- Experiencing or fear of adverse events or painful treatments.
- Stigma/embarrassment associated with illness or taking medication.
- Illness or treatment impacting social life. Fear of impact on relationships and physical attractiveness (acne, weight gain).

Individual factors

- Reduced capacity in children to evaluate treatment benefit and consequences of non-adherence.
- Reduced acceptance of diagnosis and prognosis (they may feel invincible).
- Anger at illness directed towards parents and clinicians and their imposed treatment.
- Parent–child conflict and child's desire to exert autonomy by disregarding parental advice.
- Feeling overwhelmed by responsibility of managing own health. Non-adherence is a means of exerting control of a situation in which they feel disempowered.
- Psychiatric disorder: depression (hopelessness), poor insight, ODD, ADHD (forgetting medication).
- Primary and secondary gain: avoid school, maintaining parental attention.

Parental/family factors

- Psychiatric disorder.
- Family conflict.
- Inadequate parental supervision and increased number of siblings.

Management

Open discussion of positive and negative aspects of treatment

- Psychoeducation utilizing age-appropriate information both at time of diagnosis and transition to adolescence (a time of increasing responsibility for own condition). Check understanding of child and caregivers. Is there a language barrier?
- Avoid term 'non-compliance' (suggests deliberate antagonism and implies blame).
- Do the consequences of non-adherence justify an intervention?
- Empower child and family by involvement in treatment decisions and acknowledge validity of their views on positive and negative treatment effects. Siblings can play an important part in motivating the patient.

- Discuss strategies to manage side effects.
- Consider increasing the frequency of contact to enhance therapeutic alliance.

Suggestions to facilitate discussion based on motivational interviewing techniques

- Explore the problem rather than trying to solve it. Write a list with the young person of pros and cons of treatment and no treatment. Do they assign greater importance to some factors over others? Review treatment-related fears and confidence to change.
- Who from your family most wants you to receive the treatment? Who next? What do you think the reasons are?
- How would life be different in 1 year or 5 years' (adjust time according to age of child) time without and then with the treatment?
- Elicit aspirations and visualize success. What would you need to do to achieve your goals? How would treatment influence this? Reflect discrepancy between goals and present behaviour.
- What advice would you give to a friend in a similar situation?
- Identify barriers to change and how to overcome.
- Identify who will help with change, monitor small steps, and celebrate success.
- Remember ambivalence may still be present even once change has commenced.

Practical measures

- Provide written/translated handouts/interpreter if required.
- Build a daily routine which includes medication. Daily pill dispenser (dosette box), charts/calendar, reminder apps, phone alarms.
- Simplify medication schedule (sustained-release preparations, avoid mid-day dosing, home versus school adherence).
- Switch to more acceptable alternative treatment.
- Consider different taste, mix medication with food/liquid/flavouring, liquid versus tablet preparation, less side effects. Seek advice from pharmacy.

Other

- Identify and treat mental illness.
- Liaise with hospital psychology service or CAMHS if individual or family work appropriate.
- Young people may respond better to non-professionals, e.g. support groups, online charities, contact with other young people with similar condition.

Further resources

El-Rachidi S, LaRochelle JM, Morgan JA (2017). Pharmacists and pediatric medication adherence: bridging the gap. Hosp Pharm, 52, 124–31.

Resources

Mental Health Foundation: ☎ 020 7803 1100; ℅ http://www.mhf.org.uk
Mind: ☎ 020 8519 2122; ℅ http://www.mind.org.uk

Anxiety

Anxiety UK: ☎ 0844 477 5774 ℅ http://www.anxietyuk.org
OCD Action (UK charity for OCD): ☎ 0845 390 6232; ℅ http://www.ocdaction.org.uk/

Autistic spectrum disorders

National Autistic Society: ℅ http://www.autism.org.uk

Bullying

Anti-Bullying Network (not-for-profit company): ℅ http://www.antibullying.net/
Parentline Plus (advice to parents regarding bullying): ℅ http://www.familyandparenting.org/ or
   helpline ☎ 0808 800 2222.

Child maltreatment

MOSAC (UK charity supporting non-abusing parents and carers of sexually abused children): ℅
   http://www.mosac.org.uk/

Depression

Childline (UK helpline provides a confidential telephone counselling service for children with any
   problem): ☎ 0800 1111; ℅ http://www.childline.org.uk
Get Connected (UK confidential helpline signposting to sources of help): ☎ 0808 808 4994; ℅ www.
   getconnected.org.uk
Young Minds (UK charity to improve mental health of children and young people): ☎ 020 7336 8445.
   Downloadable publications on depression: ℅ http://www.youngminds.org.uk/

Eating disorders

BEAT (UK charity): ℅ http://www.b-eat.co.uk/Home

Enuresis and encopresis

ERIC (The Children's Bowel & Bladder Charity; UK children's charity dealing with bedwetting, daytime wetting, constipation, soiling, and potty training): ℅ http://www.eric.org.uk/
Heins T, Ritchie K (1988). Beating Sneaky Poo: Ideas for Faecal Soiling, 2nd ed. Leaflet free to download at: ℅ http://www.dulwichcentre.com.au/beating-sneaky-poo-2.pdf

Learning disabilities

Challenging Behaviour Foundation (charity for children and adults with severe LDs; has information
   sheets for managing behaviour): ℅ http://www.thecbf.org.uk/
Foundation for People with Learning Disabilities: ℅ http://www.learningdisabilities.org.uk/
LD online (US website on LDs and ADHD): ℅ http://www.ldonline.org/

Parenting, conduct disorder, and oppositional defiant disorder

Incredible Years: ℅ http://www.incredibleyears.com
Family and Parenting Institute: ℅ http://www.familyandparenting.org/
Young Carers Net (UK website for <18-year-olds who look after someone in their family who has
   an illness, disability, drug/alcohol addiction, or mental illness): ℅ http://www.youngcarers.net
Parentline Plus: ☎ 0808 800 2222; ℅ http://www.parentlineplus.org.uk

Self-harm

National Self Harm Network (UK charity, has downloadable advice leaflets for young people): ℅
   http://www.nshn.co.uk

Substance misuse

Drugscope (independent UK charity): ℘ http://www.drugscope.org.uk
FRANK (independent UK government-funded website offering information and support): ℘ http://www.talktofrank.com

Tic disorders

Tourettes Action (UK charity): ☎ 0845 458 1252; ℘ http://www.tourettes-action.org.uk/

Therapies in neurodisability

Limitations are but boundaries created inside our minds.

Chinese proverb

Physiotherapy: assessment

Refer children with the following conditions to physiotherapy

- Long-term neurological, e.g. CP (see ➲ pp. 92–101).
- Syndromes, e.g. DS (see ➲ pp. 496–500), Rett syndrome (see ➲ p. 266).
- Neuromuscular, e.g. muscular dystrophy (see ➲ pp. 272–3).
- Developmental delay in gross motor skills (see ➲ p. 379).
- DCD (see ➲ pp. 146–9).
- Hypermobility (see ➲ p. 379).

Other conditions that may be treated in the community or alternatively in secondary/tertiary centres or musculoskeletal outpatient physiotherapy departments:

- Juvenile arthritis.
- Developmental orthopaedic conditions: Erb's palsy, talipes/clubfoot (see ➲ p. 376), plagiocephaly (see ➲ p. 239), torticollis, tip-toe walking.
- Long-term respiratory conditions, e.g. cystic fibrosis.

Assessment

Subjective

Abilities, concerns, and problems in the areas of:

- Impairments, e.g. pain.
- Activity limitations, e.g. mobility, self-care.
- Participation, e.g. how does child spend day, interests, sport, etc.
- Environment, e.g. equipment used.

Objective

Observation is made of the child's posture and movements in supine, prone, side lying, floor sitting, box sitting, and standing of:

- Position of head, upper limbs, lower limbs, shoulder girdle, pelvis, spine.
- Alignment of body parts to each other.
- Weight distribution.
- Symmetry/asymmetry.
- Tone, associated reactions, reflexes, involuntary movements, tremor.

Assess how child achieves the movements listed in Table 7.1 including predominant movement patterns and the ability to dissociate one movement from the rest of the body.

Range of movement/muscle power/deformity

May be measured of all muscles and at all joints but with attention to those listed in Table 7.2 for specific conditions.

Tone

- Assessed partly through observation of posture and movement in different positions.
- Through examination and palpation of muscle.
- By passive movement at different velocity.

Table 7.1 Movement assessment

Position	Movement
Supine	Head turning, lifting off supporting surface
	Upper limbs to midline and crossing midline
	Lower limb kicking, hands to feet
	Rolling over either side to prone
	Pivoting
Prone	Freeing arms
	Lifting and turning head
	Forearm prop
	Pivoting
	Pushing up into four-point kneeling
	Crawling
	Rolling over either side to supine
Side lying	Maintenance of position
	Hands to midline
Lying to sitting	How the child achieves sitting actively
	If unable to rise to sit independently, observation of pull to sit for head control; fixation of pelvis; flexibility of hips; active assistance
Floor sitting	Tailor sitting, side sitting, long sitting, and w-sitting
	Head upright, turning and control
	Maintenance with and without propping
	Movement within and outside of base of support
	Pivoting
	Bottom shuffling
Box sitting	Movement on and off box to floor
	Maintenance of position with and without hand support
	Movement within and outside base of support
	Movement into standing
Standing	Maintenance with and without support
	Crouch
	Single leg stance
	Gait
	Kick
	Run
	Hop
	Jump
	Stairs

Standardized tools for assessment
See Table 7.3.

Table 7.2 Movement/muscle range in specific conditions

Condition	Measurement/muscle
CP with lower limb involvement	Two joint muscles; rectus femoris, hamstrings, gastrocnemius
	Rotational profile; femoral neck anteversion, hip rotation, tibial torsion, foot posture
	Leg length (measured from anterior superior iliac spine to medial malleolus)
CP with upper limb involvement	Pectorals, supinators, long finger flexors, thumb abduction
CP	Individual isolated movement
Lower limb developmental orthopaedic conditions	Rotational profile as above
	Intermalleolar distance with knees touching
	Intercondylar distance with malleoli touching
Muscle weakness	Oxford scale (0–5)
	Timed rising from floor
	Timed 10 m walk

Table 7.3 Standardized assessment tools

Condition	Assessment
Talipes/club foot	Pirani score
Neuromuscular disease	North Star
CP	Gross Motor Function Measure (GMFM)
	Functional Mobility Scale (FMS)
	Chailey ability levels
	Migration percentage from hip X-ray
	Shriners Hospital Upper Extremity Evaluation (SHUEE)
	Assisting Hand Assessment (AHA)
Developmental delay	Alberta Infant Mobility Scale (AIMS)
DCD	Movement ABC-2
Hypermobility	Beighton Scale

Physiotherapy: approaches to treatment

Cerebral palsy and long-term neurological conditions

(See ➡ pp. 92–101.)

- Aim: to encourage and increase the child's ability to move and function in as normal a way as possible while preventing contracture and deformity.
- Treatment may include:
  - 24-hour postural management in lying, sitting, and standing. In the child with low ability this will be achieved through the use of suitable equipment such as sleep systems, wheelchairs, static supportive seating, and standing frames. Emphasis is on improvement of body alignment.
  - Stretches—active, passive, through use of position/equipment or orthotics. Targeting susceptible muscles.
  - Influencing tone through position, manual techniques, handling, facilitation, active movement.
  - Constraint-induced movement therapy—active use of the hemiplegic upper limb while the non-affected arm is restrained, e.g. by wearing a mitten/glove.
  - Strengthening.
  - Providing mobility aids—k-walker, rollator, tripod/quadripod sticks, or walkers that offer trunk support such as the Rifton Pacer.

Neuromuscular conditions

(See ➡ pp. 272–6.)

- Aims: slow down rate of development of contractures/deformity. Preserve respiratory function. Promotion of activity and participation.
- Treatment includes:
  - Stretches—active, passive, through position/equipment or orthotics.
  - Exercise and activity without fatigue.
  - Appropriate introduction of aids/equipment.
  - Respiratory physiotherapy.

Developmental coordination disorder

(See ➡ pp. 146–9.)

- Aims: improve core stability, hip stability, shoulder stability, bilateral integration, eye–hand coordination, eye-foot coordination, and motor planning.
- Treatment may include:
  - Strategies for both home and school to compensate for problems.
  - Direct therapy/exercises targeting problems either individually or in a group.
  - Recommendations for suitable mainstream sport/clubs to generalize skills gained through therapy.
  - Recommendations of suitable games and equipment.

Developmental delay

(See ➍ pp. 30–1.)
- Aim: promote gross motor development through play and daily activities.
- Treatment may include progression through prone development, rolling, crawling, sitting, standing, and walking.

Hypermobility

- Aim: develop co-contraction around joints to promote gross motor skills, and prevent problems such as pain and joint subluxation/dislocation.
- Treatment: muscle strengthening programmes.

Hippotherapy

- Also called therapeutic riding.
- This may be beneficial in a variety of neurological conditions such as CP.
- The three-dimensional movement of the horse's pelvis as it walks can affect a child's tone, alignment, balance, strength, and function.

Hydrotherapy

- Water properties can be used to provide an environment conducive for treating a variety of conditions.
- Water temperature, buoyancy, turbulence, and drag provide an alternative medium for treatment.
- Halliwick is a method of teaching swimming and water safety for both disabled and non-disabled children. The child is taught to achieve independence in water starting with breathing control and relaxation.

Gross Motor Function Classification System—Expanded and Revised (GMFCS-E&R)

- The GMFCS is a five-level classification that differentiates children with CP (see ➔ pp. 92–101) based on:
  - The child's current gross motor abilities.
  - Their limitations in gross motor function.
  - Their need for assistive technology and wheeled mobility.
- The GMFCS-E&R contains five age bands:
  - <2 years.
  - 2–4 years.
  - 4–6 years.
  - 6–12 years.
  - 12–18 years.
- The aim of the GMFCS-E&R is to ascertain which level best represents the child/youth's present abilities and limitations.
- Distinctions between levels are made by functional limitations, use of hand-held mobility aids, and use of wheelchairs.
- The emphasis should be on the child's usual performance in home, school, and community settings (i.e. what he/she can do), rather than what they can do at their best (i.e. capability).
- PTs and doctors do not require specific training to perform the assessment.
- Physicians and therapists familiar with a child can complete the GMFCS-E&R in <5 minutes. Those unfamiliar with the child may require 15–20 minutes to observe and then complete it.
- The GMFCS-E&R brochure can be downloaded at no cost for personal or non-commercial use.
- Using the GMFCS-E&R level is very useful in sharing with parents the treatment/management plans for their child and for shared goal setting.
- The GMFCS-E&R is enormously useful in terms of intervention planning at the level of a given child's impairment and activity.
- If the question is 'Will my child walk?', then the GMFCS-E&R, should help you provide an answer to parents/carers of a child with CP.
- A child usually remains in one level and does not change levels and, therefore, by looking ahead to the descriptor as they age, their prognosis can be determined and communicated, especially after 2 years of age as GMFCS-E&R levels mostly remain stable.
- The GMFCS-E&R need not be used at every review or clinical encounter. It needs to be used to determine their level when the child is first seen for a neurodevelopmental assessment. The GMFCS-E&R can also be used during interdisciplinary or special clinic visits or when a child is older.
- The title for each level describes the main method of a child's mobility:
  - Level I: walks without limitations.
  - Level II: walks with limitations.
  - Level III: walks using a hand-held mobility device.

- Level IV: self-mobility with limitations; may use powered mobility.
- Level V: transported in a manual wheelchair.
- Developed by Robert Palisano, Peter Rosenbaum, Stephen Walter, Dianne Russell, Ellen Wood, and Barbara Galuppi in 1997, it was expanded and revised in 2007.
- In 2002, motor growth curves for children with CP were produced by plotting the Gross Motor Function Measure (GMFM)-66 against the GMFCS.

Further resources

CanChild: ℘ https://canchild.ca/en/resources/42-gmfcs-e-r
Download GMFCS-E&R: ℘ https://canchild.ca/system/tenon/assets/attachments/000/000/058/original/GMFCS-ER_English.pdf

Gross Motor Function Measure (GMFM)

- The GMFM is an evaluation tool designed to measure changes in GM function over time or with intervention, in children with CP.
- But the GMFM has also been used in other conditions, e.g. DS (see ➔ pp. 496–500), TBI (see ➔ pp. 108–9), SMA (see ➔ pp. 550–1), etc.
- While the GMFCS-E&R is quick to use, the GMFM takes up to an hour for an experienced assessor.
- There are two versions of the GMFM. The GMFM-88 is the original 88-item measure, that scores items in five different GM activities as mentioned later.
- The GMFM-66 is a subset of the original GMFM-88. The GMFM-66 provides information regarding the level of difficulty of each item, thus helping to plan interventions.
- The basal and ceiling version uses the GMFCS to decide age and level to indicate the approximate level to begin testing. A basal level is established when three consecutive items based on difficulty order are scored as 3. Testing is continued until three consecutive items are scored as 0, determining the ceiling. A minimum of 15 items need to be scored.

Five gross motor activities/subsections

- Lying and rolling.
- Sitting.
- Crawling and kneeling.
- Standing.
- Walking, running, and jumping.

Scoring key

- 0 = does not initiate.
- 1 = initiates.
- 2 = partially completes.
- 3 = completes.

Posture management and special seating

- Many young people with complex disabling conditions, primarily neurological in origin (see p. 217), require wheelchairs (see pp. 388–9) and special seating provision to:
  - Maintain comfort.
  - Maximize function.
  - Minimize further deterioration.
  - Minimize energy expenditure.
- People with physical disabilities usually tire more quickly than able-bodied people and are less able to resist the forces of gravity. This needs to be considered when prescribing wheelchairs and seating.
- 'Off the shelf' seating systems offer a limited amount of accommodation of asymmetric body shape.
- Custom contoured seating (this is a system where a mould is taken of the body and a bespoke seat manufactured to match this; a variety of materials are available, each having specific advantageous features) is beneficial.

Posture and mobility services

In some areas, a posture, independence, and mobility service (see p. 384) encompasses the wheelchair service (see pp. 388–9). The extended services include:

- Assessment and provision of assistive technology for children (see p. 393).
- Assessing therapeutic positioning in lying, sitting, and standing.
- Considering supportive positions to restore symmetry and reduce destructive postures in the child with complex problems.

Posture and seating assessment: the key principles

- A thorough assessment requires input from:
  - Clinicians (typically OTs and/or PTs with specialist training in a seating course).
  - Clinical engineers with specialist expertise (see pp. 430–1).
- This guarantees that the costly process of designing bespoke seating is justified by good clinical outcomes such as:
  - Maximizing functioning.
  - Minimizing clinical risks such as pressure sores.
  - Minimizing pain and spasticity.
- For example, a patient with CP (essentially a non-progressive condition) will experience deterioration due to spasticity, deteriorating skin, and increased pain if careful attention is not paid to seating.

Seating provision

- Pushchairs or buggies may be more suitable for the younger child.
- Consideration is given to the postural need of the child.
- Specialist seating systems may be provided for children requiring extra postural control and support.

Principles for achieving stability in seating

- Wide base of support.
- Recruit gravity to secure a position.
- Account for established structural asymmetries, e.g. scoliosis, kyphosis, pelvic asymmetries, and hip joint range limitations, by matching body contours to support surfaces (seat cushion, backrest, etc.).
- Minimize distorting factors, e.g. gravitational pull on shoulders from weight of arms.

Principles of ideal seating position

- Feet hip width apart, ankle at 90° (right angle) and foot supported. Footrest height maintains femurs horizontal.
- Knee flexed to 90°.
- Cushion horizontal under ischial tuberosity and then ramped from gluteal crease to support the femurs horizontally.
- Sacral pad forward of back rest up to the lumbosacral junction to accommodate the greater width of the trunk at chest height.
- Trunk symmetrical; may require curved backrest with side supports.
- Head upright and in midline.

Fundamentals of posture/physical assessment

- Assessment of the pelvis is fundamental to good seating.
- The pelvis has three planes of motion:
  - Obliquity (lifting on one side).
  - Rotation (forwards on one side).
  - Tilt (the pelvis moves to either exaggerate or diminish the lumbar lordosis).
- Basic measurements at the assessment:
  - Seat width, depth, and height.
  - Armrest height.
  - Backrest height and angle.
  - Footrest height.
  - User's weight.
- For all patients, but especially those with diminished sensation, measurement of pressure at the interface between the body and the cushion is vital to minimize the risks of pressure ulceration. Pressure mapping systems are commercially available and are used in specialist seating centres.
- Typical deviations from the ideal posture:
  - Windswept hips.
  - Scoliosis (see p. 545).
  - Kyphosis.

Posture management

- It should be noted that management of posture in the wheelchair in isolation to other forms of support used in any 24-hour period is likely to be ineffective, regardless of the age of the individual (including babies!).

- Children can spend 10–12 hours of every day in their beds. If adequate support is not provided, posture in the wheelchair will be affected. As an example, for someone with flexion contractures in the hips and knees and lying on their back, the legs will tend to fall to one side or the other. This places a twist on the pelvis and the spine causing discomfort.
- The adoption of such sustained postures is likely to lead to the development of structural musculoskeletal changes and will, as a result, impact wheelchair seating provision.

Training in posture management

Clinicians who wish to become specialists in this area can follow a variety of courses ranging from, e.g. the 4-day course at the Oxford Centre for Enablement in Oxford to a major component of the Oxford Brookes University Master's degree in Rehabilitation.

Wheelchair services

- Wheelchair services are provided by local health authorities. Services, organization, and eligibility vary between locations. In some areas they are part of a posture, independence, and mobility service which may have a more all-encompassing role.
- Children generally need to be >30 months to be referred as before this age standard buggies can usually accommodate needs.
- Referrals are accepted from healthcare professionals, but some localities accept self-referral.

Role of wheelchair service

- Assessment of need.
- Recommendation of suitable chair.
- Explanation of funding options.
- Provision of chairs and accessories.
- Training in use of equipment.
- Maintenance and repair of equipment.

Assessment

Assessment for a chair will include:
- The child's condition and level of ability.
- Where and when the chair will be used.
- The child's ability to use the chair themselves or whether others will be propelling them.
- Where children have more severe disability, standard chairs may not be appropriate and more postural custom-made support will be necessary.

Types of wheelchairs and accessories

- Manual:
  - Self-propelled.
  - Attendant propelled.
- Powered, either indoor (often called EPIC: electrically powered indoor chair), indoor/outdoor (EPIOC), or outdoor (EPOC):
  - Driven by occupant.
  - Driven by attendant.
- Tilt in space, either in manual or powered wheelchairs (utilizing gravity to maintain position).
- Other forms of posturally supportive seating:
  - Armchair.
  - Workstation, e.g. for computer use, hobbies.
  - Classroom.
  - Dining.
- Accessories include mobile arm supports, arm rests, trays, cushions, head supports, and leg rests.
- Rain covers are *not* provided by the wheelchair service.

Funding options

Standard option
- Chair provided, maintained, and repaired free of charge.

Wheelchair voucher scheme
- Each local service chooses whether or not to use this scheme.
- Allows purchase of a non-NHS chair using the voucher to the value of the recommended chair and the family paying the difference.
- If this is done in 'partnership', the chair is purchased through an approved supplier. The wheelchair service will maintain and repair the chair (some of this cost will be reflected in a lower amount of the voucher).
- If the voucher is used 'independently', the family own the wheelchair and are responsible for its repair and maintenance.
- The voucher scheme increases the choice of chairs available to a child.

Training
- Training is provided for families in use of any equipment supplied, including safety issues.
- Some charities also provide skills training, e.g. Whizz-Kidz.

Maintenance and repair
- A wheelchair service has an associated approved repairer/maintenance service including deliveries, collections, modifications, and servicing.
- Service organization in UK: there are several generic small-scale wheelchair services in England, with fewer larger centres in Scotland and Wales. In addition, there are a small number of highly specialist centres with expertise in managing the most complex seating problems, e.g. the Specialist Disability Service, Oxford Centre for Enablement, Oxford University Hospitals NHS Foundation Trust, and the West Midlands Rehabilitation Centre, Birmingham Community Healthcare NHS Trust.

Further resources
Disabled Living Foundation (DLF) (impartial advice and information on all aspects of equipment): ☎ 0845 130 9177; ℰ https://livingmadeeasy.org.uk/

Fledglings (helps identify, source, and supply practical and affordable aids/equipment): ☎ 0845 458 1124; ℰ http://www.fledglings.org.uk

NHS wheelchairs: ℰ https://www.england.nhs.uk/wheelchair-services/

Occupational therapy: principles and assessment

Occupational therapy is a profession concerned with promoting health and well-being through occupation. It is the art and science of enabling people to actively participate in the day-to-day activities that are important to them despite illness, impairment, or disability.

Aim of occupational therapy

To enhance participation in activities of everyday life within the areas of:
• Work/productive activities, e.g. schoolwork (adult-directed activities).
• Play/leisure activities (child-directed activities).
• Self-care activities, e.g. activities of daily living.

Activities of daily living include

• Toilet hygiene.
• Bathing/showering.
• Personal hygiene and grooming.
• Eating and feeding.
• Dressing.
• Functional mobility.
• Sleep and rest.

Instrumental activities of daily living are more complex activities of daily living needed for adult independence such as:
• Community mobility.
• Shopping, meal preparation, and clean up.
• Home management (e.g. laundry, cleaning, household maintenance).
• Health maintenance and safety/emergency responses.
• Financial management.

Occupational therapy assessment

Ideally occurs within the child's natural environment (e.g. home and/ or school) and consists of standardized (e.g. norm-referenced tests) and non-standardized assessment tools (e.g. observation, screening tests/questionnaires, parent's/teacher's interview, review of reports of other professionals), to gain relevant information about the child's:
• Abilities.
• Performance patterns and activity limitations.
• Contexts, e.g. home, school, childcare, and community settings taking into account physical, social, and cultural factors.
• Interaction between the child's abilities and the demands of the environment.
• Concerns/priorities of the child, parents/caregivers, and teachers.

Setting collaborative occupational therapy goals

Goals/objectives of occupational therapy intervention are often linked to:
• Specific performance limitations (e.g. short-term goals).
• Participation restrictions (e.g. long-term goals).

Occupational therapy goals are developed in collaboration with the child, parents, and multidisciplinary team and outline:
• The activities the child will perform.

- The environmental conditions.
- Any environmental modifications.
- Amount and type of activity assistance (adapting activities or providing additional adult support or equipment/assistive devices). See Table 7.4.

Table 7.4 Examples of fine motor difficulties and practical suggestions for children aged <5 years. Ensure child feels successful to maintain motivation

Fine motor skills	OT recommendations
Drawing/ handwriting	Provide thicker, triangular barrelled pencils, chunky chalk, thick crayons/paint brushes, finger painting, trial of pencil grips
	Encourage drawing/writing on vertical surface (e.g. wall, easel/ chalkboard, magnetic/felt boards) or writing slope to improve wrist position for writing
	Demonstrate drawing simple shapes (increasing in complexity), e.g. vertical line, then horizontal line, circle, cross, square, and wait for child to imitate
	Appropriate handwriting programme, e.g. 'Write From the Start' or 'Handwriting Without Tears', etc.
Dressing	Encourage child to sit while dressing
	'Backward chaining' approach to dressing—adult does the first step, e.g. adult pulls sock halfway off the foot, then child finishes the task by pulling sock off foot. Gradually reduce assistance until child completes whole task
	Choose shoes with Velcro fasteners. Encourage unzipping before zipping up. Start with loose, large buttons first when child is ready (e.g. undoing pyjama/coat buttons)
Feeding	Ensure child is sitting in a stable position with feet supported, e.g. 'Tripp Trapp' chair
	Adult to steady base of two-handled cup as child brings to mouth, gradually reduce assistance then move to one-handled cup then a beaker.
	For a child aged <3 years, encourage use of either spoon or fork only using 'hand-over-hand' then move hand to child's elbow to reduce level of help
	Cut food to mouthful size and encourage child to stabilize bowl/plate with other hand
	Use child-sized built-up cutlery, e.g. 'Junior Caring Cutlery' to aid grasp. Introduce cutting with knife to cut 'Velcro fruit', 'play dough', or banana, etc.
Other play activities to develop manual dexterity	For more challenging fine motor activities, encourage child to sit at child-sized table rather than sitting unsupported on floor
	Use 'play dough'/clay to strengthen hands by rolling, squeezing, squashing, etc. before using shape cutters
	Large building blocks, e.g. 'Duplo' or magnetic or Velcro blocks before providing smaller construction toys, e.g. 'Lego'
	Inset jigsaws with large handles
	Thread beads onto dowel before threading onto shoelace/ string
	Pick up objects with tongs, teabag squeezers, etc. before snipping with scissors

Occupational therapy: aids and adaptations

Occupational therapy assessment for equipment and/or home/school adaptations, considers the following:

- Environment, space within the property, ease of moving from one room to another, door widths and thresholds, etc.
- Lifestyle and cultural context of the child/young person and family—perceptions of ease of transfers (acceptability of being lifted by parents).
- The opinions of the child/young person and family, being aware of perception of aesthetics, design, comfort, and perceived usefulness of adaptations/equipment.
- The other equipment already in use and need for complementary options.
- The cognitive abilities of the child/young person, physical stage of development, and need for appropriate positioning in line with 24-hour postural management.
- Will the proposed adaptations/equipment meet the child's needs and is it 'necessary, appropriate, reasonable and practical' as set out in the Housing Grants, Construction and Regeneration Act 1996?
- Is the family eligible to apply for a means-tested *disabled facilities grant* from the district or city council for major adaptations to a privately owned, rented, or housing association property?
- Will the child/young person be more integrated into the family life and have increased access to activities after provision of adaptations/equipment?
- Is recommended equipment adjustable for growth?

The OT works together with a range of professionals within:

- Health (e.g. paediatrician, physiotherapist (see ➔ pp. 374–6), SLT (see ➔ pp. 402–3), etc.).
- Education (e.g. teaching assistant, teacher, SEN coordinator (see ➔ pp. 656–8), educational psychology, properties and facilities for adaptations to school buildings/grounds).
- District/county council (e.g. application for a disabled facilities grant).
- Voluntary sector (e.g. charities who may provide additional funding).

OT intervention may include recommendations (Table 7.5) for:

- Standard or specialist equipment/assistive devices.
- Minor or major housing adaptations to the child's home/school environment.
- Information and advice to children and families about other sources of support.

Table 7.5 Examples of adaptations and equipment/assistive devices which may be recommended

Potential barriers	Adaptations	Assistive devices
Entrances and exits (including access to car and garden)	Grab rails Stair rails Ramps Built-up terrain to threshold height In-home lift Increase door width Door re-hinged to open in/out	Lever door handle Environmental control unit
To improve safety for children who have reduced awareness of danger	Stable doors Door handles raised to adult height Safe fencing	Sound monitors
Bathroom	Low mounted sink Level access shower with shower seat Ceiling hoist Grab rails	Toilet seat reducer Toilet step/footrest Potty chair with postural support Single-lever faucets Bath board/seat/lift Mobile over toilet/shower chair Mobile hoist Hoisting, bathing, and/or toileting slings
Bedroom	Downstairs bedroom Ceiling hoist Grab rails	Bed rails Firm mattress and/or specialized bed Mobile hoist Hoisting slings
Kitchen	Lowered countertops/cabinets Sliding drawers and organizers in cabinets	Dining seating with postural support Cutlery with built-up handles
Living room	Ceiling hoist	Seating with postural support Mobile hoist Hoisting slings

Further resources

Disabled Living Foundation (DLF) (impartial advice and information on all aspects of equipment): ℘ https://livingmadeeasy.org.uk/

Fledglings (helps identify, source, and supply practical and affordable aids/equipment): ℘ http://www.fledglings.org.uk

Occupational therapy: enabling hand function, seating, etc.

Effective use of the hands to engage in a variety of occupations depends on a complex interaction of:
- Fine motor skills (see ➔ p. 46).
- Postural mechanisms (see ➔ pp. 384–6).
- Cognition (see ➔ pp. 416–18).
- Visual perception (see ➔ p. 50).

Link between postural ability and fine motor skills

- Tasks that require concentration and accurate fine motor skills necessitate stabilizing the body, work surface, and tools. Improved postural ability with increased shoulder and pelvic girdle control, leads to increased control of fine motor skills. No one correct sitting posture exists because no position is constant, nor should it be.
- Many variables influence the choice of body position and posture including:
  - The nature of the activity.
  - Convenience.
  - Requirements of speed, precision, and strength.
- Postural and motor ability are affected by a combination of factors including:
  - The maturational level of the nervous system.
  - Sensory integration.
  - Changes in lengths of muscles.
  - Selective muscle control for posture and movement.
  - Formation of bones and joints.
  - Biomechanical forces.
  - Nutrition.
  - Health.
  - Environmental factors.
  - The activity the child is engaged in.
- Postural management equipment, e.g. specialized seating, is designed to (see ➔ pp. 384–6):
  - Promote normal motor control.
  - Support without restricting movement.
  - Improve practical ability.
  - Reduce the progression of deformity.
  - Improve the efficiency of complex cognitive tasks by reducing the need to focus attention on maintaining posture.

Sensory integration

- Sensory integration theory hypothesizes that every human action involves integrated neurological processes from sensory, motor, and other cognitive and emotional systems.
- Sensory integration knowledge can be applied in different ways to different populations for different purposes. This has resulted in difficulties in drawing conclusions about the effectiveness of sensory integration intervention; however, there is evidence in the neuroscience literature to support the use of active, engaged, sensory-motor activities to enhance neuroplasticity (and emerging evidence that they support learning, memory, and problem-solving).

Sensory processing disorder (SPD)

- Previously described as sensory integrative dysfunction—is not currently included in the DSM-5 or ICD-11; however, sensory processing difficulties are included as one of the symptoms in the diagnostic criteria for ASD (see ➲ p. 116).
- SPD is a neurological disorder characterized by poor detection, modulation, discrimination, or responses to sensory stimuli.
- This results in the brain having problems with sorting out, filtering, analysing, organizing, and connecting (integrating) sensory messages.
- When some aspect of sensory integration does not function efficiently, the child may experience stress in the course of everyday occupations because neurological processes that should be automatic or accurate are not.
- Common diagnostic groups who may exhibit signs of SPD/difficulties:
  - ASD (see ➲ pp. 114–25).
  - ADHD (see ➲ pp. 126–34).
  - CP (see ➲ pp. 92–101).
  - Genetic conditions, e.g. fragile X syndrome (see ➲ pp. 516–17), DS (see ➲ pp. 496–500).
  - Developmental delay (see ➲ pp. 30–1).
  - Visual impairment (see ➲ pp. 202–8).
  - Hearing impairment (see ➲ pp. 168–9).
  - Learning disabilities (see ➲ pp. 136–41).
  - TBI (see ➲ pp. 108–9).
  - Prematurity.
  - Environmentally deprived, e.g. in cases of abuse/neglect (see ➲ pp. 560–1).

SPD is usually manifested as either over-responsiveness (hypersensitivity) or under-responsiveness (hyposensitivity) specific to any, or a combination of the seven senses:

Over-responsiveness (hypersensitivity)—'A little feels like a lot'
- The child who is over-responsive is overwhelmed by ordinary sensory input and reacts defensively to it, often with strong negative emotion and activation of the sympathetic nervous system.

- Over-responsiveness is characterized by 'sensation avoiding' with a tendency to avoid sensations, be fearful, distressed, cautious, negative, aggressive, or withdrawn (a 'fight or flight' response).
- This condition may occur as a general response to many types of sensory input, or it may be specific to one or a few sensory systems affected, e.g.:
  - Tactile defensiveness.
  - Gravitational insecurity.
  - Over-reactions to light, sounds, odours, and tastes.

Under-responsiveness (hyposensitivity)—'A lot feels like a little'
- The child who is under-responsive frequently fails to attend to or register relevant environmental stimuli.
- The child may seem oblivious to touch, pain, movement, taste, smells, sights, or sounds.
- This is characterized by either 'low registration' with a tendency to withdraw and be difficult to engage, or 'sensory-seeking' behaviours—craving/seeking out intense sensory input, e.g. being constantly 'on the go', jumping from dangerous heights during play, preferences for very strong flavours in foods, etc.
- Children with under-responsiveness to tactile and proprioceptive input may also have difficulties postural control or praxis (ideation, motor planning, and sequencing of movements), e.g. DCD (see ➔ pp. 146–9).

Aims of occupational therapy intervention in SPD
- To help children, parents, and teachers understand SPD and its impact on the child and their everyday life.
- To provide strategies enabling the child to achieve an optimal level of alertness, facilitating more effective engagement in everyday life activities at home, school, and in the community.
- To improve child's self-esteem by empowering child and family, decreasing frustration/stress levels (by addressing sensory difficulties) and improving participation in activities (occupations).

Occupational therapy recommendations for children with SPD
▶ Occupational therapy recommendations for children with SPD should be very specific, according to the child's individual sensory profile (for examples, see Table 7.6). Parent/carers should supervise all recommended activities, allow the child to do the activities in his/her own way, build on activities chosen by the child, and stop the activity if the child becomes distressed.

Sensory modulation
Sensory modulation refers to CNS regulation of its own activity. Sensory modulation problems may be identified when children fluctuate between the two extremes of over- and/or under-responsiveness, even within the same sensory system, affecting the child's level of alertness.

Table 7.6 Occupational therapy recommendations for children with SPD

	Over-responsiveness	Under-responsiveness
Proprioception	(Not observed)	Lots of 'heavy work' activities, i.e. activities where muscles/joints are pushed/pulled, e.g. weight bearing on hands and knees, jumping on a trampoline, pushing/pulling heavy wagon, digging, hammer toys/drums, tug of war, obstacle course, etc. Provide chewy necklace/bracelet or chewy tube Offer sleeping bag or heavier blanket/duvet for sleeping
Tactile	Avoid light/sudden touch—use firm touch instead Offer firm 'bear hugs' Offer firm head massage and/or wear tight-fitting hat prior to hair washing/cutting Offer child choices for texture/type of clothing, bedding, towels, etc. and cut tags out of clothing if requested Slowly introduce messy play activities/new textures gradually	Use touch to get child's attention before speaking to him/her Provide many opportunities for messy play, plenty of different textures for hands, fidget toys, etc.
Vestibular	Encourage 'heavy work' (proprioceptive) activities prior to and following movement activities Provide opportunities for slow, regular linear movements (e.g. gentle back-and-forth motion, starting with feet on the ground first incl. rocking chair) rather than fast or jerky angular/rotatory movements	Encourage regular movement breaks throughout the day, e.g. rough and tumble play, 'animal walks', playground, trampoline, swing (including rotary swings), self-spinning toys, slide, space hopper, exercise ball, 'move and sit' cushion, etc.
Auditory	Use quiet voices and try to minimize loud, unexpected noises as much as possible Have quiet space for child to retreat to at home and school Offer ear-defenders to block out noise when needed, e.g. shopping centre, vacuum, lawn mower, etc. Carry laminated 'out of order' sign to stick on to hand dryers in public toilets if necessary	Vary tone of voice when speaking Lots of music, singing, nursery rhymes Provide opportunities to experiment with noisy toys, e.g. musical instruments, drums, shakers, whistles, etc.

Table 7.6 *(Contd.)*

	Over-responsiveness	Under-responsiveness
Visual	Uncluttered visual spaces, soft lighting, muted colours (turn off fluorescent lights) Allow child to wear sunglasses (even indoors)	Visually exciting environment, bright colours, posters/mobiles, light up/flashing toys, etc. Visual discrimination and hand–eye coordination games, e.g. batting at balloons, throwing bean bags into washing basket, popping bubbles, fishing games, visual treasure hunts/'Where's Wally?', etc.
Olfactory	Avoid perfumes, scented body lotions, and strong laundry powder Turn on fan in kitchen to disperse cooking odours	Use scented 'play dough' or pens Encourage child to smell different foods during cooking activities
Gustatory	Often oversensitivity is due to texture, i.e. touch rather than taste, commonly lumpy foods (mixed texture) are difficult to tolerate, and child may gag Encourage oral motor skills, e.g. chewing, sucking, blowing, etc. Do not pressure child into eating foods that he/she finds uncomfortable Have non-preferred foods available throughout day for child to experience on own terms (e.g. messy food play, involvement in cooking activities) rather than pressuring child to eat and increasing stress at mealtimes Provide a wide range of foods, and offer a variety of different textures and temperatures of each food Consider referral to dietician if there are concerns regarding nutritional intake or to speech and language therapist if there are concerns regarding drooling/chewing/swallowing	Offer crunchy/chewy foods and/or foods with strong flavours, e.g. grapefruit juice, peppers, adding herbs/spices Try an electric toothbrush

Occupational therapy resources for parents

- *The Out of Sync Child: Recognizing & Coping with Sensory Processing Disorder* by Carol Stock Kranowitz (revised edition 2006; new edition due 2022).
- *Sensational Kids: Hope and Help for Children with Sensory Processing Disorder* by Lucy Jane Miller (revised edition 2014)
- *The Out-of-Sync Child Has Fun: Activities for Kids with Sensory Processing Disorder* by Carol Stock Kranowitz (2006)
- *The Ultimate Guide to Sensory Processing Disorder: Easy, Everyday Solutions to Sensory Challenges* by Roya Ostovar (2010)
- *Raising a Sensory Smart Child: The Definitive Handbook for Helping Your Child with Sensory Processing Issues* by Lindsey Biel and Nancy Peske (2009).
- SPD Foundation website: ℘ http://spdfoundation.net/index.html

Speech and language therapy: aims, approaches, and conditions

Aims

- To promote comprehension and clear expression of language.
- To enable child to communicate with others.
- To develop oral feeding skills (see ➔ pp. 444–6).

Approach

- Work is carried out either 1:1, in groups, or with parents, carers, and other professionals to help the child develop their skills.
- Increasingly SLTs work through people who are in daily contact with the child, providing training and treatment programmes for them to carry out.
- Services are split into early years and school age:
  - Preschool SLTs work primarily in clinics, children's centres, and early years settings.
  - School-age SLTs visit children at school and services are generally restricted to those children who have a SEN (see ➔ pp. 656–8).
  - Children with complex needs may have specialist staff who visit at home or in mainstream or special schools (see ➔ p. 656).

Prevalence

- Approximately 7% of 5-year-olds entering school have significant difficulties with speech and/or language. The majority of these children have expressive language delay.
- Approximately 1% of 5-year-olds have the most severe and complex speech, language, and communication needs. These children have limited comprehension and expression.
- In socially disadvantaged areas, it is possible that up to 50% of children at nursery age could have significant language delays.

Descriptions of speech and language conditions

- *Language delay*: delayed development of comprehension or expressive skills (see ➔ p. 56).
- *Language impairment*: atypical development, e.g. expressive skills appear in advance of comprehension, or severe delay of either or both.
- *Speech (phonological) delay*: pronunciation similar to that of a younger child, e.g. no use of consonant clusters ('poon' for 'spoon').
- *Speech (phonological) impairment*: atypical pattern of development or use of sounds; or severe speech delay.
- *Articulation disorder*: difficulty in moving tongue, lips to create sounds:
  - Mild: lisp ('th' for 's'), difficulty with 'sh', 'ch', 'r', or 'l'.
  - Severe: dysarthric type oral motor difficulty affecting articulation, e.g. slow laboured speech.
- *Verbal dyspraxia*: difficulty in the motor planning of articulatory movements, leading to limited number of sounds and sound sequences produced or copied (see ➔ pp. 402–3).

- *Disorders of nasal resonance*: hypernasal quality to speech or at worst, inability to make oral consonants such as 'b/d' instead producing 'm/n'. This could be as a result of cleft palate, submucous cleft, or velopharyngeal insufficiency (short soft palate, increased dimensions of nasopharynx post adenoidectomy, or poor motor control).
- *Dysfluency*: stammering in ~1% of population. Prevalence of ~5% in children <6 years have been reported.
- *Voice disorders*: hoarse or breathy voice, generally due to vocal abuse such as excessive shouting or structural abnormalities/pathology, e.g. laryngeal webbing/vocal fold palsy or dysarthric type motor difficulty, e.g. in CP (see ⊃ pp. 92–101).
- *Social communication disorders*: ASDs or pragmatic disorders, i.e. difficulty in use of language to communicate (see ⊃ pp. 114–25).

Speech and language therapy: assessment

The following areas are assessed to aid diagnosis:

Attention and listening skills

- Attention span and ability to switch attention from play to speaker is noted.
- Ability to attend to activities that are adult directed are observed.

Play skills

- The ability to show functional use of objects (e.g. brush for hair, cup for drinking) is a precursor to pretending and develops by 12 months.
- The presence of pretend play is linked with early language development. It emerges from about 15 months.
- The ability to sequence play actions to create a story line is also observed (this develops by 3 years).

Social interaction skills

- The ability and desire to interact with others.
- Using appropriate eye contact.
- Facial expression.
- Gesture.
- Pointing.
- Use of language to request, comment, respond to questions, ask questions, direct, and retell events.
- Conversational skills and joint play skills.

Verbal comprehension skills

- Verbal comprehension skills are assessed using increasingly complex instructions that require a motor response, i.e. selection of objects or pictures by pointing, or moving toys.
- This enables differentiation between children with purely expressive difficulties and those with comprehension and expressive problems.
- Tests start with single-object label recognition, verb recognition, then testing 2–4 key word level instructions as well as concept and grammatical understanding.

Expressive language skills

- Counting number of words/signs/symbols used by child to communicate.
- Types of words, i.e. nouns, verbs, adjectives, prepositions, etc.
- Length of phrases. These phrases must be flexible and not rote learned as 'chunks', e.g. here-it-is.
- Grammatical complexity of sentences, e.g. use of pronouns he/she/they; use of verb tenses fell/washed. Use of sentences linked with and/because/that.
- Functional use of expressive language, e.g. to make requests, comment, ask and answer questions, describe, converse.
- Formal testing involves eliciting specific responses to pictures, toy materials or questions.

- Informal testing involves transcribing child's language during relaxed play or interaction. This often results in a more reliable sample of child's language but is more time-consuming.

Speech/articulation skills

- Speech is assessed by presenting target pictures which contain all the sounds of speech in different word positions.
- The child's system of simplification (phonological system) can then be analysed.
- Typical patterns of error in development include:
  - *Stopping*, i.e. f, s, sh, ch all substituted by b/d. Generally resolves by 3 years.
  - *Fronting*, i.e. k/g substituted by t/d. Can be as late as 4 years.
  - *Consonant blend deletion*, i.e. sp becomes p, bl becomes b. Generally, correct by 4½ years.
- Child's ability to copy different speech sounds in isolation is also tested. This will show if any articulation difficulties with specific sounds exists.
- *Dyspraxic* children struggle to copy consonant vowel sequences. Many have limited range of vowels and consonants and would have made very slow progress with speech development (see ➋ pp. 402–3).
- If *dysarthria* is suspected, DDK rates (diadochokinesis—the speed at which sounds such as p/t/k can be repeated) can also be tested and the difference between connected speech (longer strings of words) and single-word naming compared. In dysarthria, there is often a tiring effect with worsening intelligibility as the sentence continues or over a longer word.

Resonance

Hypernasal speech may suggest some structural abnormality such as cleft or submucous cleft palate or some neuromuscular condition affecting control of the velopharyngeal sphincter. (The velopharyngeal sphincter elevates the soft palate to close the nasopharynx so as to allow oral airflow.)

Voice

- Persistent hoarse or breathy voice needs ENT investigation and may require follow-up therapy to teach more effective and less damaging voice use.
- Dysphonia in children is often due to vocal abuse (i.e. shouting) but actual pathology is important to rule out, e.g. abnormalities such as webbing, unilateral cord palsy, nodules, or polyps.

Fluency

- Dysfluency (stammering) is an issue for a small percentage of children.
- For most it is a transient stage as linguistic output increases.
- If it persists for >6 months, referral to SLT is essential.
- Good outcomes exist for children <5 years using programmes such as *Lidcombe Therapy* which reinforces fluency in work with mother and child.

• Assessment includes type of dysfluency experienced, history of dysfluency, measures of amount of stammering in several minutes of speech and differences across different situations, and secondary behaviours associated with stammer, e.g. blinks, gestures, word switching, and avoidance.

Assessment tools

See Table 7.7.

Table 7.7 Common assessment tools used by SLTs

Area assessed	Name of test	Age range tested
Comprehension	Assessment of comprehension/expression	
	Bracken test for concepts	6–11 years
	British Picture Vocab Scales-3	3–7 years
	CELF-Preschool 2	3–16 years
	CELF-5	3–6 years
	Derbyshire Language Scheme	5–21 years
	Test of problem-solving	1–4½ years
	TROG-2	6–11 years
	New Reynell Developmental Language Scales	4–18 years / 2–7½ years
	PLS-5	0–6 years
Expression	Derbyshire Language Scheme	1–4½ years
	Renfrew Action Picture Test	3½ years–8 years and 5 months
	Renfrew Bus Story	3–8 years
	Renfrew Word Finding	3–9 years
	STASS	3–7 years
	CELF-Preschool 2	3–6 years
	CELF-5	5–17 years
Speech	STAP	3+ years
	DEAP	3–7 years
	Nuffield Dyspraxia assessment	3–6 years
Social interaction	Pragmatics Profile	All ages
	Social Communication Profile	All ages
	Social Use of Language Programme	All ages

CELF, Clinical Evaluation of Language Fundamentals; DEAP, Diagnostic Evaluation of Articulation and Phonology; PLS-5, Preschool Language Scale (PLS-5), fifth edition; STAP, South Tyneside Assessment of Phonology; STASS, South Tyneside Assessment of Syntactic Structures; TROG-2, Test for Reception of Grammar, Version 2.

Speech and language therapy: treatment strategies

For verbal comprehension

- Observe, watch, listen (OWL) and follow child's lead in play and conversation, reduce language complexity to child, and use descriptive commentary.
- Repetitive practice of target words/concepts in play and everyday situations.
- Use of photos, pictures, and real objects.
- Practise listening to increasing amounts of information.
- Teach conceptual vocabulary such as size, position words, colours, numbers, and grammatical items: pronouns, tenses, why, because, etc.
- Use of signs (e.g. Makaton) or photos/pictures to augment spoken communication.

For language expression

- OWL and follow child's lead in play and conversation.
- Repetitive input of target words in play and everyday situations.
- Use of a descriptive commentary, i.e. talk about what child is doing while he/she does it to input appropriate language models.
- Reduce number of questions to child as these produce limited response or are too stressful for some children.
- Add one word to what child says, i.e. expansion.
- Model phrase child needs to copy.
- Use signs and/or picture prompts to promote longer phrases.
- Teach noun, verb, adjective vocabulary, setting up games and activities for repetitive practice.
- Teach grammatical aspects, e.g. pronouns, tenses and use of linking words such as 'and', 'because', etc.

For speech

- Practise with target sounds, listening to meaning differences (minimal pair work, e.g. tea/key).
- Practise of target sounds in words, phrases, and connected speech.
- Options are to target one process, e.g. fronting—making all sounds at the front of mouth, or to target one sound at a time.
- Use of visual representation of sounds (pictures, letters) to aid sequencing of sounds—particularly useful in dyspraxia.
- Work on improving intelligibility of highly motivating words.
- Cued articulation—use of hand gestures to prompt specific articulatory movements.
- In dysarthric children, practise with oral movements to increase range, speed, accuracy of tongue articulation and use of pacing to improve intelligibility.

For social interaction/pragmatic use of language

- Interactive play including turn taking, action songs, peek-a-boo, etc.
- Specific work to teach rules of conversation.
- Modify environment to promote requests and comments (e.g. stop automatic provision of items for child, use of waiting for child to respond, introduce novelty or bizarre events).
- Use of picture exchange communication system to develop functional ability to request and comment.
- Use of AAC to support communication (see ➔ pp. 212–14).

For resonance

Practise producing oral consonants and use of visual feedback to encourage self-monitoring of nasality.

For dysfluency

- General advice to parents/carers regarding strategies to create a relaxed communication environment (e.g. reduce number of questions and demands for verbal responses).
- Practise relaxed ways of producing difficult words or sounds (methods generally use slowed articulation or use specific breath control techniques).
- Practise of these in increasingly difficult situations.
- Cognitive behavioural approaches to anxiety created by stammering (see ➔ p. 339).
- *Lidcombe therapy* is widely used in younger children. This teaches children to approach difficult words in a more relaxed way and reinforces fluency in activities carried out with the parent and child together.
- In older children, the psychological impact of having a stammer is addressed in group therapy as well as tackling the stammering behaviour itself by using relaxed articulation, slowed speech, or breathing techniques.

For voice

- Therapy for vocal misuse involves teaching the child to use better breath support for voice and less tension to produce volume (to 'yell well') as well as advocating lessening of shouting.
- Children with neurological conditions may need help to practise stronger voice or use better breath control to maintain voice during speech.

Autism Diagnostic Observation Schedule (ADOS)-2

- As its predecessor (ADOS), ADOS-2 is a semi-structured, standardized assessment of communication, social interaction, play, and restricted and repetitive behaviours, to assess anyone over 12 months of age, suspected of having ASD/autism (see ⊃ pp. 114–25).
- ADOS-2 has updated protocols, revised algorithms, a new 'Comparison Score', and a Toddler Module. Together it can provide a very precise picture of a child's/young adult's current symptoms.
- ADOS-2 is considered as a 'gold standard' in observational assessment of ASD. It is designed to be a complementary assessment to the Autism Diagnostic Interview.
- ADOS-2 can be administered to children at the whole range of developmental levels, i.e. from children with no language to those with fluent, full adult grammar.
- It presents various activities and 'social presses' (planned social situations) that can elicit behaviours directly associated to a diagnosis of ASD. By observing and coding these behaviours, one can acquire information that informs diagnosis, treatment planning, and educational placement.
- There are five modules in ADOS-2. However, an individual is administered only one module, chosen according to the child's expressive language ability and chronological age. The modules are:
  - Toddler Module (for ages 12–30 months. Provides 'ranges of concern for ASD' rather than 'cut-off' scores).
  - Module 1 (31 months and older).
  - Module 2 (any age, verbally not fluent/phrase speech).
  - Module 3 (verbally fluent, child/adolescent).
  - Module 4 (verbally fluent, older adolescent/adult).
- Social interaction is assessed in the ADOS-2 under two headings:
  - Communication.
  - Reciprocal social interaction.
- Aspects of communication assessed are:
  - Frequency of vocalization directed to others.
  - Stereotyped/idiosyncratic use of words or phrases.
  - Use of other's body to communicate.
  - Pointing.
  - Gestures.
  - Amount of social overtures.
  - Conversation.
- Aspects of reciprocal social interaction assessed are:
  - Unusual eye contact.
  - Facial expressions directed to others.
  - Shared enjoyment in interaction.
  - Showing.
  - Spontaneous initiation of joint attention.
  - Response to joint attention.
  - Quality of social overtures.

- Quality of social response.
- Amount of reciprocal social interaction.
- Overall quality of rapport.

Useful contacts

- AFASIC supports parents and carers of children with speech language and communication needs. Operates a parents' helpline: 🔗 https://www.afasic.org.uk/
- Communication Matters is a national organization providing information and symposia on AAC: 🔗 https://www.communicationmatters.org.uk/
- ICAN supports children with speech language and communication needs and provides information and training for parents and professionals: 🔗 https://ican.org.uk/ and 🔗 https://ican.org.uk/i-cans-talking-point/
- Royal College of Speech and Language Therapists is the professional body for SLTs in the UK and Ireland: 🔗 http://www.rsclt.org

Psychology: assessment and management of behavioural problems

Assessment of behavioural problems

Involves understanding the purpose and function of the behaviour by functional analysis (ABC analysis):

Antecedents
• What triggers it? Situation, timing, place, people present, environment.

Behaviour
• Detailed description of the behaviour. Nature, frequency, severity, duration.

Consequences
• What occurs after the behaviour? How is it managed? Child gets their immediate wants/attention, change in demands/expectation of child.
• Information gathering methods:
  • ABC diaries kept by parents.
  • Direct observation at home/school.
  • Videos of behaviour.

Treatment or behavioural modification

This is based on the idea that patterns of behaviour are reinforced by the response they elicit.

Desirable behaviours can be increased by
• Positive reinforcement: rewards, praise, star charts, adult positive attention, privileges.
• To be most effective, rewards should be given as soon as possible after desired behaviour (unlike bribes which are offered in advance), consistently given, tangible, in proportion to achievement, and readily achievable so child experiences early success.
• But the threshold for receiving a reward should increase with time until eventually the desired behaviour is achieved and maintained without need for reward.

Undesirable behaviours decreased by
• *Remove/change antecedent stimuli*: e.g. taking hyperactive child to park rather than staying indoors all day.
• *Extinction*:
  • Removing unintended reward (e.g. attention) for undesirable behaviour, ignoring undesired behaviour (behaviour may temporarily escalate in attempt to elicit response).
  • Not appropriate for serious bad behaviour.
• *Time out*:
  • Child taken away from context where behaviour occurred to quiet place for agreed period of time (e.g. a few minutes) and child should be calm before coming out.
  • Should be undertaken as part of behavioural programme.

- Rules must be clear, warning given, and alternative behaviour should be offered to child before removing them.
- Time-out place should be free of stimulus/entertainment.
- Parent should supervise but not interact with child.
- *Punishment*:
  - E.g. telling off, withholding rewards, loss of privileges.
  - Must be immediate, time-limited, proportionate, and perceived as negative by child.
  - Child can habituate quickly to punishment and so use only sparingly if behaviour unacceptable/dangerous.
  - Must be coupled with explanation and lots of positive reinforcement of desirable behaviour.
  - Avoid trap of unwittingly giving child too much attention for negative behaviour.

Setting up behavioural programme

- It is easy to become overwhelmed so initially focus on one or two behaviours, that can relatively easily be achieved—helps build confidence in child and parents.
- Specify target behaviour precisely and agree desired outcome in precise behavioural terms. Focus on formulating positive desired behaviours rather than stopping negative behaviours.
- Share understanding of the behaviour (ABC analysis) and impact on child/family with parent and child, emphasizing possibility for change.
- Establish system of rewards, time out, etc. as previously described.
- Parents should minimize anger when enforcing rules.
- Once target behaviour has been established, threshold for reward is increased and frequency of rewards decreased until target behaviour firmly established when rewards should cease.
- A new behaviour may then be targeted if necessary.

Clinical neuropsychology

Introduction

- Clinical neuropsychology is practised by clinical psychologists who require additional ('Qualification in Clinical Neuropsychology') training in neuropsychology.
- The primary concern of clinical neuropsychology is to elucidate brain–behaviour relationships.
- Assessments may be diagnostic, therapeutic, or serve as a baseline against which to measure developmental trajectory, recovery, or change following treatment.
- Following a detailed clinical interview (with the child and family) and examination of relevant medical and educational records, age-appropriate tests are typically administered over a period from 1 to 4 hours, with breaks as necessary.
- Questionnaire measures designed to screen and/or quantify behaviour, psychological or physical symptoms, and quality of life may also be given.
- A neuropsychology assessment should yield:
  - A formulation of whether the observed clinical presentation and cognitive profile are consistent with any known neuropsychological syndrome, developmental/congenital disorder, neurological illness/injury, or other medical/psychiatric condition.
  - Whether clarification of presenting difficulties are 'organic' and/or 'functional', and/or whether there are any social or mental health difficulties.
  - Detailed feedback of findings to parents and/or child and discussions/advice regarding implications for likely future developmental trajectory, education/training, social–emotional adjustment, behaviour management, etc.
  - Recommendations for education, therapy, further investigation, or assessment.
  - If appropriate, short psychological interventions (see ➔ pp. 366–7) for acute mental health issues (i.e. CBT, supportive counselling).
  - If appropriate, time-limited outpatient case management/monitoring.
  - Ongoing liaison with education (see ➔ Chapter 13) and any other relevant health professionals.

Rough guide to cognition

- All skills are dependent on age and environment (including education and familial factors, especially with verbal skills).
- All skills are mediated by arousal, disposition, effort, mood, and attention (see ➲ p. 126).
- Consider carefully if there is a GDD or LD/ID (see ➲ pp. 136–41); clues may include:
  - Indolent early development.
  - Features of medical history.
  - Pervasive school failure (see ➲ pp. 650–1).
- If GDD/LD, then most if not all cognitive domains are likely, by definition, to be similarly delayed. LD may present as 'poor memory/ concentration', 'slow learning', or 'poor school attainment'; there may, however, also be islands of relative ability (i.e. rote memory, motor skills).

If GDD/ID is unlikely, consider cognition in terms of 'domains'

Language expression and comprehension

(Dominant brain hemisphere.)
- Problems may present as:
  - Inability to understand what is said reliably (with no contextual clues).
  - Difficulty in naming objects/pictures, repeating sentence/word and/ or expressing self.
  - Poor prosody, semantics, syntax, or articulation (also see ➲ p. 405).
- Try 'open-ended' questions (e.g. 'What do you enjoy doing when you are not at school?').

Spatial skills

(Non-dominant brain hemisphere.)
- Problems may present as:
  - Left–right disorientation.
  - Getting lost easily.
  - Inability to read analogue clock face.
  - Putting clothes on wrong way round.
  - Putting shoes on wrong feet.
  - Inability to tie shoelaces.
  - Inability to write without lines to guide.
  - Inability to read maps/graphs.
- Ask the child to copy simple shapes, i.e. most can draw a circle at 3 years, a square at 4 years, a triangle at 5 years, and a diamond at 7 years (also see ➲ p. 46).

Memory/new learning skills

(Medial temporal lobes, diencephalic.)
- Neuropsychologists generally refer to 'long-term' rather than 'short-term' memory. Broadly equivalent to storage of information on a computer 'hard drive'; requires both adequate registration and retrieval skills. Fractionation may include the following:

- 'Remote' memory is memory for events some years ago and/or memories that pre-date the index illness/injury.
- 'Prospective' memory refers to planning for/remembering future events.
- 'Semantic' memory refers to fact-based knowledge.
- 'Autobiographical' memory refers to personal memories.
- 'Episodic' memory refers to memory for events placed in time.
- The younger the child, the less able to recall spontaneously; their recognition recall, or cued recall is better.
- Verbal recall is mediated by adequate language skills.
- Executive skills may mediate recall.
- In GDD/ID, word-finding difficulties or certain executive deficits may present as 'problems with memory'.
- Problems with 'long-term memory' may present as:
  - Forgetting activities, conversations, or events day-to-day.
  - Losing the thread of meaning while reading a book or watching TV programme.
  - Inability to recount favoured TV episodes.
  - Repeating self or questions.
  - Getting lost.

Attention and executive skills
(Prefrontal and frontostriatal.)
- 'Meta-cognitive' (e.g. mediating the use of language, attention, spatial and memory skills) executive skills continue to develop up to, and through the adolescent years.
- They correlate highly with IQ until ~8 years (and remain weak in GDD/ID).
- Until 7–8 years distractibility and disinhibition are hallmark features of a 'dysexecutive' syndrome.
- A dysexecutive' syndrome can be cognitive and/or behavioural.
- These skills are heterogeneous and difficult to assess in structured situations.
- They can include difficulties with organization, attention, and the self-regulation of behaviour (i.e. poor impulse/affect control).
- Disinhibition or 'inappropriate' behaviour is defined contextually; 'normal' adolescent adjustment may appear dysexecutive.
- Auditory attention span (i.e. digit span) is sometimes referred to as 'working' memory broadly equivalent to 'random access memory' (RAM) on a computer.
- Ask the child to repeat back a 2-, 3-, 4-, or 5-digit sequence (e.g. 6–7/4–3–7/5–7–3–2/ etc.), read at the rate of one per second. Then ask for same spans (but different digits) repeated back in reverse (i.e. 8–9–4 repeated back as 4–9–8).

Speed of information processing
- Problems with slowed mentation; sometimes confused with psychomotor speed.

- Can present as problems with divided attention or multitasking (e.g. keeping more than one 'ball in the air' cognitively).
- Figuratively, like the speed of the processor on a computer.

Dexterity
- Problems can present as clumsiness and/or poor writing (see ➡ pp. 146–9).
- Consider handedness (note: switching preferred hand till 4 years is not uncommon; 70% of left-handers are left hemisphere dominant).
- Gross motor skills: cycling, swimming, catching, running, sports (see ➡ p. 42), etc.

Attainments
These are learned, not necessarily innate skills.
- Problems with literacy and/or numeracy; single word/sentence reading, reading comprehension, spelling, adding, subtracting, times tables, etc.
- Referred to as 'dyslexia' (see ➡ p. 142) and 'dyscalculia' (see ➡ p. 142).
- There are many reasons why children have difficulties in reading—for *dyslexic* diagnosis, poor reading should normally be within a context of relatively well-preserved general intellectual skills.
- A *selective* dyscalculia is very rare.

Neuropsychology: referral considerations and indications

Indications from observations and reports

- Younger children may not complain of cognitive problems explicitly, especially if slow developing or chronic; it may need to be indirectly inferred from school observations or concerns of maladaptive behaviour (i.e. aggression, withdrawal, disorientation).
- Parental perspective needs to be weighed carefully (consider: are there older sibs for comparison? The perspective of extended family? Any relevant sociocultural factors? Parental expectations, presentation, occupation, education and mental health). Seek/consider *both* parents and/or extended family's perspective on problem.
- Corroboration from school needs to be weighed carefully (consider pedigree and specificity of school report, compliant children may be overlooked, ethnicity, language, literacy level, parental involvement). Consider whether major transitions at school (i.e. primary to secondary, exams) are unmasking underlying weaknesses. Seek continuity of opinion from school.
- What do reports from others in the health or educational sector say?
- Your own observations and consideration of all available evidence is crucial.

Medical indications

Any injury, illness, or congenital condition that may have compromised normal brain function could be a potential referral to neuropsychologists. These conditions generally present with abnormal neurology or physical malaise. The following list is illustrative rather than exhaustive.

- Traumatic: acceleration–deceleration (road traffic accidents, falls, non-accidental injury) (see ➡ pp. 108–9), missile wound, birth trauma, CP (see ➡ pp. 92–101).
- Cerebrovascular: stroke, haemorrhage, arteriovenous malformation (see ➡ pp. 270–1).
- Seizure disorder (see ➡ pp. 248–55): poorly controlled, absences, status epilepticus, nocturnal, subclinical activity, Rasmussen's.
- Space-occupying lesion: neoplasms, hydrocephalus (see ➡ p. 420).
- Infection: meningitis, encephalitis, abscess, herpes, HIV, syphilis.
- Neurotoxic: metals (lead, mercury), solvents/fuels (glues, paints) pesticides, carbon monoxide.
- Metabolic disorder (see ➡ pp. 152–7): hypoxia, diabetes, PKU.
- Environmental/social: severe neglect/abuse (see ➡ pp. 560–1), fetal alcohol spectrum disorder.
- Pervasive developmental disorders: ASD (see ➡ pp. 114–25), Rett syndrome (see ➡ pp. 518–19).
- Other neurodevelopmental disorders: e.g. ADHD (see ➡ pp. 126–34), Tourette (see ➡ pp. 304–5) syndrome.
- Genetic (see ➡ pp. 484–5): i.e. Williams, fragile X, Turner, Prader Willi, Angelman syndromes.
- Iatrogenic: radiotherapy, chemotherapy, medications (anticonvulsants, i.e. valproate), postoperative cognitive disorder (cardiac surgery, kidney dialysis, chronic anaesthetic neurotoxicity).

Issues to consider before a referral to neuropsychology

General considerations

- Consider whether involvement of neuropsychology would in any way advance the care of the child/young adult. If in doubt, seek guidance from the clinical neuropsychologist.
- Consider school/parental concerns and medical indications (see ➔ p. 420).
- Children with a GDD/ID (typically defined as a child with global intellectual abilities at or below 2 SD below the mean, i.e. IQ <70) should normally be referred to local Learning Disability Services. At the extremes of the normal distribution of ability (i.e. either very able or disabled), the efficacy and utility of neuropsychological assessment diminishes as the 'ceiling' or 'floor' of age-appropriate tests is reached.
- If there is no medical or psychiatric dimension, general difficulties at school are often best dealt with by educational psychology services (see ➔ pp. 666–7).
- If there is no neurological dimension, then referral to CAMHS may be more appropriate in the event of general behavioural or social–emotional problems (see ➔ p. 288).

Age considerations

- The extent to which cognition can be usefully fractionated depends upon age.
- With children younger than ~3 years, general developmental scales (i.e. assessment of gross and fine motor skills, language, social, and adaptive skills as, e.g. in the BSID-4 or Griffiths-III) need to be employed. The results of any cognitive assessment at this age will be a poor predictor of later intellectual skills.
- With preschool (3–6 years) children, assessment will generally be confined to verbal and non-verbal general intellectual skills, psychomotor/processing speed, attention and language skills; there are also measures of more selective skills (i.e. memory, attention/executive, spatial skills), though these are less commonly available outside specialist centres and may be less reliable.
- Until children first start to be exposed to school disciplines many are not familiar with or biddable to sitting down and completing tests over a period of time, which is required for successful neuropsychology assessments.
- All raw scores on the neuropsychology tests administered to children are referenced against a normal population of same-age peers and reported in terms of SD from the mean scores for that age band. Scores may be expressed as:
  - Percentiles.
  - T-scores (where the mean = 50, SD 10).
  - Standard scores (mean = 100, SD 15).
  - Age-scaled scores (mean = 10, SD 3).
  - 'Mental-age' equivalents.

Neuropsychology: advice to parents and school

- If a programme of 'cognitive rehabilitation' is offered, consider carefully:
  - Has there been a proper neuropsychological formulation of the quality and distribution of any cognitive impairment?
  - Is there a sound, peer-reviewed evidence base for the intervention?
  - Is it costly?
  - Is it onerous for the child?
  - Is there a sport or activity which the child could engage in pleasurably which might be of equal benefit and have incidental social value?
  - Does it purport to 'retrain', 're-organize', or 'recover' lost brain function? If so, treat with caution.
  - Does it purport to educate (i.e. understanding distribution of strengths and weaknesses correctly), support (i.e. re-establish self-confidence and insight), and/or maximize external and organizational aids (i.e. calendars, mobile phones, mechanical/electronic aids to recall, organization of function)? If so, it may be helpful.
  - COGMED Working Memory Training is one computerized cognitive training programme of working memory for which there is a reasonable, independent evidence base. The programme is suitable for children aged 4 years and older. There are peer-reviewed studies available, which suggest that COGMED training might improve some features of 'working memory', with some sustained and generalizing benefit. It is, however, a commercial programme which requires considerable commitment from parents and children over several weeks.
- Recovery or rehabilitation (see pp. 422–3, p. 535, pp. 533–4, p. 110, and p. 110) is often more about maximizing adaption, accommodation, and insight than restoration of lost function.
- Restore normal daily routines as far and as quickly as possible given the nature and severity of illness/injury.
- Encourage peer social activities whenever possible and/or appropriate.
- Consider carefully whether it is better to 'work' on lost skills which may never fully recover or focus instead on residual strengths (NB: the importance of self-confidence and self-esteem in adaption and recovery).
- Be aware of recovery gradients:
  - Following acute injury/illness. recovery takes up to 2–3 years with the rate of recovery diminishing over time; recovery in year 1 is much more marked than years 2–3.
  - Cognitive development can 'plateau' with new skills still being acquired but not at the same rate as age-related peers. For example, following radiotherapy the younger the child, the greater and more quickly any deleterious effects are apparent. In children >7/8 years effects are more subtle and take longer to be expressed—often in speed of information processing and/or attention.
  - Recovery can be 'stepwise' when interrupted by treatment or complications.

- The evidence for delayed emergence of cognitive or behavioural deficits (i.e. 'executive' deficits in adolescence following a frontal injury/illness in infancy) is very weak if there has been no manifestation of the deficit in intervening years. Pre-existing deficits can, however, be *exacerbated* or exaggerated by adolescent adjustment.
  - Extent of impaired awareness/cognition acutely does not always correlate with longer-term neuropsychological outcome.
- Age-related vulnerability/plasticity. There is some evidence to suggest that at approximately:
  - 0–12 months: confers increased vulnerability to brain insult (which outweighs beneficial effects of potential plasticity).
  - 1–6 years: vulnerability is less but there is still plasticity, which may lead to greater recovery potential.
  - 6–7 years: the evidence for true brain plasticity (i.e. ability to spontaneously reorganize or recommit skills to non-damaged brain area) can be limited.
- In adolescence, maladaptation to chronic or serious acute illness/injury (see p. 354) is more common than in the younger or middle years of childhood.

Orthotic management of neurodisability

- *Orthoses*, often referred to as splints or braces, are externally applied medical devices that compensate for impairments in the musculoskeletal (see ➔ Chapter 10) or neurological systems (see ➔ Chapter 5).
- *Orthotists* are the allied health professionals specifically trained to advise on whether and how an orthosis can be designed and made.
- Orthoses are prescribed to achieve clinical objectives such as to prevent deformity or to improve functioning (see ➔ p. 426).
- Orthoses are usually custom moulded from plastics, such as polypropylene, and incorporate judiciously placed straps and padding in order to achieve their goals.

Biomechanical principles

- The means by which orthoses work is biomechanical, through the application of force and lever systems.
- Typically, the forces that orthoses apply are 'reaction' forces generated in response to gravity, where muscles are weak, and/or to counter forces of muscle imbalance, as in the case of spasticity.
- Key biomechanical principles underpinning orthotic management are that using longer lever arms means less force is required; and that applying forces over large surface areas means less pressure is applied to the body. For stability, the centre of mass of the body must be within the base of support.
- An appreciation of gait analysis (see ➔ p. 530) is necessary to understand how orthoses can improve the efficiency of walking.

Terminology

- Terminology for orthoses can be confusing. The standard system is to describe an orthosis by the joints that are encompassed in the device. For example, an orthosis enclosing the ankle and foot but finishing below the knee is an ankle–foot orthosis, with the acronym AFO. Similarly, a spinal orthosis encompassing the thoracolumbar and sacral spine is referred to as a TLSO.
- Sometimes the aim of the orthosis is included in the name, such as hip abduction orthosis.
- Confusion can occur when orthoses are named after people or places or referred to by trade names. Terms such as dynamic are vague and should be avoided.

Foot orthoses

- Insoles, supportive footwear, and shoe modifications can all be used to increase stability during standing and walking.
- Mild plano-valgus or varus deformities (see ➔ p. 553) can be controlled by foot orthoses that are designed to encourage better skeletal alignment.
- Foot orthoses occasionally extend just above the ankle to gain greater control, and these designs are termed supra-malleolar orthoses (SMOs).
- Insoles can also be moulded to redistribute plantar pressure under the foot.

Ankle–foot orthoses

- To control equinus (see ➔ p. 540) or calcaneus deformity, or moderate to severe valgus or varus deformities, an orthosis needs to encompass the ankle and foot and extend to just below the knee.
- AFOs provide longer leverage and control in the sagittal plane. AFOs may be trimmed to be flexible or incorporate hinges to allow dorsiflexion, or made rigid to provide maximum control.
- AFOs are widely prescribed for children with CP (see ➔ pp. 92–101), spina bifida (see ➔ pp. 278–9), and other neuromuscular conditions (see ➔ pp. 272–6) to improve gait efficiency.
- AFOs are also used to control foot position and prevent deformity in non-ambulant children.
- Sometimes AFOs are used at night, although this should not be pursued if this interferes with sleeping.

Knee–ankle–foot orthoses (KAFOs)

- A KAFO extends from the thigh and includes the ankle and foot; a hinge is usually included at the knee to enable flexion during sitting but these are often designed to be locked in extension for standing and walking.
- Children with neuromuscular conditions such as muscular dystrophy (see ➔ pp. 272–3) or SMA (see ➔ p. 273) may find that KAFOs enable them to stand and walk; however, KAFOs are rarely used with children with CP.

Hip–knee–ankle–foot orthoses (HKAFOs)

- HKAFOs can enable children who are unable to maintain standing unaided to stand and become mobile.
- HKAFOs extend from the trunk and control the whole lower limb. Children with spina bifida or paraplegia can learn to use custom-fitted modular orthoses such as the Swivel Walker or ParaWalker.

Thoracolumbar sacral orthoses

- Spinal orthoses (TLSOs) are used to control scoliosis (see ➔ pp. 278–9) in children with a variety of neuromuscular conditions.
- Although orthoses may not prevent progressive scoliosis, TLSOs are often used to reduce the rate of progression and delay the need for surgical stabilization, or when surgery is not possible.

Upper limb orthoses

- Orthoses are used to position the arm, wrist, and hand to improve upper limb functioning and/or manual ability (see ➔ p. 547).
- Wrist–hand orthoses usually hold the wrist in extension, and may extend to control thumb posture to promote a functional position.
- 'Paddle' type designs of wrist–hand orthoses may be used to resist flexion deformities in the wrist and fingers.

Head orthoses

- A protective helmet may be indicated when a child is prone to falling, for instance, during seizures (see ➔ pp. 248–55), or injuring themselves.
- Helmets vary in design; some are constructed from dense foams while other designs have hard exteriors.

Lycra-based orthoses
- There has been increasing interest in fabric orthoses that use Lycra-based materials to control body postures.
- These types of orthoses can be designed to fit different parts of the body.
- However, there is limited evidence that Lycra-based orthoses are effective, or to inform patient selection.

Summary
- Orthoses can be very useful to improve functioning in children with neurodisability and may reduce the rate of progressive deformity.
- However, orthoses can occasionally create skin problems due to pressure or friction, and repairs may be required. Therefore, families should be able to easily access an orthotist directly, and the fit of an orthosis should be checked by an orthotist as necessary.
- Typically, a child grows out of their orthosis between 6 and 14 months, and so reassessment and replacement of the orthosis needs to be considered.
- There can be stigma associated with using equipment that identifies children as different to their peers. Therefore, the benefits of orthoses for individual children should be carefully assessed and re-evaluated over time.
- An orthotist with an understanding of the nuances of neurodisability should be an integral member of the MDT (see ➜ pp. 526–8).

Prosthetics

What is a prosthesis?

A prosthesis replaces a part of the body, e.g. a missing limb. It should be distinguished from an orthosis, which is a device to hold part of the body in a more correct or desirable position (see pp. 424–6).

What is a prosthetist?

Prosthetists and orthotists are the health professionals trained to design and manufacture these devices. They are dual trained in the two roles but generally specialize in one or the other later.

Prosthetics in childhood and adult life

- The requirement for a prosthesis is rare in early childhood and is usually the consequence of a congenital abnormality, often, for instance, a trans-radial deficiency resulting in an absent hand.
- In childhood other causes of limb deficiency accumulate: trauma, cancer, and increasingly frequently as a result of a child surviving sepsis.
- This contrasts dramatically with adult-onset limb deficiency which is overwhelmingly the result of vascular problems due to diabetes, smoking, and atherosclerosis.

Some key principles

- Use play to help the child to want to wear the prosthesis, e.g. encourage them to wear it while a story is being read aloud or particular toys are being played with.
- Enable the child to reach their developmental milestones on time, e.g. have the prosthetic leg ready for learning to walk.
- Children are infinitely adaptable; they find ways around limb deficiencies very often, e.g. using the elbow flexion of an arm with no hand, to replace the hand. This can make encouraging them to use the artificial hand very difficult. The residual limb has good sensation, whereas the prosthesis has none.
- Make sure the prosthesis is functionally useful at that time for the child. An upper limb device is more of a tool than a hand, e.g. to hold a bicycle handlebar, or play with a particular toy.
- Involve the child's carers or parents in the process of learning to use a device.
- Parents of children who lose a limb through trauma are often overwhelmed by feelings of guilt and may themselves need a chance to spend time with a counsellor.
- For parents of a child with a congenital limb deficiency the major impact comes at a much earlier stage in the child's life, even before they are born if the deficiency has been identified on a scan.
- Deciding to remove parts of a residual limb that get in the way of making prosthetic progress is an agonizing and protracted process, e.g. removing a deformed and inappropriately placed foot in proximal femoral deficiency.

- Using other body parts to replace a missing hand, e.g. using the mouth and teeth as a surrogate hand, can have significant consequences for the part that is used later in life—such as wear and tear on teeth, or painful joints if feet are used as hands.
- The prosthetic user will have lifelong contact with a prosthetic service, with differing needs at different stages of life.
- Children with limb deficiencies will benefit greatly if there is close liaison with the school or nursery, to educate staff and other children, and ensure appropriate adaptations are made. Points of transition are particularly important, e.g. starting science laboratory lessons, going on school trips away from home.

About prostheses

- The first prosthesis tends to be very simple mechanically.
- As the child grows, there is space for a more sophisticated component.
- As the child ages, different priorities apply, e.g. cosmesis over functioning at a stage in the early years of adolescence onwards, the need to ride a bike at an earlier stage.
- An upper limb prosthesis is really a tool to do tasks and children may need several devices to carry out different tasks.

Clinical engineering

Clinical engineers work across a wide spectrum of areas to provide a technical solution to clinical problems. They also work as part of the clinical team in elucidating the nature of the problem and in planning technical solutions.

Diagnostics

Gait lab
- The gait lab is used to analyse a client's gait pattern and posture.
- Engineers work on analysing the gait and collaborate with orthopaedic surgeons (see ➜ pp. 533–4), orthotists (see ➜ pp. 424–6), and PTs (see ➜ pp. 374–6) in planning surgical and therapy interventions to improve gait and posture.

Clinical measurement
Examples of this include:
- Interface pressure mapping, e.g. for wheelchair seating (see ➜ pp. 388–9).
- Monitoring of sensory and motor signals along the spinal cord during spinal surgery.

Technical solutions for clinical problems

Wheelchairs and special seating
Clinical engineers work with PTs (see ➜ pp. 374–6) and OTs (see ➜ pp. 390–1) in assessing posture and pressure areas to provide seating which maximizes functioning and minimizes the risk of pressure sores.

Environmental control units (ECUs)
- A child with complex impairments (see ➜ pp. 108–9 and pp. 92–101) that severely restrict his/her independence can be helped to achieve a much higher degree of independence by the provision of an ECU system.
- The fundamental requirement is for the client to have one reliable means of signalling—this can be as little as a reliable head or mouth movement.
- The ECU is designed by the engineers around the client's abilities and wishes, enabling them to do things independently such as:
  - Open a door which has been set up to respond.
  - Turn on lights.
  - Turn on or off other electronic devices.
  - Drive electronic wheelchairs.
- Setting up a system in a single room can cost in the region of £3000.
- Specialist centres are located in Bristol at the Frenchay Hospital, Birmingham at the Regional Rehabilitation Unit, and Oxford at the Oxford Centre for Enablement.

Computer access
- There are a wide variety of both hardware and software which enable the client to make use of computers.

- Hardware examples include:
  - Keyboards having guards to avoid pressing multiple buttons at once.
  - Alternative mouse to match limited hand function, e.g. to cope with tremor.
  - Screens which respond to eye gaze as a means of control.
- Software can be provided to allow improved speed and response where limited movement and limited cognition are in evidence.
- Increasingly, use is being made of commonly available equipment such as smart phones, tablet PCs, and 'apps'.

Communication aids
(Also see ➲ pp. 212–14.)
- There is a huge range of equipment. Examples include:
  - Touch pads with letters that can spell out words or phrases using an electronic voice.
  - Letter boards (ETRAN) to spell out words using eye movements.
  - 'Litewriter' which has a keyboard input and displays the output visually or audibly.
- Clinicians seeking a technical solution are advised to contact a specialist centre as the range of technology is huge.

Functional electronic stimulation (FES)
- If a client has a foot drop, causing a tendency to catch the toes against the ground resulting in a trip, the FES device can be set up to follow the gait cycle and trigger the foot dorsiflexors to act, reducing the trip risk.
- FES devices cost in the region of £700–£5000 according to the degree of sophistication.

Contacting a clinical engineering department
Specialist services can be contacted at Oxford University Hospitals NHS Foundation Trust (Oxford Centre for Enablement), Kings College Hospital in London, Birmingham, Manchester, and Leeds.

Care of the child with a disability

Gastroenterological care of children with disabilities

GI problems are encountered in at least one-third of children with CP. These include:
- Oral motor dysfunction or dysphagia.
- Gastro-oesophageal reflux (GOR).
- Constipation.
- Abdominal pain.
- Nutritional deficiencies.

Oral motor dysfunction/dysphagia

- Effective oral feeding requires the coordination of sucking, swallowing, and breathing and is the most complex sensorimotor process the newborn infant undertakes.
- Dysphagia occurs as a result of impairment of one of the phases involved in the swallowing process: oral, pharyngeal, or oesophageal phases.
- The foregut, from mouth to duodenum, is the part of the GI tract most severely affected in children with CP, because of its great density of extrinsic innervations.
- Dysphagia (50% of children with CP) is closely related to the severity of the neurological impairment.
- Children with the most severe motor deficit (GMFCS level IV–V) have the most severe degree of dysphagia.
- Dysphagia in CP is associated with significant morbidity and mortality; major consequences include:
  - Poor feeding: excessive food spillage, excessive time taken to feed.
  - Dehydration.
  - Nutritional and growth deficits.
  - Aspiration.

Management strategies for oral motor dysfunction

- The aim of management is to reduce the risk of aspiration, dehydration, and poor nutrition.
- Involvement of a SLT and OT to formulate an eating and drinking plan is essential.
- This will ensure optimum positioning of the child and carer during feeding by:
  - Maximizing stability and minimizing abnormal reflexes to give a good head control and seating position.
  - Establish consistent and appropriate feeding techniques.
  - Utilize oral control techniques to aid lip closure and jaw stability.
  - Determine the optimum texture of food and drink to ensure a more efficient and safer swallow.
  - Determine the choice of suitable utensils to achieve efficient and effective safe feeding.
  - Advise on appropriate oral sensorimotor therapy and desensitization especially in the hypersensitive orally aversive child.
  - Address behavioural issues such as food refusal and ensure good communication between carer and child.

Assessment of the disabled child with feeding difficulties

MDT input is essential and includes:
- Community or neurodisability paediatrician, paediatric gastroenterologist, paediatric surgeon, paediatric radiologist, SLT, dietician, clinical nurse specialist, OT, PT, play therapist, psychologist, and social worker.
- Open channels of communication with the child's GP, school, HV, and community nurse are essential.

Medical history

Include information on:
- Underlying neurological condition.
- Current neurological status including mobility, activities of daily living, communication, cognition, etc.
- Severity of general and oral-motor impairment.
- Presence and severity of comorbid conditions and medications.
- Epilepsy, GOR, chronic cough, and constipation.
- Recent hospitalizations.

Feeding history

- Food intake should be recorded, including information regarding quantities and consistencies of food ingested and spillage.
- Duration of mealtimes and mode of feeding are important.
- Most of the scientific literature on dietary intakes in CP children have used a 3-day food diary.
- Ask about mealtime respiratory symptoms such as coughing, choking, gagging, wet/gurgly respiration, or rattly chest.
- There is often limitation in obtaining an accurate feeding history as families tend to overestimate intake and underestimate spillage.

Growth history

- The child health record, hospital, community, or school records can provide an accurate weight history.
- Given the difficulties in obtaining accurate height measurements in children who cannot stand, it may not be possible to obtain previous accurate height recordings.

Physical examination

To identify factors interfering with feeding ability, complications of feeding difficulties, and evidence of malnutrition:
- Muscle tone, truncal stability, and head control.
- Contractures, spasms, and abnormal movements all impact feeding ability and increase energy consumption.
- Chronic lung disease resulting from chronic aspiration.
- Peripheral circulation and skin condition help identify those at risk of nutritional deficits such as anaemia and vitamin and mineral deficiencies.
- Oral examination is essential as caries is often present in children due to difficulties in poor oral hygiene and GOR.

Anthropometry and nutritional status

Obtaining accurate weight and (especially) height measures is difficult in children with severe neurological impairment due to inability to stand, scoliosis, and contractures.

- Body weight measurement may require the use of wheelchair, sitting or hoist scales; weighing a child along with a parent and subtracting parental weights is an alternative option.
- BMI or weight-for-height are frequently used to estimate nutritional status, yet they are poor predictors of body fat percentage.
- Triceps skinfold thickness is a relatively easy measurement to perform; given the tendency of children with CP to store fat centrally, reduced triceps skinfold thickness may not necessarily mean low fat stores.
- Supine length is only useful if the child can lie in a straight position with appropriate limb alignment.
- Forearm length (ulnar length), lower leg length (tibial length), and knee height are appropriate alternative height measurements.
- Measurements should be plotted on an appropriate sex-specific growth chart; CP-specific growth charts are available (see ◊ http://www.lif eexpectancy.org).

Oral motor skills

Evaluation of oral motor movements both at rest and during feeding and management of jaw movements with input from a SLT are central to any feeding plan:

- Assessment of jaw stability and movement of the lips, cheeks, and tongue.
- Tonic biting, tongue thrusting, and retraction makes spoon-feeding difficult.

Investigations

These will be determined by the history and examination and may include:

- Videofluoroscopy:
  - Invaluable in the assessment of feeding and risk of aspiration.
  - Provides useful information on optimum feeding position, rate of feeding, and suitable textures.
- Blood tests:
  - Blood tests are less reliable indicators of nutritional status; poor sensitivity and specificity.
  - May be useful to identify specific micronutrient deficiencies: ferritin, zinc, copper, vitamins A and D.
  - Abnormal serum calcium, phosphate, alkaline phosphatase, and vitamin D levels may reflect poor bone mineral status.
  - Lower oesophageal pH monitoring and oesophageal impedance.
  - Where there is concern about GOR and gastrostomy feeding is contemplated.

Note that despite normal clinical history and preoperative radiological and lower oesophageal pH studies, GOR can become apparent in neurologically impaired children after gastrostomy tube placement.

Gastro-oesophageal reflux

- GOR occurs in up to 75% of children with neurodisabilities. Causes include:
  - Oesophageal dysmotility.
  - Hiatus hernia.
  - Prolonged supine position.
  - Increased intra-abdominal pressure secondary to hypertonia, scoliosis, or seizures.
  - Poor head control and low truncal tone.
  - Antro-duodenal dysmotility.
- Recurrent regurgitation and vomiting is an objective hallmark of GOR (occurs in >80%). Other clinical signs and symptoms include:
  - Haematemesis.
  - Retching.
  - Poor sleep.
  - Epigastric pain.
  - Dysphagia.
  - Peptic oesophagitis.
  - Food aversion or food refusal.

Management of GOR

Feeding regimen

- If tube fed then change from bolus to continuous pump feeding and use of whey-predominant enteral milk formulae which have been shown to be associated with faster gastric emptying and (more controversially) less reflux.
- Raising the head of the bed, reducing weight, and avoiding spicy foods, fatty foods, and chocolate can reduce the frequency and severity of GOR.

Drug therapy

- Proton pump inhibitors, e.g. omeprazole, lansoprazole.
- Histamine type 2 receptor antagonists (H2RAs), e.g. ranitidine.
- Reducing stomach acid levels even if the reflux occurs reduces symptoms and prevents damage.
- H2RAs become ineffective after 6 weeks of treatment (tachyphylaxis), so not a viable long-term option.
- Proton pump inhibitors are superior to H2RAs as they reduce meal-induced acid secretion which H2RAs do not.
- Although widely prescribed, evidence for the efficacy of prokinetic agents such as domperidone in reducing the frequency of GOR is lacking and should not be routinely prescribed.

Surgical approaches

These approaches are usually required when there is an indication for gastrostomy feeding (see later in topic) and/or presence of significant GOR not responding to pharmacology and non-pharmacological measures:

- Nissen fundoplication is the standard surgical option (now routinely performed laparoscopically).

- However, the complication rate and redo operation rate in children with neurological impairments are significantly higher than in the general population; hence, judicious use of the approach is needed.
- Surgical jejunostomy (endoscopic gastrojejunostomy) can be considered as an alternative to fundoplication.

Delayed gastric emptying (DGE)

- DGE occurs in 28–50% of cases of GOR in children.
- Has been demonstrated in typically developing children and children with neurological impairment.
- More at risk of developing gas bloating and persistent retching after fundoplication.
- Treating GOR without addressing DGE may be one of the reasons why GOR treatments fail.

Management of DGE

- Gastric scintigraphy is considered to be the most accurate method of diagnosis.
- As gastric emptying depends to some extent on food type, a change to a whey-predominant feed may be helpful.
- Consider a surgical gastric emptying procedure (e.g. pyloroplasty) for significant DGE.
  - NB: carries a risk of precipitating dumping syndrome (as a result of food reaching the small intestine too rapidly).

Further resources

British Association for Parenteral and Enteral Nutrition (BAPEN): ☎ 01527 457850; ℘ http://www.bapen.org.uk

PINNT (a support and advocacy group for people on home artificial nutrition): ℘ https://pinnt.com/

Constipation

- Constipation is a common comorbidity in CP (prevalence of 24–74%).
- Represents a significant therapeutic challenge and standard treatment regimens may prove to be insufficient.
- Contributory factors include:
  - Prolonged immobility.
  - Skeletal abnormalities.
  - Hypertonia.
  - Generalized hypotonia.
  - Abnormal bowel motility associated with certain neurological lesions.
  - Diet: low fibre and fluid intake (often due to associated feeding difficulties).
  - Drugs: anticonvulsants, opioids, antispasmodic, antihistamines, or aluminium antacid medications.
- Chronic constipation has been associated with:
  - Impaired quality of life.
  - Urinary symptoms.
  - Poorly voiding bladder, recurrent urinary tract infection.
  - GI manifestations.
  - Recurrent vomiting.
  - Chronic nausea.
  - Chronic or recurrent abdominal pain.
  - Early satiety.

Management of constipation

Management of chronic constipation aims to evacuate retained faeces followed by maintenance therapy to ensure defecation is regular and painless.

Medical treatment

If mild constipation and no evidence of megarectum or soiling, ensure regular passage of soft stool:

- Dietary manipulations to increase fluid and fibre intake.
- If gastrostomy fed, use a formula with added fibre.
- Drug therapy may also be needed.

Stool softeners (e.g. lactulose)

Use of preparations containing polyethylene glycol (e.g. Movicol™). Paraffin oil should be used with great caution in children with neurological abnormalities and GOR due to the significantly increased risk of aspiration.

Stimulant medications (e.g. senna)

- To ensure defecation occurs at least three times a week.
- Docusate sodium has both stool softening and stimulant properties.
- In children with rectal impaction and megarectum, disimpaction should be attempted:
  - Consider sodium citrate or sodium acid phosphate enemas before commencing stool softeners and stimulant medication.

Surgical treatment

Surgery is usually reserved for patients who have failed medical management especially those with spinal cord lesions:

- Malone antegrade continence enema procedure.
- Antegrade continence enema procedure has an 80% reported success rate.
- Best results are achieved in children aged >5 years with a neuropathic bowel or anorectal malformation who are highly motivated to remain continent.

Further resources

Colostomy Association: ☎ 0800 328 4257; ♂ http://www.colostomyassociation.org.uk
Ileostomy & Internal Pouch Association (IA): ☎ 0800 0184 724; ♂ http://www.the-ia.org.uk

Management of nutritional compromise in the child with a disability

- Nutritional intervention should aim to achieve:
  - Appropriate nutrition and growth within the limits of the child's neurological condition.
  - Improved overall growth and not simply improved weight should be the goal.
  - Increased weight due to fat alone has negative impact on general health and increases carer burden.
- Formulate individualized care plans taking account of:
  - Nutritional status.
  - Feeding ability.
  - Degree of motor impairment.
  - Energy requirement.
- Intervention is required when there is evidence of poor nutrition and/ or growth failure. This may involve:
  - Dietary supplementation with glucose polymers and/or long-chain triglycerides.
  - Hypercaloric or high-energy-density feeds.
- Gastrostomy tube feeding is indicated:
  - If oral feeding is unsafe.
  - When nutrition cannot be maintained orally (e.g. dependence on nasogastric tube feeding).
  - Daily feeding time is prolonged (>3 hours per day).
- Careful tailoring of nutritional requirements is important with gastrostomy tube feeding in children with severe motor impairment who are particularly vulnerable to overfeeding.
  - Consider use of low-energy dense, micronutrient complete, high-fibre feed.
- Regular reassessment is necessary to gauge response to nutritional intervention:
  - Infants and younger children require more frequent assessment.
  - Yearly assessment may be sufficient in older children.

Further resources

British Association for Parenteral and Enteral Nutrition (BAPEN): ☎ 01527 457850; ⅋ http://www.bapen.org.uk

PINNT (a support and advocacy group for people on home artificial nutrition): ⅋ https://pinnt.com/

Energy and nutritional needs of children with disabilities

The lack of normative growth data for children with CP and the variable contribution of individual factors to growth make the assessment and management of growth problems in CP challenging. This also applies to estimates of energy intake requirements:

- Accurately determining the energy requirement of a child with a complex neurological disability is challenging.
- The energy recommendations and equations used to estimate energy requirements for healthy children cannot be confidently applied to children with a neurodisability.
- Differences in body composition and energy expenditure mean that standard reference data for ideal nutritional input and optimal growth do not apply to children with CP.

The body composition of the child with severe CP differs from that of the average child

- A decrease in body cell mass accompanies an expansion of the extracellular fluid volume.
- The relative immobility of the child with severe CP reduces fat-free mass as well as energy expenditure.
- The reduced energy expenditure of children with CP is reflected in a lower dietary energy requirement—around 80% of current recommendations for typically developing children.

These body composition and energy requirements differences have consequences for nutritional management:
- Previous studies of children with CP have pointed to a positive energy balance associated with reduced energy expenditure and both high body fat mass and low muscle mass even if the children are fed with 80% of the estimated average requirements for energy.
- Most feeds used for enteral nutrition via gastrostomy are high-energy proprietary feeds (1.0 or 1.5 kcal /mL) that are not formulated to meet the nutritional needs of immobile children with severe neurological impairment and its associated motor and neurological deficits:
  - Thus, overfeeding becomes a real possibility especially in gastrostomy fed children who receive such energy dense feeds.
  - Low-energy (0.75 kcal/mL) gastrostomy feeds have been shown to improve nutritional status without adversely affecting body composition.

❶ It is important that paediatric enteral feeds are formulated to meet the macro- and micronutrient requirements of children who are reliant on them to supply a major proportion of their intake.
- Any attempt to 'dilute' the existing proprietary feeds in order to reduce the calorie intake to a level commensurate with the energy expenditure of a child with a disability is likely to have an adverse impact on micronutrient intake.
- This also applies to attempts to use liquefied family diet (blended diet) as a gastrostomy feed where both macro- and micronutrient intake may be compromised by the 'watering down' required to administer the feed through the gastrostomy tube.

Feeding difficulties: assessment and management from a SLT perspective

SLTs assess a child's ability to eat foods and drink fluids orally and swallow safely. They then advise on modifying textures and feeding techniques to ensure optimum feeding and safety.

The following aspects are assessed:

Child's oral motor ability

Oral phase
- Coordinated movements of lips and tongue to break up food, collect bolus, and ready it for swallow.
- Developmentally, this progresses from:
  - Suckle: tongue moves in and out of mouth in forward–backward motion (from birth).
  - Tongue movements: in up-and-down squashing action on hard palate (~6–8 months).
  - Lateral tongue movements with chewing (~9–12 months).

Pharyngeal phase
Initiating and completing swallow without gag, choke, cough, or aspiration.

Ability to tolerate different textures

- Puree: when weaning at 4–6 months.
- Thick semi-solid: 6–8 months.
- Mashed or lumpy consistency: 8–10 months.
- Soft solids, e.g. cooked root vegetables: 8–12 months.
- Easy chew, e.g. casseroled meat: 12 months.
- Hard to chew, e.g. raw apple: 15 months.
- Mixed textures, e.g. mince with vegetables, soup with chunks: from 12 months.

Points to note
- Textures must be matched to the child's oral motor development. Feeding with inappropriate textures can lead to risk of choking or aspiration.
- The International Dysphagia Diet Standardisation Initiative (IDDSI) is a global standard to describe texture-modified foods and thickened drinks for individuals with swallowing difficulties of all ages, in all care settings. The framework comprised of eight levels; drinks are measured 0–4, foods are measured 3–7; with cross over for levels 3 and 4. Each level has specific standards with clear characteristics and specifications. Levels can be identified by text labels, numbers, and colour codes.
- It enables clear descriptions of textures based on evidence and rigorous test rather than subjective descriptions. The standardized descriptors allow for consistent production and testing of thickened drinks and texture-modified foods.
- More information is available at ℘ http://www.iddsi.org

Feeding position

- This is a particular issue for children with neurological conditions with hypotonia or spasticity.
- Inappropriate feeding position (e.g. reclining or head in extension) can result in risk of choking and aspiration.
- Feeding upright and with the head in midline can inhibit abnormal reflexes seen in CP (e.g. tongue thrust, gagging, jaw extension, bite reflex) and enable the child to feed more normally.

Features that should cause concern

- Gagging: on lumps is relatively common in children between 9 and 15 months but diminishes as better ability to chew and sort mixed textures is developed. It is also seen in GOR or neurological conditions such as CP where heightened oral reflexes exist.
- Choke/cough.
- Pharyngeal residue: audible 'bubbly' breathing which is not cleared by swallowing or coughing.
- Aspiration which can be audible or silent.

Investigation

Videofluoroscopy carried out by a radiologist and a SLT and is the gold standard assessment for aspiration and should be considered if the following is evident:

- Watering of eyes when swallowing.
- Excessive gagging.
- Effortful or slow swallow (i.e. swallow slow to initiate).
- Pharyngeal residue (bubbly breathing).
- History of chest infections.
- Weak or absent cough.

Sensory aversion

- Condition where children refuse oral food and sometimes this extends to toys or teethers.
- It is often seen after prolonged periods of reflux, nasogastric tube, or force feeding but can also follow difficult feeding experiences, e.g. early breathing difficulties or in children with poor oral motor/sensory control.

SLT treatment strategies

- *Positioning* in midline to suppress abnormal reflexes and to prevent choking due to the opening of airway (if head extended) or gagging in neurological intact children.
- *Pacing* of bottle feeding or feeding with solids to allow child time to breathe and deal with each mouthful/clear residue.
- Use of *appropriate textures* for child's level of development.
- *Thickening fluids* often aid swallowing as bolus moves more slowly to allow time to trigger safe swallow—aspiration of thin fluids is more common than thicker semi-solids.

- *Practice chewing* with teethers (e.g. Chewy Tube) held if necessarily by carers between premolars/molars.
- Use of *dissolvable food* placed between premolars to stimulate chewing movements.
- *Messy play* with food and 'gooey' textures such as 'play dough' and 'finger paint' can help with sensory aversion.
- Encouragement for child to *feed themselves* is often very effective in children who have sensory issues.

Respiratory care of children with disabilities

Children with developmental disabilities have a high degree of respiratory morbidity and mortality because of the following factors:
- Feeding/swallowing difficulties.
- Aspiration of oral secretions.
- Ineffective cough/clearance of secretions.
- GOR.
- Obstructive sleep apnoea (OSA).
- Muscle weakness leading to chronic hypoventilation.
- Chest wall deformities causing restricted lung expansion.
- Predisposing factors, e.g. lowered immunity in DS, chronic lung disease in prematurity, immobility after TBI causing orthostatic pneumonia, etc.
- Medications, e.g. antiepileptic drugs causing sedation.
- Comorbidities, e.g. intractable seizures.

Obstructive sleep apnoea
Conditions associated with increased risk of OSA
- Tonsillar and adenoidal hypertrophy.
- Achondroplasia.
- Craniosynostosis.
- Neuromuscular e.g. DMD, SMA.
- CP.
- Syndromes, e.g. DS, Beckwith–Wiedemann syndrome, Prader–Willi syndrome, Treacher Collins syndrome.
- Obesity.
- MPS.
- Hypothyroidism.
- Choanal stenosis.

Consequences of OSA
- Sleep fragmentation (decreased intellectual functioning, decrements in dexterity, daytime sleepiness, disorientation, confusion, irritability, anxiety, etc.).
- Increased work of breathing (failure to thrive).
- Pulmonary hypertension.
- Intermittent hypoxaemia (reduced ventricular function, neuronal apoptosis, hampers neurocognitive potential—no one is sure of the mechanism—this is the same as sleep fragmentation).

Management
- *History taking* (enquire about snoring, gasps, heroic snorts in sleep, unusual sleeping position, headaches, behaviour, etc.).
- *Physical examination* (examine nasal passages, size of tonsils, palate, plot height, weight, BMI, blood pressure, listen for loud P2).
- *Investigations*: nocturnal polysomnography (PSG) is the gold standard, night-time oximetry, ENT referral for nasopharyngoscopy/laryngoscopy, ECG, and echocardiography—rarely.

- *Treatment*: tonsillectomy and adenoidectomy (T&A). This resolves great majority of OSA.
- *Follow-up*:
  - Weight reduction.
  - PSG 6–8 weeks after T&A—if snoring persists.
  - Intranasal steroids, montelukast, continuous positive airway pressure/ bilevel positive airway pressure have been used to address OSA.

Aspiration

- Could be:
  - Antegrade (while feeding/swallowing) or
  - Retrograde (secondary to GOR).
- Consequences of aspiration:
  - Bouts of coughing, gagging, and/or vomiting.
  - Exacerbation of wheeze.
  - Lower respiratory tract infections (LRTIs).
  - Repeated silent aspirations lead to chronic bronchitis, bronchiectasis, and/or reduction in lung function.
- *Antegrade* (excessive oral secretions, poor swallow, etc.):
  - Swallowing requires coordination of oral, pharyngeal, laryngeal, and oesophageal muscles.
  - Aspiration can result from impaired coordination of any of the above-mentioned muscles.
  - It could occur before, during, or after a swallow.
  - Aspiration can occur even when the child is nil by mouth.
  - Videofluoroscopy is the investigation of choice to detect antegrade aspiration and establish safe swallow.
  - Management could include small frequent feeds, thickening liquids, positioning head/neck, oral sensory therapy, stopping oral feedings, and temporary nasogastric tube placement. Placement of a gastrostomy tube is a safe and effective medium/long-term solution.
  - A gastrostomy tube helps in reducing feeding times, attaining satisfactory growth, and reducing silent aspirations and LRTI. Children who require gastrostomy should undergo tests for GOR. Those positive for reflux could have antireflux surgery (e.g. Nissen's fundoplication) and gastrostomy tube placement at the same time.
- *Retrograde* (secondary to GOR, see ➜ pp. 438–9).

Ineffective cough/airway clearance

- *Conditions* commonly associated with inadequate clearance of secretions:
  - Neuromuscular diseases, e.g. DMD, SMA, etc.
  - Severe kyphoscoliosis causing restrictive lung function.
  - CP.
  - Intractable seizures with depressed consciousness.
- *Signs and symptoms*:
  - Abnormal breath sounds (crackles, wheeze).
  - Abnormal respiratory rate, rhythm, and depth.
  - Shortness of breath.

- Excessive secretions.
- Hypoxaemia/cyanosis.
- Ineffective or absent cough.
- *Consequences* of ineffective cough:
  - Repeated LRTIs, bronchiectasis (rarely), loss of lung volume, hospitalizations.

Investigations
- Lung function tests; serial measurements to monitor.

Management
- Avoid infections where possible and treat infections promptly.
- Vaccinate against seasonal flu. Other vaccinations as schedule to minimize respiratory morbidity from other causes, i.e. infections.
- Postural management (optimize positioning).
- Suctioning.
- Chest physiotherapy.
- Manual cough assist (caregiver pressing on upper abdomen as you cough).
- Cough assist machine.
- Treat thoracic deformities where possible.

Drooling

- About 1–1.5 L of saliva can be produced/day; 65–70% of it is produced by the submandibular glands alone; 20% is produced by the parotid glands.
- Considered normal in children <4 years; ~30% of patients with CP have difficulties with drooling.

Conditions
Normal amount of saliva production
- Cognitively impaired children (impaired attention, motivation, understanding).
- CP (poor lip seal, tongue thrusting, impaired swallowing, open bite, poor neck/head control, etc.).

Excess saliva production
- Medications (e.g. anticonvulsants, tranquilizers, etc.).
- GOR.
- Gingivitis and caries could increase drooling.

Consequences of drooling
- Anterior (frequent change of bibs, soiling of teaching/communication aids, barrier to social interactions, dehydration, skin breakdown around mouth, burden on caregivers, etc.).
- Posterior (coughing, gagging, vomiting, silent aspirations, repeated LRTIs).

Management
- History:
  - Frequency (occasional/frequent/constant drooling).
  - Severity (mild/moderate/severe (soiled clothing)/profuse (clothing, equipment, tray soiled)).

- Number of bibs/day.
- Impact on quality of life (barrier to social interaction, soiled IT equipment, etc.).
- History of consequences as previously described.
- Examination:
  - Identify factors contributing to drooling (poor head control, tongue thrust, large tongue).
  - Head/neck control, perioral hygiene, tongue thrusting behaviours, size of tonsils, open bite, caries, gag reflex, examine ENT and cranial nerves.
- Treatment:
  - Treat if any of these is compromised (hygiene, comfort, social interaction, and respiratory system).
  - Non-medical measures (oral motor training, behavioural therapy) if child/carer motivated and adequate cognitive function in child. Time-consuming. Not much data about effectiveness.
  - Medical, e.g. benztropine, scopolamine, and glycopyrrolate. Effective to a great extent. But antimuscarinic side effects common. Botulinum toxin injections into submandibular gland—very effective, but requires repeat at periodic intervals.
  - Surgical, only after trying above-listed measures for 6–12 months. Includes re-routing of submandibular gland, excision of submandibular, and/or parotid duct ligation to address drooling. Submandibular duct re-routing could worsen aspiration into lungs especially in presence of unsafe swallow.

Pneumonia

- Pneumonia is the commonest reason for children with CP to require hospital admission.
- Predisposing factors include:
  - Aspiration of saliva or food/fluid.
  - GOR.
  - Poor cough.
  - Increased secretions (e.g. secondary to benzodiazepines).
  - Immobility.
  - Severe scoliosis.
- It is usually impossible to distinguish viral from bacterial aetiology based on specific signs and symptoms. Hence, treatment with antibiotics is recommended where pneumonia is suspected clinically.
- Penicillin or amoxicillin covers the commonest bacterial cause—*Streptococcus pneumoniae*. Where there is the possibility of aspiration pneumonia (anaerobes likely) or for pneumonia following influenza infection (*Staphylococcus aureus* more common), then co-amoxiclav provides a cover. Additional treatment for atypical organisms (e.g. *Mycoplasma pneumoniae*) should be considered in the event of severe disease or treatment failure.
- Recurrent infections are very rarely due to immunological problems.

Dermatological care of children with disabilities

- Children with disabilities and complex care needs are at least as susceptible to ordinary skin diseases as the rest of the child population.
- Furthermore, their individual circumstances can make them prone to additional problems such as pressure injuries and ulcers.

Pressure injuries and ulcers

- Defined as localized damage to the skin and underlying soft tissue usually over a bony prominence or related to a medical or other device. The injury can present as intact skin or an open ulcer (pressure ulcer) and may be painful. The injury occurs as a result of intense and/or prolonged pressure or pressure in combination with shear.
- Risk for pressure ulcers is higher in children who are admitted to secondary or tertiary care for prolonged periods or those with risk factors associated with disability such as significant limited mobility, inability to reposition themselves, significant loss of sensation, nutritional deficiency, significant cognitive impairment, or previous or current pressure ulcer.
- Commonly affected areas include back of skull, ear lobes and sacrum, heels, scapula, spinal processes, and ischial tuberosities.
- Medical devices most associated with pressure injuries are non-invasive ventilation facemasks, tracheostomy tubes, and ties, casts, and orthotics.

Principles of management of pressure injuries and ulcers
General
- Prevention by removal of the pressure.
- Adequate repositioning.
- Adjustment and proper fitting of devices.
- Frequent checking of contact sites with equipment.
- Pressure-reduction mattresses.
- Soft linen.
- Care for the skin includes keeping it clean with avoidance of excess moisture or dryness.
- Caregiver education.

Specific
- Support from tissue viability team.
- Irrigation and debridement if needed.
- Wound dressing.
- Treatment of any infection.
- Pain management.

Dermatological problems associated with gastrostomy

Hypergranulation tissue (granuloma)

- Granulation tissue protruding beyond skin level, caused by friction due to the tube moving too freely.
- Can have associated green, yellow, or serosanguinous discharge making it look like it is infected.
- Check that the external fixator is not too loose or too tight. Correct positioning of the external retention device can reduce the risk of overgranulation.
- Consider the use of an absorptive dressing such as Tegaderm™ Foam or Lyofoam®. This should be used for a minimum of 2 weeks to determine if it has been effective.
- A steroid-based, antibiotic or antifungal cream may be prescribed, e.g. Maxitrol® eye ointment, Fucidin® H, etc.
- If unsuccessful, consider cauterization using silver nitrate or in severe cases surgical excision.

Skin irritation around stoma

- May be a consequence of hypergranulation tissue, leakage of feeds and fluids, or secretions from gastric mucosa.
- Can be treated by applying barrier cream.

Infections

- Tenderness often is the first sign, although it is not recognized in neurologically impaired patients. Other signs are redness, increased purulent and/or foul-smelling discharge, pustule formation, etc.
- Pinpoint rash (satellite lesions) may indicate fungal infection.
- Fever could indicate severe or systemic infection.
- Treat by cleaning site and drying or warm saline compresses.
- Consider topical antibiotic and/or antifungal creams after taking a swab for culture.
- In case of systemic illness, consider enteral antibiotics.

Bone health in children with disabilities

- Children with CP have low bone mineral density (BMD). This leads to an increased risk of fragility fractures.
- In children, the diagnosis of osteoporosis is based on two criteria: (1) the presence of low BMD defined as z-scores less than −2.0 on a DXA scan; and (2) the presence of a significant fracture history (long-bone fracture of the lower extremities, vertebral compression fracture, or two or more long-bone fractures of the upper extremities).
- Although 'osteopenia' is a term used with adults, it is more challenging to define in a paediatric context, and the term 'low BMD' is more appropriately used in children.
- Risk factors for low BMD and fragility fractures (osteoporosis) in children with CP include decreased weight bearing, the use of anticonvulsants, poor nutrition, and decreased exposure to sunlight.
- Prevalence rates for fragility fractures have been estimated at 20% in non-ambulatory children and young adults with CP. The incidence of fractures in children with severe CP has been reported to be between 7% and 9.7% per year.
- The most common area for fractures in children with CP is the distal femur.
- Recognition of the risk factors for low BMD and prevention is essential.

Investigations

Children with one or more risk factor(s) or recurrent fractures or known low bone density should have the following investigations:
- FBC, erythrocyte sedimentation rate.
- Urea, electrolytes, creatinine.
- Liver function test.
- Calcium, phosphate, alkaline phosphatase.
- Parathyroid hormone.
- Coeliac screen.
- Vitamin D levels.
- Thyroid function tests.
- Consider bone density measurement using DXA scan.

Treatment

- If possible, any underlying cause of secondary osteoporosis should be addressed.
- Weight bearing should be encouraged although effectiveness of weight-bearing interventions to improve or maintain BMD and prevent fragility fractures in children and young people with CP and low BMD is conflicting.
- Vitamin D and calcium are possibly effective in improving BMD.
- Many children are not exposed to sufficient sunlight, and dietary intake and/or supplementation is required to maintain healthy vitamin D levels.
- The recommended daily requirement of vitamin D for healthy children is 600 IU/day; however, some bone health specialists have recommended that a higher dosage, such as 800–1000 IU, should be considered in children with CP. This allows the body to maintain

adequate stores and to achieve levels of 25-hydroxyvitamin D (25(OH) D) above 50 nmol/L (vitamin D sufficient state). Many recommend that the vitamin D intake be titrated to maintain the 25(OH)D levels in the high-normal range between 70 nmol/L and 100 nmol/L in children with CP.

- Calcium intake should be assessed at baseline by reviewing a dietary history and comparing intake with recommended norms. It can be enhanced through modifications to the diet or by calcium supplementation. If possible, dietary enhancement is the route of choice, as this form of calcium is more soluble, there is better compliance, and there is less risk of constipation.
- If a calcium supplement is used, it should be taken on an empty stomach to enhance absorption, which is affected by foods that are fatty, acidic, or high in oxalates. One of the potential side effects of vitamin D and calcium supplementation is an increase of calcium in the urine (hypercalciuria), which increases the risk of renal stones or nephrocalcinosis.
- Bisphosphonates, when given in conjunction with vitamin D and calcium, are probably effective in improving BMD in children with CP and are possibly effective in reducing fragility fractures in children who have a history of fractures.
- Possible adverse effects of IV bisphosphonate therapy include transient flu-like symptoms and occasional hypocalcaemia. There were also radiographic reports of metaphyseal bands developing in the growing bones of children on bisphosphonate therapy but the clinical impact of these bands on growing bones is unknown.
- Experts recommend bisphosphonates only after the child sustains a fragility fracture. Bisphosphonates are not recommended for use in children with low BMD as a preventative measure until further research is available to guide practice.
- Bone deformities may improve with growth and medical treatment of the underlying condition but may otherwise require corrective surgery.

Gynaecological care in children with developmental disabilities

- The period between 12 and 25 years of age is essential for human sexual development and includes physical changes, masturbation, dating, beginning intimate relationships, and sexual experiences. This applies to people with and without physical disabilities or chronic illnesses. Having CP or a disability does not mean one cannot enjoy an active sex life or go on to have a family.
- Children with developmental disabilities have similar sexual desires as their non-disabled peers.
- A literature review of young people with physical disabilities noted three developmental phases of adolescence; each of these phases can bring about specific problems related to relationships and sexuality:
  - In the early phase (11–13 years), adolescents are concerned about physical (pubescent) development, such as development of secondary sex characteristics and a changing outward appearance.
  - In the middle phase (14–16 years), the contacts with peers become central as they learn and share about dating and sexual experiences with peers.
  - In the final stage (17–19 years), developing long-term intimate relationships, questions about fertility and pregnancy become more prominent.
- Puberty could be early (e.g. neurofibromatosis, hydrocephalus), delayed (e.g. Prader–Willi syndrome), or less vigorous and less sustained (e.g. DS). Hence feelings of sexual adequacy, and doubts of ability to reproduce and parent can arise.
- Adolescents with disability are likely to have more risk-taking behaviours as they may want to prove that they are 'normal'.
- Children with disabilities are at increased risk of sexual harassment, sexual abuse, and incest.
- Dependence on parents can make it difficult for some young people to develop the adult roles that are important for building a relationship necessary for experiencing intimacy.
- Gynaecological care includes:
  - Managing menstruation.
  - Education about fertility, contraception, and pregnancy.
  - Regular cervical smears (Pap smear) and human papillomavirus (HPV) vaccine as required.
  - Information appropriate to their developmental ability regarding sexuality, dating, sexual abuse, sexually transmitted diseases, self-care, hygiene, etc.

Factors complicating gynaecological care

Child factors

- Reduced cognitive abilities making it difficult to explain treatment and obtain consent.

- Increased communication difficulties.
- Other issues, e.g. feeding tubes, colostomy, catheters.
- Variations in timing of pubertal changes.
- Orthopaedic problems, e.g. spasticity, joint deformities, kyphoscoliosis.
- Neurological factors, e.g. seizures, antiepileptic medications.

Parental factors
- Lack of knowledge regarding sexual health aspects.
- Refusal to engage.
- Overprotection leading to lack of independence.
- Considered as a low priority when compared to other aspects of care, e.g. feeding, managing seizures, etc.

Societal factors
- Myth that children with disabilities have no sexual needs.
- Myth that they do not require sexual education.

Physician/health professional's factors
- Lack of training in this area.
- Fear of upsetting parents by bringing up the topic of sexual health.
- Considered as low priority when compared to other medical needs.

Management
- The GP and/or paediatrician are well placed to identify and address the sexual and gynaecological needs and issues, but this takes time and creativity to fit into a busy practice or clinic. Enquire about issues such as sexual activity, contraception, menstruation, masturbation, etc. with sensitivity as part of the routine health reviews.
- Provide appropriate information and signpost/refer.
- Refer to:
  - GP, e.g. contraception, HPV vaccine.
  - Gynaecologist, e.g. amenorrhea, menstrual problems.
  - Sexually transmitted disease clinic, e.g. screening for sexually transmitted diseases and treatment.
  - School health nurse/teacher, e.g. education about emergency contraception, hygiene, etc.
  - Special counsellor, e.g. issues about sexuality, sexual dysfunction, past history of abuse.
- Provision of access to these resources will maximize their life chances.
- Holistic care should be extended to all—capable or incapable.

Assessment and management of pain

NICE guidelines recommend that when assessing pain in children with long-term conditions, tool selection should be based on age-appropriateness, developmental stage, and the child's communication ability.

It is also important to consider:

- Possible causes of pain (musculoskeletal, neuropathic, dental, visceral, dystonia, tissue viability) and any specific treatments available to manage these.
- Regular assessment for potentially recurring pain/distress.
- Individualized management plans, including pharmacological and non-pharmacological treatments to capture the biopsychosocial dimensions of symptoms.

Assessing pain

- Ask the child (supplement questions by using body charts, pain scales, 'faces scale'); younger and intellectually disabled children may not be able to describe pain easily but direct report is the most accurate when possible.
- Ask caregivers for their interpretation of the child's comfort/distress behaviours, including potential contributory factors (position, feeding, bowel habit, passing urine, tone, concurrent illness).
- Assess directly: observe heart and respiratory rate, pallor, sweating, quietness or crying, and social withdrawal, compared to the child's normal behaviour; being mindful that children with complex neurodisability may have atypical autonomic and behavioural responses. Consider using FLACC (face, legs, activity, crying, and consolability) scale. A modified FLACC scale exists specifically for children with cognitive impairment.
- For long-term assessment of chronic pain/distress, consider using a behaviour rating scale such as the Paediatric Pain Profile (PPP) as many children with neurodisability have intellectual impairments making communication more difficult.

Managing pain in children

Modification of environmental factors (noise levels, light levels, calm atmosphere), basic care consideration (clean nappy or pad, well fed, warm, comfortable position, reassured) and non-pharmacological measures (distraction, stories, films, music, and pleasurable activities alongside more formal psychological and physical therapies) have a large role to play, alongside conventional analgesics. A child presenting in distress may of course not only be in pain, and it is important to consider causes such as primary agitation, frustration, and anxiety alongside physical pain. The biopsychosocial model of pain supports the use of multiple modalities to address its management.

Psychological treatments

In children with chronic pain, psychological management through CBT and related interventions (such as behavioural therapy and relaxation therapy) may be used. These can be delivered either face to face, remotely, or with a combined approach.

Physical treatments

Physical therapies can also be used alone or in combination with other modalities and tend to reduce functional disability related to chronic pain.

Pharmacological treatments

- Simple analgesics (such as paracetamol) are a sensible starting point, once reversible causes and non-pharmacological strategies have been considered. These may need to be given regularly rather than 'as required' in some situations.
- Consideration of adjunctive drugs for inflammatory (non-steroidal anti-inflammatories) or neuropathic pain (e.g. gabapentin) is important.
- It may be necessary to use stronger pain killers such as morphine in some situations. It is important to avoid using ever-escalating doses of opiates to manage chronic pain. Referrals to a multidisciplinary chronic pain service including physiotherapy, occupational therapy, and psychology is essential in the face of chronic pain (see earlier in topic).
- If children with neurodisability need a longer-term regular dose of strong pain relief, the partial agonist buprenorphine can be a good choice. This can be administered as a transdermal patch, has slower development of tolerance, and is felt to cause less constipation. All children started on background opiates should be kept under regular review by a team with expertise in pain management.

Further resources

Harrop E, Brombley K, Boyce K (2017). Fifteen minute consultation: practical pain management in paediatric palliative care. Arch Dis Child Educ Pract Ed, 102, 239–43.

Hunt A, Goldman A, Seers K, et al. (2004). Clinical validation of the paediatric pain profile. Dev Med Child Neurol, 46, 9–18.

Likar R (2006). Transdermal buprenorphine in the management of persistent pain – safety aspects. Ther Clin Risk Manag, 2, 115–25.

Liow NY, Gimeno H, Lumsden DE, et al. (2016). Gabapentin can significantly improve dystonia severity and quality of life in children. Eur J Paediatr Neurol, 20, 100–7.

Malviya S, Vopel-Lewis T, Burke C, et al. (2006). The revised FLACC observational pain tool: improved reliability and validity for pain assessment in children with cognitive impairment. Pediatr Anaesth 16, 258–65.

Merkel SI, Voepel-Lewis T, Shayevitz JR, et al. (1997). The FLACC: a behavioural scale for scoring postoperative pain in young children. Pediatr Nurs 23, 293–7.

National Institute for Health and Care Excellence (2016, updated 2019). End of Life Care for Infants, Children and Young People with Life-Limiting Conditions: Planning and Management. NICE guideline NG61. London: NICE. Available at: 🔗 https://www.nice.org.uk/guidance/NG61

World Health Organization (2021). Guidelines on the Management of Chronic Pain in Children. Geneva: WHO. Available at: 🔗 https://www.who.int/publications/i/item/9789240017870

Incontinence in children with developmental disabilities

Problem

- Control of bladder and bowel function is influenced by genetic, neurodevelopmental, social (parental expectations), environmental (starting preschool), and physiological (ability to sit) factors. Most children are continent by 3 years of age.
- Late toilet training in children with disabilities is associated with increase in urinary incontinence and child's reluctance to engage with toilet training later.

Causes

- Central: CP, IDs, acquired brain injury, cerebral malformations, neurometabolic disorders.
- Local: spina bifida, spinal cord defects, myelomeningocele, Hirschsprung's disease, anal atresia/stenosis.
- Behavioural: ASD (see → pp. 114–25) and ADHD.
- Consider sexual abuse (see → pp. 584–5) as a possibility.

Contributory/predisposing factors

Constipation

- Causes: poor diet, reduced fluids intake, decreased mobility, non-erect positioning, low tone, inability to communicate pain/discomfort, medications, etc. all contribute towards establishment of significant and long-standing constipation.
- Consequences: pain, bleeding, anal fissures, poor feeding and fluid intake, behavioural problems, social stigma (overflow incontinence), psychological distress to family, megacolon, urinary incontinence, and bowel obstruction.

Poor fluid intake

- Causes: swallowing difficulties, inability to communicate thirst, reduced access to drinks, inability to fetch a drink, considered a low priority (versus medications, feeds, etc.), lack of appreciation of importance of fluid intake in parents/carers, etc.
- Consequences: insufficient hydration over a period causes small capacity bladder (bladder deficit) leading to urinary incontinence; there is good correlation between maximum voided volume and bladder continence; also, poor hydration can contribute to constipation.

Consequences of incontinence

- Impact on the child: low self-esteem, social isolation and exclusion, long-term psychological consequences.
- Impact on family: stigmatization, parental stress, siblings' discord, significant burden of care.
- Impact on society: huge financial implications from provision of additional carers and aids.

Toilet training

- The issue of when and how to begin toilet training can be particularly challenging for parents.
- Toilet training works best when parents have access to the guidance, instruction, and encouragement of their paediatrician, other trained professionals, or support groups.
- The first step to take is to determine whether the child is ready to begin.
- Is the child aware of the difference between being wet and being dry?
- Can he/she stay dry for at least 2 hours at a time?
- Can he/she sense when he/she needs to urinate or have a bowel movement?
- Steps of toilet training:
  - Sitting on the toilet (or potty) regularly especially after meals.
  - Addressing well-balanced diet and good drinking habits.
  - Toilet habits—pulling pants up/down, sitting on the toilet, handwashing.
  - Moving on to washable underwear and trainer pants.
  - Rewards, praise, encouragement for using the toilet.
- Techniques:
  - Shaping (increasing proximity to toilet).
  - Fading (reducing presence of nappy).
  - Operant conditioning (modification of voluntary behaviour by positive or negative reinforcement).
  - Other measures: soft music and distractions, blowing balloons, etc. while seated on toilet.

Management

- General measures: adequate fluids and balanced diet are essential.
- Normalization of fluid intake has good correlation with bladder continence.
- Multidisciplinary liaison:
  - OT: advice on access to toilet, seating, clothing, self-care skills, etc.
  - Continence nurse advisor: can help with fluid intake charts, behavioural modification, toilet training methods, supply of absorbent products, advice on bedding, enuresis alarms, etc.
  - Psychologist: address low self-esteem in child, psychological support to the family.
  - SLT: use of social stories and picture exchange communication system to communicate needs around toileting.
  - School: consistency and good communication between home and school.
- Medical measures: treat constipation with laxatives (e.g. lactulose), stimulants (e.g. senna), and osmotic agents (e.g. polyethylene glycol/ Movicol®).
- Surgical measures: appendicocaecostomy—Malone antegrade continence enema (MACE) procedure for chronic treatment resistant constipation.
- Adaptations: clothing alterations, nappies/diapers, or pull-ups.

- Aids: nappies/diapers or pull-ups. The choice depends on the level of independence in toileting, discreteness in changing, fit, appearance, etc. Pull-ups can assist with toileting and pad changes. Nappies/diapers are easy to change especially if child has calipers, adapted footwear, etc. Since nappies/diapers are more absorbent, they are preferred for night-time use.

Prognosis

- Likelihood of continence is directly proportional to the degree of LD and degree of physical immobility.
- Children with moderate LD and moderate disability in mobility can be expected to be continent by 3–4 years.
- Children with severe to profound disability in learning and mobility are less likely to become continent after 8 years.

Further resources

Bladder and Bowel Community: ℘ https://www.bladderandbowel.org/

ERIC (The Children's Bowel & Bladder Charity; UK children's charity dealing with bedwetting, day-time wetting, constipation, soiling, and potty training): ☎ 0845 370 8008; ℘ http://www.eric.org.uk

Dental health in children with developmental disabilities

Problem

- Children with a disability are four to five times more likely to have dental problems versus non-disabled peers.
- They are less likely to receive preventive and restorative dental care.
- Dentists report communication problems and carers report non-cooperation of the child as significant barriers to oral care.
- Dentists must adapt their approach to provide oral care to children with a disability. Learning appropriate skills and techniques to meet their unique oral health needs will help the dentists in delivering successful care.

Predisposing factors to poor dental care

- Child factors: fear of examination, inability to comprehend the need for treatment, dry mouth (e.g. mouth breathing), oral medications, difficulty in swallowing/feeding, GOR, inability to communicate sensation in the mouth, involuntary tongue thrusting, sensory integration difficulties with brushing.
- Parent/carer factors: competing priorities with other health needs, lack of awareness of importance of early dental care, difficulty in accessing suitable services.
- Dental service-related factors: lack of training in special needs, lack of adequate number of dentists in special needs dentistry, negative attitudes, inadequate provisions for socially excluded groups.

Common dental conditions in children with special needs

- Halitosis: caused by mouth breathing, chronic sinusitis, bronchitis, GI disturbances, periodontitis (gum disease), certain foods, etc.
- Malocclusion: crowding, misalignment, gap between upper and lower set of teeth.
- Dental caries: secondary to inadequate brushing, poor hygiene, medications containing sugar, GOR.
- Tooth anomalies: delayed or late-onset, variations in shape, size, and number of teeth.
- Xerostomia (dry mouth): mouth breathing, medications, inadequate fluid intake.
- Bruxism (habitual grinding and clenching of teeth): secondary to boredom, anxiety, pain, malocclusion, spasticity, and dystonia.
- Oral trauma: secondary to falls, seizures, lack of protective reflexes, etc.
- Periodontitis: caused by plaque formation.
- Infections: oral thrush (*Candida albicans*).
- Bleeding gums: nutritional deficiencies (scurvy), bleeding disorders, phenytoin use.
- Pica: eating of non-edible substances can damage teeth and gums.

Consequences of poor dental health

- Inability to receive adequate nutrition.

- Halitosis, missing teeth, and periodontal disease become a further barrier to social interaction/acceptance.
- Build-up of bacteria in the mouth can impact general health.
- Frequent dental pain can have impact on sleep, behaviour, general well-being, and quality of life.

Prevention

- Good oral care: twice-daily brushing after meals, dental floss, and mouthwash or rinsing with plain water.
- Start brushing after the first tooth eruption; use fluoride toothpaste.
- Involve OT and/or SLT to help with positioning, equipment, and oral desensitizing techniques.
- Resistance to brushing could be overcome by good support, comfortable head position, well-lit location, using brush with soft/ultra-soft bristles, brushing while seated in front of a mirror, brushing as a family, letting the child play with brush, oral massaging, lots of praise, being patient, etc.
- Regular dental check-ups; fear of dental practices can be managed by gradual introduction to the premises to get familiarized, shorter appointments, etc.
- Preventive dentistry could minimize the need for dental extractions and later operative interventions.
- Balanced diet, sugar-free medications, and physical activity where possible.
- Education of patients and parents/carers.

Management

- CBT in selected cases could address dental phobias.
- Measures to restrain should be explained and agreed with parents/carers before the procedure.
- Good analgesia and use of conscious sedation should be offered when required; small proportion of children might require general anaesthesia.
- Sealants for dental cavities, tooth extraction, and restoration for dental caries.
- Consider artificial saliva for dry mouth.
- Herpes simplex virus stomatitis: analgesic mouthwashes/spray (e.g. Difflam®) and oral aciclovir would help.
- Candidiasis: treat with nystatin pastille, suspension, or gel.

Further resources

Association for Rehabilitation of Communication and Oral Skills: ℘ http://www.arcos.org.uk
British Society for Disability and Oral Health: ℘ https://www.bsdh.org/
National Institute of Dental and Craniofacial Research, National Institute of Health: ℘ http://www.nidcr.nih.gov
Oral Health Foundation (formerly known as the British Dental Health Foundation): ℘ https://www.dentalhealth.org/
Scope (disability equality charity): ℘ http://www.scope.org.uk

Sleep disorders and management

- Approximately 30% of preschool-aged children have sleep-related problems.
- Sleep disturbances such as sleep initiation, sleep maintenance, and sleep scheduling are more common and more severe than in children without disabilities; prevalence can be as high as 80%.
- Process of sleep regulation and sleep consolidation is influenced by a combination of biological, behavioural, environmental, and neurodevelopmental factors.

Types of sleep disorders

- Primary sleep disorders:
  - Dyssomnia (a disturbance in the quality, quantity, or timing of sleep): e.g. bedtime resistance, delayed sleep onset, frequent awakenings, hyperarousal, etc.
  - Parasomnias (deviated behavioural or physiological events that occur during sleep), e.g. sleep walking, night terrors, nightmares.
  - Periodic limb movements in sleep (arms and legs move frequently and involuntarily during sleep).
  - Restless leg syndrome (leg pain, crawling feeling in the legs, urge to move the legs when settling to sleep).
  - Circadian rhythm disorder (disruption to the circadian rhythm resulting in sleep timing out of alignment with routine activities).
- Sleep disorders secondary to medical conditions, e.g.:
  - CNS: CP, epilepsy.
  - Respiratory: asthma, OSA.
  - Cardiovascular system: pulmonary oedema due to heart failure.
  - GI: colitis.
  - Skin: atopic dermatitis.
  - Skeletal: arthritis.
  - Eye: blindness.
- Sleep disorders secondary to neurobehavioural and psychiatric conditions: e.g. anxiety, depression, phobias, post-traumatic stress disorder, ADHD, ASD, etc.
- Substance-induced sleep disorders: e.g. alcohol, cocaine, opioids, amphetamines, caffeine, sedatives, etc.

Causes of behavioural sleep disorders

Can be classified into:
- Child factors, e.g. behavioural difficulties, pain, seizures, etc.
- Parental factors, e.g. poor parenting, poor sleep hygiene, maternal depression, etc.
- Environmental factors, e.g. noisy neighbourhood, overcrowded household, shared bedroom, etc.

Consequences of sleep disorders/deprivation

- *Child*:
  - Short term: irritability, tiredness, daytime somnolence, hyperactivity, behavioural problems, prone to accidental injuries.

- Long term: negative impact on neurocognitive functioning, learning, educational attainments, emotional and behavioural disorders, overweight/obesity, drug abuse.
- *Family*: significant impact on family functioning, parental well-being, marital discord, increased incidence of child neglect and abuse.
- *Society*: reduced chances of employment; family breakdowns, antisocial behaviours.

Assessment

History taking

- What exactly is the problem (e.g. bedtime refusal, difficulty in falling asleep or staying asleep, daytime behaviour/sleep, etc.)?
- Enquire about severity (hours of sleep), frequency (number of awakenings/per night/per week), and duration of the sleep difficulties (months/years etc.).
- Explore predisposing factors (e.g. developmental delay), precipitating factors (e.g. recent house move, illness in family, etc.) and perpetuating factors (poor sleep hygiene, erratic routine).
- Elicit the impact/consequences of the sleep disorder.
- Child (concerns from nursery/preschool, behaviour, daily routine, medical problems).
- Parent (education, motivation, behavioural techniques, co-sleeping, mental health).
- Family (number of persons in household, relationships, number of bedrooms, family routine).
- Environment (room temperature, access to TV/computer games/toys in bedroom, noise, light, activities of siblings, neighbours, etc.).
- Comorbidities (ADHD, ASD, LD, epilepsy, etc.).

Physical examination

- Growth (height, weight, OFC).
- Look for dysmorphic features, craniofacial anomalies, neurocutaneous signs, signs of metabolic disorders.
- Complete system review including chest and neurology.
- Developmental assessment; note: behaviour, affect, alertness/attention.
- ENT (size of tongue, tonsils, etc.).

Investigations

- Review 'sleep log/diary'.
- Request audiovisual recording, e.g. capture snoring, night terrors on home video/mobile phone.
- PSG: overnight sleep study which measures body physiological parameters including sleep staging as well as cardiorespiratory data and leg movements.
- Multiple Sleep Latency Test (MSLT): objective testing of daytime sleepiness which is useful in cases of suspected narcolepsy.
- Actigraphy: recording from a wrist device which has an accelerometer which estimates rest–wake cycles.

Management of sleep difficulties

Behavioural

Evidence based and effective.

- Establish good sleep hygiene:
  - Consistent bedtime/awake time in the morning; night-time indicator clocks such as Gro-Clock or products such as a sunrise lamp available on the market; these can be used in conjunction with a reward system.
  - Consistent sleep routine (giving warm bath, soft music, read a book in bed/bedtime story, 'lights off', quiet time/low noise activities for 1–2 hours preceding, no TV/computer games 1–2 hours prior to sleep).
  - White noise and pink noise apps; pillow with iPod-type devices all allow sound to be played throughout the night as a sleep signaller.
  - Aromatherapy oils such as lavender can be helpful.
  - Using an object of reference (e.g. placing a teddy sprayed with mum's perfume or using a pair of dad's old pyjamas) may help if there are sleep association difficulties and co-sleeping.
  - Daytime physical activity/exercise is likely to have a positive effect.
  - Diet: avoid caffeine; avoid heavy meal just before bed.
- Sleep programmes:
  - Graduated extinction (involves ignoring bedtime crying for increasing length of time).
  - Unmodified extinction (involves putting child to bed at a predetermined time and letting child develop self-soothing skills and falling asleep).
  - Scheduled awakening (involves parents waking up the child before the child's expected awakenings and gradually withdrawing this over time).

Pharmacological

- Consider only after or with the above-mentioned behavioural interventions.
- To be considered only for children with neurodevelopmental disabilities or medical problems and not for typically developing children.
- Use for short-term periods to help establish sleep routine.
- Medications are used 'off-label'.
- Medications: melatonin-used to treat circadian rhythm disturbances in children with neurodisability; evidence suggests a decrease in sleep latency but no increase in overall sleep.

Referrals

Referrals to following professionals may be required:

- Neurologist (narcolepsy, frontal lobe epilepsy).
- Respiratory physician (asthma, chronic lung disease, sleep apnoeas).
- ENT (OSA syndrome, floppy larynx, macroglossia).
- Psychiatrist (ASD, depression, substance abuse).
- Psychologist (CBT, behavioural programmes).

Transition: moving from paediatric to adult services

- Transition from children's to adults' services can be a complex process, spanning a range of agencies and specialisms. Transition is defined as a purposeful and planned process of supporting young people to move from children's to adults' services. But making this move can be difficult or provoke anxiety in young people and their carers. See Box 8.1.
- Practitioners should start transition planning for adulthood from year 9 (age 13 or 14) at the latest.
- There is a wealth of policy and guidance on agreed principles in respect of good transitional care, but there is also evidence that these principles are often not reflected in practice.
- The absence of a coordinated approach to providing services across health, education, and social care can result in ineffective communication, poor engagement, and discontinuity of care. This can be disruptive for young people, particularly during adolescence when they are at a higher risk of psychosocial problems.
- Adults' and children's services need to come together to pool funding, addressing the structural and cultural barriers that prevent them from achieving this. Transitional care should become a shared priority, despite the current pressures on public funds.
- Families and carers often feel left out once the young person moves to adults' services, which can cause them considerable distress and uncertainty. The young person may themselves ask for their family not to be involved so families may also undergo a 'transition' in their involvement in the care of the young person.

Box 8.1 Good transitions: what young people say they want

- Active management of transition. Plan early and prepare for leaving children's services.
- Take account of how attitudes, thinking, and behaviour vary between individual young people.
- Involve young people in service design and delivery: provide opportunities to ask questions, express opinions, and make decisions.
- Provide accessible information about services, share information between services, and ensure multiagency working, coordination, and accountability
- Stress the importance of a trusted adult who can challenge and support them, act as advocate, and help develop self-advocacy skills.
- Establish a shared philosophy between adult and paediatric care.
- Adopt an individualized honest approach.
- Address loss of continuity of care at transition; ensure new relationships are established.
- Train professionals in adolescent health in both paediatric and adult sectors.

Source: Transition: getting it right for young people, Department of Health/Department for Education and Skills 2006.

Overarching principles

- Ensure transition support is developmentally appropriate, taking into account the person's maturity, cognitive abilities, psychological status, needs in respect of long-term conditions, social and personal circumstances, communication needs, etc.
- Ensure transition support is strengths based and focuses on what is positive and possible for the young person rather than on a predetermined set of transition options.
- Use person-centred approaches to ensure that transition support treats the young person as an equal partner in the process and takes full account of their views and needs; involves the young person and their family or carers, primary care practitioners, and colleagues in education, as appropriate; supports the young person to make decisions and builds their confidence to direct their own care and support over time; and addresses all relevant outcomes, including those related to education and employment, community inclusion, health and well-being, including emotional health and independent living and housing options.
- Help the young person to identify a single practitioner—who should act as a 'named worker'—to coordinate their transition care and support.
- The named worker should be someone with whom the young person has a meaningful relationship. The named worker could be, depending on the young person's needs, a nurse, youth worker, or another health, social care, or education practitioner, an allied health professional, the named GP, or an existing keyworker, transition worker, or personal adviser.
- Discuss the transition with the young person's parents or carers. Understand their expectations about transition. This should include recognizing that the young person's preferences about their parents' involvement may be different and should be respected, taking into account the young person's capacity, following the principles of the Mental Capacity Act and other relevant legislation, as necessary.
- The parents and/or carers should help the young person develop confidence in working with adults' services by giving them the chance to raise any concerns and queries separately from their parents or carers.
- Adults' services should take into account the individual needs and wishes of the young person when involving parents or carers in assessment, planning, and support.

Running a transition clinic

The pattern described here follows a routine developed for a paediatric transition clinic covering Oxfordshire.

- The 'Clinic Paediatrician' familiarizes with the history before the clinic, and preferably would also have spoken with the paediatrician referring the patient to the clinic. The history to date is reviewed and summarized with the patient and their family participating as much as possible.
- Observation suggests that this process of reviewing and summarizing is itself therapeutically beneficial, allowing time to reflect on and reassess critical events such as operations, or periods of crisis such as hospital emergency admissions.

- Adult disability specialists attending might include a whole range of therapists, depending on the individual patient's needs.
- The clinic runs in roughly two halves; firstly summarizing past events and reviewing current problems, followed by a consideration of what adult services are available that might be helpful.
- It is essential to offer follow-up to avoid the feeling of abandonment, which is inherent in this process of transition. An offer of a follow-up appointment with the adult medicine physician in a few months' time and a phone number to call if there is a crisis is helpful.

Schedule for a transition clinic

- Introductions.
- Explanation of the purpose of the clinic.
- Review of medical history especially key events.
- Review and list all agencies currently involved.
- Review of current, active problems. A 'biopsychosocial model' is paramount: medical, educational, social, and psychological matters are all considered.
- Referrals to appropriate agencies (e.g. tertiary specialist colleague, Connexions, counselling, wheelchair services, etc.).
- Arrangements for follow-up.
- Summary letter copied to agencies involved (with consent).

What needs to be addressed in transition clinic?

The philosophy of the clinic is a '*biopsychosocial approach*' for alleviation and enablement of the adolescent.

The clinic should consider all of the following *social concerns*, according to the ability of the young person:

- Educational needs.
- Relationship issues.
- Accommodation plans for the future.
- Driving.
- Vocation, plans to work, etc.
- Hobbies and interests.

Medical issues might include the following:

- Referrals to a wide range of adult clinics including neurology, specialist epilepsy services, and spasticity clinic.
- Wheelchair and special seating review.
- Women's health services.
- Assessment of fitness to drive.
- Assessment of mental capacity relating to financial and other key matters.
- Liaison with LD services.

Palliative care for children

Paediatric palliative care is defined as an active and total approach to care, embracing physical, emotional, social, and spiritual elements, which focuses on enhancements of the quality of life for the child and support for the family and includes the management of distressing symptoms, provision of respite, and care through death and bereavement.

Specialized palliative care services for children may be delivered in a variety of settings:

- Consultant-led teams may be found within some children's hospices, as well as in tertiary children's hospitals, and occasionally within community-based services.
- Hospices and community services offering a specialist service will often 'in-reach' to local hospitals, as well as supporting palliative care in hospice, in school, and at home.
- Core palliative care skills exist in many community paediatric teams, among children's community nurses, and general paediatricians/GPs.

Specialist palliative care is provided to children with life-threatening or life-shortening conditions who have an extremely wide range of diagnoses (in excess of 300), and there is a very significant overlap with those with severe disabilities and complex needs.

However, a significant proportion of children with palliative care needs (up to 15%) do not have a definitive underlying diagnosis.

Unlike adult practice, oncology makes less than half of the workload for most specialist paediatric palliative care services, with inherited metabolic disease, neuromuscular diseases, and acquired brain injury making up a significant proportion.

Talking to children and families about life-limiting illness

When a child is diagnosed with a life-threatening condition, one of the most challenging tasks facing healthcare professionals is how to communicate this to the child, and to their parents or caregivers. The Following points can be very useful in practice:

1. *Prepare yourself*: examine your own comfort levels and ensure that when you meet the child and family, you can present a calm impression. Build a relationship with the child and family and be prepared to listen first.
2. *Prepare the parents*: discuss the importance of communicating with the child about significant changes in their health.
3. *Prepare information*: plan what you need to communicate and prioritize key information.
4. *Prepare the environment*: identify a quiet and private area. Consider who needs to be with the child and make plans for other siblings.
5. *Development*: consider the age of the child and any neurodevelopmental issues or communication impairments.
6. Pay attention to *emotional understanding* and allow them to express their feelings.
7. Ask the child and parents what they have *understood*.
8. *Make a plan* for what will happen next.

Vulnerability assessment tools—knowing who to refer

Around two-thirds of children and young people with palliative care needs also have an impairment causing limitations to activity, such as intellectual problems or restricted mobility.

Despite this, <25% of children with CP die in childhood and it can thus be a challenge to identify those most in need of palliative care.

Vulnerability assessment tools exist to guide clinicians.

Box 8.2 is an evidence-based guide to the sort of vulnerability factors that make a child with CP (or other static neurological conditions) likely to most benefit from a palliative care referral (and meet the criteria of such a service).

Box 8.2 Evidence-based guide to vulnerability factors that may indicate benefit of a palliative care referral

Respiratory factors
- Frequent or increasing numbers of LRTIs.
- Paediatric intensive care unit (PICU) admission for LRTI.
- Requirement for long-term oxygen therapy or non-invasive ventilation at home.
- Tracheostomy and/or 24-hour ventilation.

Feeding factors
- Gastrostomy.
- Jejunostomy.
- Severe uncontrolled reflux despite maximum treatment.
- Losing weight due to feeding difficulties.
- Pain/distress associated with feeding, necessitating progressive feed reduction.

Seizure-related factors
- Epileptic activity needing medication.
- Poor seizure control despite numerous drugs.
- Frequent use of rescue medication (daily basis).
- Episodes of status epilepticus requiring intensive treatment (IV infusions/PICU).

Locomotor factors
- Spastic quadriplegia/total body involvement.
- Poor head control/fixed spinal curvature.
- Dependent on a wheelchair driven by a carer.
- Difficulty with maintaining sitting position (GMFCS-E&R level V).

Other neurological vulnerability to consider
- Other evidence of severe bulbar involvement (worsening swallow, cough, gag reflex).
- Baclofen pump (as a marker of severe hypertonia/very difficult spasms).
- Ventriculoperitoneal shunt (particularly with frequent need of review).
- Severe sensory impairment, including blindness.

In the light of these factors, would you be surprised if the child was still alive at the age of 18 years?

Key principles for delivering paediatric palliative care

- Involve the child in the planning process in as much as they feel able.
- Use 'parallel planning'—it is often not possible to predict when a significant deterioration or death will happen; children are very resilient. *'Hoping for the best and planning for the worst'* can be a useful strategy.
- Every family is different, has different priorities, and responds differently to new information; support needed may be medical, emotional, or practical and may vary over time.
- Parents who have a relationship directly to each other rather than 'through the child' and who sustain this are best equipped to cope in the long run.
- Provision of respite will help parents' physical and mental health, as well as supporting their ability to meet the needs of siblings.
- Use the MDT—including the full range of therapists, chaplains, and social workers.
- Regularly review the sources of support available to families. Consider social services-provided respite, continuing healthcare packages, charity funded help, and ensure that the sum total of the care provided allows for a manageable quality of life for the family.
- The dying of a child is a journey for the whole family, including siblings and grandparents, aunts and uncles, whose needs for support must also be addressed (both before and after bereavement); details of support organizations are provided later in this chapter (see pp. 481–2).
- Families should be encouraged to express a preferred place of care for a child when death is a possible outcome. This may be an acute hospital, but wherever preferred they should be supported to receive care in a children's hospice or at home, with access to nursing care and back-up support from a consultant in paediatric palliative care.
- If a child is in hospital and dependent on life-sustaining technological care, have open discussions with the family about the burdens and benefits of all treatments and the impact that they may have on achieving their preferred place of care.
- Consider ambulance transfer to home or hospice if withdrawal of life-sustaining treatment is being discussed, as long as this can be safely achieved.
- Remember the emotional impact of caring for children at the end of their lives on the multiprofessional healthcare team and ensure adequate opportunities for debriefing and support.
- After the death of a child, it is important to sensitively contact all those caring for the child and family, in education, social care, as well as in the wider healthcare team.
- Healthcare professionals wishing to increase their knowledge of topics relating to paediatric palliative care can access free online modules (available in many languages) via the International Children's Palliative Care Network (ℵ http://www.icpcn.org/icpcns-elearning-programme/).

Advance care planning

An advance care plan (ACP) is the record of a discussion between an individual (where possible), their professional caregivers, and those close to them about their future care. It forms a core element of good palliative care.

- One example of a suitable document is the 'Children and Young Person's Advance Care Plan' (ℜ http://cypacp.uk/).
- When performed well, the advance planning process provides all those involved with the opportunity to talk honestly about the future, allowing children and their families to retain autonomy and to influence how they are looked after.
- It typically covers the concerns and wishes of C&YP and their carers about their treatment, including what should be done, where, how, when, and by whom.
- Importantly, while ACPs also consider what should not be done, it is vitally important that healthcare professionals know that an *ACP is NOT an automatic statement of intent not to treat.*
- While most child deaths still occur in acute healthcare settings, evidence suggests that most families do not want their child to die in hospital.
- A local audit of the deaths of children who had an ACP in place, within the Thames Valley (UK), showed that three-quarters died out of hospital. This suggests that the impact of careful, supportive planning can help achieve more out-of-hospital death.
- Children who die after being admitted to a PICU are increasingly likely to do so after a prolonged period of ventilation. The modes of these deaths are increasingly likely to involve withdrawal of life-sustaining treatment.
- Without an effective ACP in place, this may involve the prolongation of treatments which prove futile and burdensome for the child and family, as well as having clear resource implications.

When should an ACP be written?
- Ideally at a time that best suits the family—or at least involving some choice for them.
- Sometimes following a natural 'trigger' (PICU admissions, progression in condition, changes in goals of care, stopping chemotherapy).
- Planning can begin before birth following antenatal diagnosis of life-limiting conditions.

How should an ACP be written?
- The initial conversation may just be a 'warning shot across the bows' with information provided about the process (such as the parent/carer leaflet available on the Child and Young Person's Advance Care Plan Collaborative website (ℜ http://cypacp.uk/), or a copy of the blank care plan), followed by a plan for the next meeting.
- Even if the initial offer is declined, it may stimulate further reflection for the family.
- In situations where parents find it unbearable to open the conversation, it can be helpful to offer to fill in a draft form reflecting the views of the MDT, on a best-interests basis. This can be shared with the family either during a consultation or for them to reflect on in private with the option of adding comments of their own.
- There are of course situations where time is short, and decision-making between families and healthcare professionals needs to happen more rapidly. In these cases, it is probably helpful to fill in only the parts of the ACP that are immediately relevant and to offer to revisit the remainder of the document at a later date.

- If the conversation stalls, it can be helpful to offer to talk through possible scenarios, in the context of the child's underlying illness and current clinical condition. It is important to help children and families to understand the difference between potentially reversible deteriorations (such as infections) and the relentless progression of an underlying disease, which is less likely to be amenable to intervention.
- The benefits and burdens of treatments considered need to be carefully weighed.
- It is important to try to understand what motivates parents towards particular choices. In this context, it can be helpful to ask 'what they still hope for' and 'what they most fear'.
- Lastly, it is important to stress that an ACP stating that the child is for full resuscitation can still be very useful. Firstly, it is likely to contain other useful information about individualized care plans for acute deterioration and the family's wishes in the wider care context. Secondly, if a modified resuscitation plan would eventually be more appropriate for the child, the very act of making the initial ACP will shape future thinking for the child and family. This may allow for a more individually tailored resuscitation plan to be agreed at the next revision.

Who should write it?
- Ideally, the person completing the ACP should both have expertise in the process and know the child and family well.
- That person should have had the opportunity to consult other healthcare professionals involved in the care of the child and to gauge their views on issues such as quality of life and rate of disease progression.
- Any appropriately experienced doctor or nurse can contribute to an ACP[1] although some hospitals stipulate that a particular grade of doctor is required to countersign a decision to limit treatment/resuscitation.

Pitfalls
- Once a draft ACP is agreed, it is helpful to test-drive the content by considering all the settings in which the plan may be activated. This can typically include home, school, hospice, respite centre, and hospital.
- If treatment plans within the ACP are impossible in any of the settings, there may need to be some clarification, or subtle changes.
- Some care settings may have less access to healthcare professionals able to make a decision about whether or not to initiate resuscitation. Schools may have local procedures requiring that an ambulance is called whenever a child becomes acutely unwell.
- An ACP is a record of decisions made about treatment. The signatures on the document are an acknowledgement that the form has been seen and reviewed by those who have signed it. It is not a legal contract that sets in stone a particular treatment decision—parents *can* change their minds and should not feel that they are 'signing anything away'.

In conclusion, a well-written ACP acts as a 'passport' to personalized care in the face of an unexpected deterioration, rather than acting as a treatment limitation order.

Symptom management

The recognition and management of symptoms in children and young people approaching the end of life can be difficult for even experienced paediatric palliative care practitioners due to their wide variety of clinical presentation.

- Environmental measures and non-pharmacological interventions have a huge role to play in managing symptoms.
- Many different medications help, not just the obvious things like opiates and anxiolytics; the Association for Paediatric Palliative Medicine produces a formulary to guide prescribing (℞ https://www.appm.org.uk/guidelines-resources/appm-master-formulary/).
- Anticipatory prescribing of medication 'as required' is very helpful for community palliative care. The medications can be detailed in the form of a symptom management plan, covering issues such as:

Pain

Assessment and management of pain is discussed on ➜ pp. 458–9. It is important to ensure that a non-verbal child is not in pain before assuming that agitation is primary.

Agitation

Children approaching the end of their lives may become agitated, shown by restlessness, irritability, aggressive behaviour, or other distress. They may also show signs of delirium, such as confusion, disrupted attention, disordered speech, and hallucinations. Consider causes such as pain, anaemia, dehydration, urinary retention, or constipation, as well as psychological factors such as fear, anxiety, or depression. Environmental calming and non-pharmacological measures such as reassurance should be used first line. If this is not adequate, medication such as benzodiazepines or neuroleptics (haloperidol or levomepromazine) may be needed, initially at low doses.

Seizures in palliative care

Distressing seizures in a dying child can be managed using subcutaneous infusions of benzodiazepines or phenobarbitone, if enteral medication is no longer effective.

Respiratory distress

If a child approaching the end of their life has respiratory distress, consider treatable causes such as anxiety, physical discomfort, accumulated airway secretions, infection, and bronchospasm. Environmental measures, such as opening a window, using a hand-held fan, or reducing overstimulation, can be very helpful. Supplemental oxygen may help symptomatically, but should not be used with normalized oxygen saturation as a goal. Antisecretory medication (hyoscine or glycopyrronium) may be helpful, and low doses of benzodiazepines or opioids may provide symptomatic relief.

Recognizing the dying child

Experienced clinicians often claim that there is an art to recognizing when a child or young person is dying which develops with experience and requires a particular set of skills. This may be true, but it is clearly the case that a better understanding of signs and symptoms associated with the dying process will also help professionals to recognize that a child or young person may be approaching the last days of life. While it is important to recognize signs and symptoms relevant to dying, it is also important to consider that some symptoms may be reversible given proportionate intervention, and that there are some signs which need to be investigated further before attributing them to the dying process. It is also important to benchmark any of the signs and symptoms listed to the child's own baseline, which may deviate from standard ranges:

• A change in breathing pattern (noisy, laboured, irregular).
• Impaired peripheral perfusion (pale or grey appearance, temperature instability).
• Loss of interest or inability to tolerate food and drinks.
• Marked and unexplained fall in urine output.
• Altered level of awareness (reduced consciousness, less responsiveness, increased sleeping, confusion).
• Intractable seizures despite optimal management.
• New onset of a profound weakness.
• Rapid increase in pain and need for analgesia.

Additionally, it is often said that a child whose deterioration can be observed from week to week may only have weeks or short months to live, and that similarly a child who changes clinically on a daily basis may die within days or short weeks. There is little evidence on which to base this, but the opinion of healthcare staff used to working with dying children is often one of the best guides to timescale. When asked to offer an estimate by families it is important to emphasize how inaccurate this may be and to continue with parallel planning.

Care around the time of death

The time immediately after the death of a child requires a complex mixture of compassionate support and legal processes. In the case of an expected death, if the child dies at home outside of working hours, the family should have been given a contact number to call. There is no prescribed timescale for confirmation of death, and this may be undertaken by a doctor or an appropriately trained nurse. The child's body can be moved only once death is confirmed. A medical certificate for the cause of death will also need to be completed by a doctor who is a regular part of the child's care, and a cremation form may be needed in addition if this is the family's preference.

This is a highly sensitive time for all concerned and it is important to:
• Respect the family's wishes, which will ideally have been recorded in their ACP.
• Be aware that tissue donation, such as heart valves and corneas (but not solid organ donation), is still possible for children who die in the community in some circumstances.
• Allow them to grieve and to prepare for burial or cremation in their own way, but consider offering practical support.
• Provide the family with support in navigating the required statutory processes mentioned previously (talking to them about this process beforehand can be helpful when a death is anticipated).

- Explain the Child Death Overview Process and any other reviews that may be appropriate, such as the LeDeR (Learning Disabilities Mortality Review) process. The LeDeR process seeks to ensure that the individual has had access to the same services as anyone else and that reasonable adjustments were made for them. It applies to all those with LDs over the age of 4 years.
- Ensure that they have an allocated keyworker to support them as a single point of call for the initial period after the bereavement.
- Do not say 'you must' or 'you should do' particular things, e.g. hold or see the body.
- Explore families' own preferences and traditions with them with respect to funeral preparation.
- Be aware that some families may wish to use a bereavement suite (an air-conditioned room with a cooling mattress or cot) available in many hospices, which allows them to spend time with the child after death. The room is maintained at around 4–8°C, meaning that the child can still be a tissue donor, if preferred, following their death in hospice (usually the next working day). A child's body can generally be kept in a cool room for up to 5 days, with this time used to offer acute bereavement support and support with practical arrangements needed following death.

The charity Together for Short Lives has produced a useful guide covering many of the issues arising at this time in more detail (https://www. togetherforshortlives.org.uk/resource/guide-end-life-care/).

Support for grief and loss

- Parents or carers of infants, children, and young people approaching the end of their life need support for grief and loss when their child is nearing the end of their life and after their death.
- This will help parents, carers, and siblings to cope better before and after the death of the child. It can help to reduce emotional distress, anxiety, and depression. This in turn limits relationship issues within the grieving family.
- It is also important to support families in knowing how to talk to their wider family about what has happened and to ensure that they have adequate practical support.
- Families vary greatly in their preferences for ongoing bereavement support. Alongside statutory provision, help is available via children's hospices, as well as a number of disease-specific charities (see below).
- It is important to remember the specific needs of siblings and grandparents.

Support organizations

- Bliss (supports the families of babies born premature or sick): https://www.bliss.org.uk/parents/coping-with-loss/bereavement
- Care for the Family (support for bereaved parents including a befriending service and Facebook community): https:// www.careforthefamily.org.uk/family-life/bereavement-support/ bereaved-parent-support

- Child Bereavement UK (supports families and educates professionals when a baby or child of any age dies or is dying, or when a child is facing bereavement): ℘ https://www.childbereavementuk.org/
- Child Death Helpline (supports anyone affected by the death of a child): ℘ http://childdeathhelpline.org.uk/
- Child Funeral Charity (assists families financially in England and Wales who have to arrange a funeral for a baby or child): ℘ https://www.childfuneralcharity.org.uk/
- Compassionate Friends (support for bereaved parents and their families): ℘ https://www.tcf.org.uk/
- Daisy's Dream (supports children and their families who have been affected by the life-threatening illness or bereavement of someone close to them): ℘ https://www.daisysdream.org.uk/
- Hope Again (supports bereaved children and young people): ℘ https://www.hopeagain.org.uk/
- Lullaby Trust (confidential bereavement support to anyone affected by the sudden and unexpected death of a baby or young child): ℘ https://www.lullabytrust.org.uk/bereavement-support/
- SANDS (supports families facing stillbirths and neonatal death): ℘ https://www.sands.org.uk/
- Winston's Wish (counselling and support for grieving children after the death of a parent or sibling): ℘ https://www.winstonswish.org/

Reference

1. Harrop E, Edwards C (2013). How and when to refer a child for specialist paediatric palliative care. Arch Dis Child Educ Pract, 98, 202–8.

Further resources

Association for Paediatric Palliative Care (2020). Master formulary, 5th ed. Available at: ℘ https://www.appm.org.uk/guidelines-resources/appm-master-formulary/

Hain R, Goldman A, Rapoport A, et al. (eds) (2021). Oxford Textbook of Paediatric Palliative Care, 3rd ed. Oxford: Oxford University Press.

Harrop E, Brombley K, Boyce K (2017). Fifteen minute consultation: practical pain management in paediatric palliative care. Arch Dis Child Educ Pract Ed, 102, 239–43.

National Institute for Health and Care Excellence (2016, updated 2019). End of Life Care for Infants, Children and Young People with Life-Limiting Conditions: Planning and Management. NICE guideline NG61. London: NICE. Available at: ℘ https://www.nice.org.uk/guidance/NG61

Stein A, Dalton L, Rapa E, et al. (2019). Communication with children and adolescents about the diagnosis of their own life-threatening condition. Lancet, 393, 1150–63.

The Children's and Young Person's Advance Care Planning Document. Available at: ℘ http://www.cypacp.com

Together for Short Lives (2019). Caring for a child at the end of life. Available at: ℘ https://www.togetherforshortlives.org.uk/resource/guide-end-life-care/

Genetics and syndromes in neurodisability

There is only one pretty child in the world, and every mother has it.

Chinese proverb

Introduction to clinical genetics

Clinical genetics is a specialty that integrates all aspects of medicine. It deals with both common and rare childhood and adult disorders which may have a genetic origin. It is involved in the use of basic sciences to understand the origin and progression of a disease, which helps the development of screening guidelines and therapeutic options, when appropriate. With the advances in use of new testing technology and bioinformatics, the opportunities for early diagnosis and therapeutic intervention are becoming more realistic.

Role of a clinical geneticist

A clinical geneticist is a medical doctor trained in paediatrics and adult medicine.

The main role of a clinical geneticist is to:
- Make a diagnosis (syndromic or non-syndromic).
- Discuss the natural progression and prognosis of the condition.
- Recommend screening and treatment measures.
- Counsel the family regarding reproductive risks.
- Discuss preconceptual advice, prenatal testing, and other appropriate reproductive options (such as artificial insemination by donor, egg donation, and preimplantation genetic diagnosis), where appropriate.
- Interpret complex results identified through genetic testing such as comparative genomic hybridization (CGH) or next-generation sequencing.

Which patients to refer?

Many patients seen in a community paediatrics clinic have shared care with a clinical geneticist.

The common reasons for referral are:
- Developmental delay: may be global or be limited to specific skill areas (see ➜ pp. 30–1).
- Facial dysmorphism.
- Congenital structural abnormalities: including cardiac, palatal, limb, brain, kidney, skeletal, skin, and bowel abnormalities.
- Growth abnormalities: proportionate or disproportionate growth restriction, or overgrowth.
- Neurological abnormalities: hypotonia or hypertonia (see ➜ pp. 112–13), microcephaly or macrocephaly (see ➜ p. 238), seizures (see ➜ pp. 248–55), movement disorders (see ➜ pp. 246–7), SNHL (see ➜ p. 520), visual anomalies (see ➜ pp. 202–8), and cranial nerve abnormalities.
- Behavioural problems: including sleep disturbances (see ➜ pp. 466–8), ADHD (see ➜ pp. 126–34), and ASD (see ➜ pp. 114–25).
- Family history of an inherited disorder (see ➜ pp. 150–1).
- Any patient identified to have variant of unknown significance following genetic testing.

Chromosomes and genes

Within each of our cells, in the nucleus, there are double-stranded DNA segments which represent our genes. There are ~25,000 pairs of genes in each of our cells, which are packaged into chromosomes. Chromosomes also come in pairs (one maternal and the other paternal) and there are 23 pairs of chromosomes in each of our cells (except the gametes). The pairs are numbered 1–22 according to their size and banding pattern and these are known as autosomes. The remaining pair of chromosomes is comprised of the sex chromosomes. 46XX is the usual karyotype in females and 46XY in males.

Modes of inheritance

Autosomal dominant

- AD disorders are caused by abnormalities (mutations or deletions) in genes encoded on the autosomes.
- A mutation in one copy of the gene is often sufficient to cause the phenotype.
- There is a 50% chance in each pregnancy that the offspring may inherit the mutation, as we pass on only one copy of each of our genes through the egg or the sperm.
- Examples include NF1 (see ➔ pp. 512–13), Noonan syndrome, tuberous sclerosis (see ➔ pp. 513–14), achondroplasia, etc.

Autosomal recessive

- AR disorders are caused by mutations in genes on the autosomes.
- Mutations in both copies (maternal and paternal copies) of the same gene are needed in order to cause the disorder.
- AR disorders are caused when both parents carry a mutation in one copy of the same gene (they are called carriers).
- When both parents are carriers, there is a one in four chance (25%) in each pregnancy that the baby may be affected.
- The healthy sibling of an affected individual is at a two in three risk of being a carrier.
- More common in consanguineous families as a shared common ancestor may pass on the same mutation to both parents.
- Some AR disorders may be common even in the absence of consanguinity if the carrier frequency in the general population is high, e.g. cystic fibrosis with a carrier frequency of 1 in 20 or SMA with a carrier frequency of 1 in 50.
- Examples include many metabolic disorders (MPS, organic acidurias, glycogen storage disease, etc. (see ➔ pp. 150–1)), cystic fibrosis, SMA (see ➔ pp. 550–1).

X-linked recessive

- XLR disorders are caused by abnormalities of genes on the X chromosome.
- As females have two copies of the X chromosome, abnormalities in one copy of the gene cause mild or no symptoms; hence they are called carriers.
- In males, as there is only one copy of the X chromosome, abnormalities of the XLR gene are manifested and males are affected.
- Although a female carrier does not usually have any symptoms herself, she can have affected sons (there is a 50% risk in each pregnancy that any son she has will be affected) and carrier daughters (there is a 50% risk in each pregnancy that any daughter she has will be a carrier).
- Males with an XLR disorder cannot pass the disorder to their sons as they will pass on the Y copy of their sex chromosome to them; all their daughters will be obligate carriers as they will have to pass on the X chromosome which carries the abnormality.

- Examples include fragile X syndrome (see ➔ pp. 516–17), DMD (see ➔ pp. 548–9), ATRX (alpha-thalassaemia/mental retardation syndrome) (see ➔ pp. 136–41), etc.

X-linked dominant

- X-linked dominant disorders are also caused by abnormalities of genes on the X chromosome.
- Typically, males are more severely affected, even resulting in spontaneous loss of pregnancy or neonatal death.
- Females are affected but tend to survive.
- When an affected female goes on to have children, there is a 33% risk of having an affected female baby as affected males are less likely to survive.
- Examples include Rett syndrome, incontinentia pigmenti, etc.

Imprinting disorders

- Genomic imprinting is the normal mechanism by which certain genes are selectively expressed from the maternal or paternal copy of the chromosome.
- When this mechanism is disrupted (by uniparental disomy (UPD) where both copies of a chromosome are inherited from the same parent, or by a defect in the imprinting centre), an imprinting disorder may be caused.
- Examples include Angelman syndrome (see ➔ pp. 517–18) caused by paternal UPD15, Prader–Willi syndrome (see ➔ p. 518) caused by maternal UPD15, Russell–Silver syndrome caused by imprinting alterations on chromosome 7 or 11, Beckwith–Wiedemann syndrome caused by loss of methylation of *KvDMR* or *UPD11*, etc.

Mitochondrial

- Mitochondrial DNA is a double-stranded circular DNA which encodes 13 proteins all of which are subunits of respiratory chain complexes.
- Tissues with a high energy demand, e.g. skeletal muscle, cardiac muscle, CNS, pancreatic islet cells, liver, and kidney, are most likely to be affected.
- Mitochondrial disorders are usually inherited from the mother as the fraction of paternal mitochondria in the fertilized egg is very small (0.1%) and is eliminated in early embryogenesis.
- When the mutation is present in only some mitochondria in a cell, it is termed 'heteroplasmy' and when the mutation is present in all the mitochondria in a cell, it is termed 'homoplasmy'.
- Mitochondrial mutations show a threshold effect, i.e. there is a threshold beyond which heteroplasmy causes disease.
- The threshold varies between different mitochondrial disorders, e.g. Leigh syndrome, NARP (neuropathy, ataxia, retinitis pigmentosa) (see ➔ p. 256), and MELAS (myopathy, encephalopathy, lactic acidosis and stroke).
- Some mitochondrial disorders are caused by nuclear genes which regulate the function of the mitochondria, e.g. some AR forms of cerebellar ataxia (see ➔ pp. 256–8).

Multifactorial

- This type of inheritance is seen in isolated disorders such as:
  - Cleft lip and palate (see p. 520).
  - Learning difficulties (see pp. 136–41).
  - Behavioural problems (see pp. 362–3 and pp. 412–13) etc.
- They occur as a result of an interaction between environmental and genetic factors.

Genetic testing

- Different genetic tests are used depending on whether the chromosomes or the genes are being tested.
- Genetic testing should be carried out with appropriate counselling and consent of the patient/parent as the results may have implications for not only the proband but also for other family members. Care should be taken to maintain confidentiality.
- Genetic testing is offered to children for diagnostic purposes or if genetic testing will provide guidance for screening measures in children at risk of a familial disorder, e.g. bowel screening in children at risk of developing familial adenomatosis polyposis.
- Predictive testing of adult-onset conditions is not recommended in children, e.g. myotonic dystrophy, hereditary motor-sensory neuropathy, etc.

Chromosome tests

Comparative genomic hybridization or microarray CGH

- This is the first-line test by which submicroscopic chromosomal aberrations (deletions or duplications) can be identified. However, these abnormalities are not always considered to be pathogenic, as some small aberrations may represent a normal variant or a recurrent copy number variant (CNV) that indicates a neurosusceptibility locus.
- Parental testing may be needed to clarify the pathogenicity of the finding and clarify recurrence risks.

Fluorescent in situ hybridization (FISH)

- This is the test that uses specific fluorescent probes which align to a part of a particular chromosome.
- It is used when a specific chromosome deletion or duplication is suspected, e.g. 22q11 deletion in DiGeorge syndrome (see pp. 506–7), but this can also be picked up by microarray CGH.
- It is used for parental testing of array abnormalities (a repeat sample from the child may be needed for validation of the FISH probes).

Karyotype

This is the basic chromosome test looking at the number and arrangement of chromosomes. It is the test used to identify balanced chromosomal re-arrangements, e.g. translocations.

Molecular tests

These tests are done when a single gene disorder is suspected. Either mutations (nucleotide substitution, deletion, or insertion) or abnormal copy numbers (whole gene deletions or duplications) in a single gene can account for a disorder.

Sequencing of a gene

- This is the test by which mutations in specific genes are looked for, e.g. gene mutations in tuberous sclerosis (see pp. 513–14), NF1 (see pp. 512–13), Rett syndrome (see pp. 518–19).
- In order to request this test, the gene for the suspected condition should be known and testing should be available either in an NHS laboratory or in a research laboratory.

- Caution should be exercised in the interpretation of results when the mutation is reported as a variant and the pathogenicity of the mutation is not clear. The American College of Medical Genetics guidelines are currently used in all laboratories nationally to determine the pathogenicity of a variant.[1]

Polymerase chain reaction (PCR)

- This is the technique by which a specific sequence of DNA from the patient is amplified using primers, DNA polymerases, and DNA precursors and compared against that of a standard DNA sequence by running them both on a gel.
- A discrepancy in the size of the PCR product indicates a mutation or deletion of the gene, e.g. in fragile X syndrome (see pp. 516–17) or myotonic dystrophy (see p. 273).

Multiplex ligation-dependent probe amplification (MLPA)

- This is a multiplex PCR method by which gene deletions or duplications are detected. Many single gene disorders may be caused by a complete or partial deletion of the gene in a proportion of patients.
- Hence, when no mutation is identified in a clinically suspected disorder, MLPA should be considered to detect abnormal copy numbers, e.g. in a patient clinically suspected to have CHARGE syndrome but with no mutations detected in the *CHD7* gene.

Whole exome sequencing

- This is the technique by which the coding sequences (exomes) of all known human genes are sequenced with an aim of finding the causative mutation/s in a gene.
- This test is currently used primarily where rapid results are needed to determine the management of the patient, e.g. in the NICU or PICU setting. Prenatal (fetal) exomes are also now becoming available for scan findings of multiple anomalies.
- Both a gene-agnostic approach and testing of panels of genes based on phenotype may be carried out on the data generated.
- Trio exome sequencing (parents and child) is likely to have a higher diagnostic yield.
- The limitation of this test is that it misses mutations in introns and structural variations which may account for a patient's phenotype.

Whole genome sequencing

- This is also a new technique by which the entire genome (exons and introns of all genes) of a patient is sequenced with an aim of finding the causative mutation/s.
- Trio sequencing is likely to have a higher diagnostic yield. Genomic sequencing normally identifies 4 million variants. Filtering of parental variants increases the chances of reaching a diagnosis particularly in *de novo* cases. Confirming the pattern of inheritance (for AR and X-linked disorders) is easier.
- Theoretically, CNVs, short tandem repeats, and chromosomal rearrangements can also be identified using this technique.

In England, the National Genomics Test Directory (https://www.england. nhs.uk/publication/national-genomic-test-directories/) provides guidance regarding eligibility for genomic testing and the availability of different genetic tests based on disease group.

Approach to evaluation of a child with dysmorphism, congenital malformation, and/or developmental delay

Facial dysmorphism and other minor physical anomalies can be a helpful clue to the clinical diagnosis in several syndromes. In some syndromes, e.g. DS, the facial features are typical and affected individuals resemble one another (see ➡ pp. 497–9). In other syndromes, the dysmorphic features may be more subtle or non-specific. Associated structural abnormalities and neurodevelopmental problems will provide further clues to the diagnosis in these cases.

Definitions of terms used

- *Syndrome*: a set of developmental abnormalities occurring together in a consistently recognizable pattern, e.g. DS, Noonan syndrome, etc.
- *Sequence*: a pattern of developmental abnormalities occurring as a consequence of a primary defect, e.g. Pierre Robin sequence, a triad of a wide U-shaped cleft palate, small chin, and relatively large tongue (glossoptosis), occurs as a consequence of a small chin, which prevents the normal-sized tongue from descending and obstructs the closure of the palatal processes.
- *Association*: a non-random collection of developmental anomalies that occur together more frequently than expected by chance, e.g. VACTERL (vertebral anomalies, anal atresia, cardiac anomalies, tracheo-oesophageal fistula, (o)esophageal atresia, renal anomalies, and limb defects).
- *Malformation*: a structural abnormality that occurs due to an abnormal developmental process, i.e. a primary error in morphogenesis (e.g. cleft lip).
- *Deformation*: a distortion of normally programmed structures by a physical force, e.g. talipes caused by oligohydramnios.
- *Disruption*: the abnormality caused by destruction of normally programmed structures, e.g. limb defects caused by amniotic bands.
- *Dysplasia*: refers to the abnormal cellular organization within a tissue which results in structural changes, e.g. renal cystic dysplasia.

History taking in dysmorphic syndromes

- *Family history*: three-generation family history with a special focus on congenital abnormalities and neurodevelopmental problems; history of miscarriages, terminations, stillbirths, and neonatal deaths.
- *Pregnancy and delivery*: maternal health, bleeding, medications, alcohol/drug intake, investigations, fetal movements, liquor volume, gestation, and mode of delivery.
- *Neonatal history*: Apgar score; birth weight, length, head circumference; feeding difficulties, admission to special care baby unit, medical problems, congenital anomalies.
- *Growth*: height, weight, and head circumference.
- *Childhood medical problems*: hearing, vision, seizures, regression of milestones, involuntary movements, and constipation/diarrhoea.

- *Developmental history and schooling history*: developmental delay and additional educational needs.
- *Behavioural issues*: social interaction and communications skills, obsessive or ritualistic behaviour, hyperactivity, poor attention span, sleep disturbances, self-harming, and involuntary laughter.

Examination

- *Face*: asymmetry, e.g. Goldenhar syndrome, CHARGE syndrome, etc.
- *Hair*: texture, e.g. curly, coarse hair in Noonan syndrome; colour, e.g. blonde hair in Angelman syndrome; alopecia, e.g. ectodermal dysplasia; premature greying, e.g. Waardenburg syndrome.
- *Skull*: shape, e.g. craniosynostosis in Apert syndrome, Crouzon syndrome; size, e.g. microcephaly in Angelman syndrome, macrocephaly in Noonan syndrome.
- *Ears*: shape, e.g. cup-shaped ears in CHARGE syndrome; size, e.g. microtia in Treacher Collins syndrome; position, e.g. low-set ears in DS, posteriorly rotated ears in Noonan syndrome; preauricular pits and tags, e.g. branchio-oto-renal syndrome.
- *Eyebrows*: deficiency, e.g. absent in ectodermal dysplasia, interrupted in Kabuki syndrome; synophrys, e.g. Cornelia de Lange syndrome, Waardenburg syndrome.
- *Eyes*: deep-set eyes, e.g. Angelman syndrome; prominent eyes, e.g. Crouzon syndrome; everted eyelids, e.g. lateral eversion in Kabuki syndrome; structural abnormalities, e.g. microphthalmia, anophthalmia; periorbital puffiness, e.g. Williams syndrome; epicanthic folds, e.g. DS; upslanting palpebral fissures, e.g. DS; downslanting palpebral fissures, e.g. Noonan syndrome.
- *Nasal bridge*: flat, e.g. DS, Stickler syndrome; prominent, e.g. AR microcephaly.
- *Nose*: short, e.g. fetal alcohol syndrome, Williams syndrome; hypoplastic alae nasi or pinched, e.g. 22q11 deletion syndrome; anteverted nares, e.g. Cornelia de Lange syndrome; prominent nasal tip, e.g. tricho-rhino-phalangeal syndrome; protruding nasal columella, e.g. Rubinstein–Taybi syndrome.
- *Philtrum*: length, e.g. short in Mowat–Wilson syndrome, long in fetal alcohol syndrome; smoothness, e.g. smooth in fetal alcohol syndrome.
- *Cheeks*: malar flattening, e.g. DS, Treacher Collins syndrome; prominent cheeks, e.g. Williams syndrome.
- *Lips*: thickness, e.g. thin upper lip in fetal alcohol syndrome; shape, e.g. cupid's bow shape in Smith–Magenis syndrome.
- *Chin*: size, e.g. micrognathia in Pierre Robin sequence; prominence, e.g. Angelman syndrome, Sotos syndrome.
- *Neck*: webbing, e.g. Noonan syndrome, Turner syndrome; sinus/fistulae, e.g. branchio-oto-renal syndrome; low posterior hairline, e.g. Noonan syndrome, Turner syndrome.
- *Thorax*: size, e.g. small in Jeune syndrome; shape, e.g. bell-shaped in Jeune syndrome; skeletal abnormalities, e.g. pectus excavatum in Marfan syndrome.
- *Abdomen*: protuberant abdomen, e.g. Beckwith–Wiedemann syndrome; umbilical hernia, e.g. Beckwith–Wiedemann syndrome.

- *Back*: spine abnormalities, e.g. scoliosis, lordosis.
- *Upper and lower limbs*: asymmetry, e.g. Beckwith–Wiedemann syndrome; disproportion, e.g. skeletal dysplasias; brachydactyly, e.g. short fourth and fifth fingers in pseudohypoparathyroidism; arachnodactyly, e.g. Marfan syndrome; camptodactyly, e.g. distal arthrogryposis; clinodactyly, e.g. Russell–Silver syndrome; abnormal thumbs, e.g. Rubinstein–Taybi syndrome; polydactyly, e.g. Bardet–Biedl syndrome; wide sandal gap, e.g. DS; nail hypoplasia, e.g. in fetal alcohol syndrome; unusual palmar or plantar creases, e.g. single palmar crease in DS, deep plantar creases in mosaic trisomy 8.
- *Skin*: hypopigmentation, e.g. ash leaf macules in tuberous sclerosis; hyperpigmentation, e.g. café-au-lait patches in NF1; hirsutism, e.g. Coffin–Siris syndrome; eczema, e.g. Dubowitz syndrome; photosensitivity, e.g. chromosomal breakage disorders.

▶ It is the facial gestalt and the pattern of associated abnormalities that guides the clinician to the diagnosis rather than a single dysmorphic feature. The list of features is by no means exhaustive.

Reference

1. Richards S, Aziz N, Bale S, et al. (2015). Standards and guidelines for the interpretation of sequence variants: a joint consensus recommendation of the American College of Medical Genetics and Genomics and the Association for Molecular Pathology. Genet Med, 17, 405–24.

Common chromosomal syndromes: aneuploidy

Refers to abnormalities in the number of chromosomes, e.g. DS (trisomy 21), Edwards syndrome (trisomy 18), Patau syndrome (trisomy 13), and Pallister–Killian syndrome (tetrasomy 12p).

Down syndrome or trisomy 21

Incidence

Approximately 1 in 1000 live births. Approximately 60,000 people with DS are living in UK.

Aetiology

- DS may be caused by:
  - Full trisomy 21, i.e. maternal meiotic non-disjunction in 94% of patients.
  - Mosaicism in 2.4%.
  - Translocations in 3.3%; ~75% of the unbalanced translocations are *de novo*, and ~25% result from familial translocation.
- Advanced maternal age remains the only well-documented risk factor for maternal non-disjunction. The chance of having a child with DS increases with increasing maternal age:
  - At 35 years: 1 in 385.
  - At 40 years: 1 in 106.
  - At 45 years: 1 in 30.

Diagnosis

Prenatal screening

- A combination of the following three factors is used for screening in the general population to calculate the chance of having a child with DS:
  - Maternal age.
  - Ultrasound findings (thickened nuchal fold, shortened long bones, hypoplastic nasal bone, echogenic bowel, etc.).
  - Maternal serum markers (low alpha-fetoprotein, raised human chorionic gonadotropin, low unconjugated oestriol (uE3)).
- If the screening result suggests an increased risk, then the following (invasive) tests are offered for more definitive answers:
  - Amniocentesis (performed at 14–16 weeks, >99% accurate).
  - Chorionic villus sampling (performed at 10–13 weeks, >95% accurate).

Postnatal studies

- FISH studies: for rapid diagnosis on the postnatal ward.
- Karyotyping: is essential to provide risk of recurrence and for genetic counselling.

Effects of extra chromosome 21

- Increased fetal loss, spontaneous abortions (reduced prenatal viability).
- Increased postnatal morbidity.
- Reduced physical growth (short stature, follow second centile on normal growth charts).
- Delayed cognitive development.
- ID.

- Dysmorphic physical features (see ➔ pp. 497–9).
- Increased chance of congenital malformations.
- Increased risk of autoimmunity.
- Reduced humoral and cell-mediated immunity.
- Abnormal physiological functioning.
- Premature senescence (cataracts, Alzheimer disease, etc.).

Clinical features

Well over 100 features have been described in DS.
- Cardiac:
  - Atrioventricular septal defect.
  - Ventricular septal defect.
  - Atrial septal defect.
  - Patent ductus arteriosus.
  - Tetralogy of Fallot.
  - Other complex congenital heart diseases.
  - Pulmonary hypertension.
- Respiratory:
  - Tracheo-oesophageal fistula.
  - Repeated aspiration (see ➔ p. 449).
  - Frequent chest infections (>10× increase in pneumonia (see ➔ p. 451)).
  - Airway obstruction secondary to glossoptosis, large tonsils/adenoids (leading to arterial hypoxaemia, alveolar hypoventilation, pulmonary hypertension).
- GI:
  - Duodenal atresia/stenosis.
  - Oesophageal atresia.
  - Anal atresia/stenosis.
  - GOR (see ➔ pp. 438–9).
  - Hirschsprung's disease.
  - Meckel's diverticulum.
  - Increased risk of coeliac disease (reported prevalence 5–15% in DS population).
  - Chronic constipation (see ➔ pp. 440–1).
- Orthopaedic/musculoskeletal:
  - Atlanto-axial instability.
  - Short long bones.
  - Hypoplasia of the middle phalanx (clinodactyly).
  - Short and broad fingers and toes.
  - Increased space between first and second toe (sandal gap).
  - Hyperextensible (increased range of movements in most joints).
  - Joint instability (hips, patella).
- Neuropsychiatric:
  - ID (IQ range in DS 20–85; normal range 80–110) (see ➔ pp. 136–41).
  - Delayed cognitive development.
  - Seizures (5–10% of DS, infantile spasms are common during infancy) (see ➔ pp. 248–55).
  - Depression (see ➔ pp. 330–2).
  - Dementia (early onset, Alzheimer's type).

- Behavioural problems (obsessive tendencies, oppositionality, etc. (see ➔ pp. 362–3)).
- Increased prevalence of autism and ASD (see ➔ pp. 114–25).
- Increased incidence of congenital SNHL (see ➔ p. 520), ADHD (see ➔ pp. 126–34), etc.
- ENT:
  - Hypoplasia of maxillary sinuses.
  - Frequent upper respiratory tract infections (both viral and bacterial).
  - Middle ear effusions (OME) (see ➔ pp. 184–5).
  - Conductive HL (secondary to the above).
  - Large adenoids, tonsils with hypotonia of neck musculature.
  - OSAs (sleep difficulties) (see ➔ pp. 448–9).
- Eye:
  - Increased incidence of congenital cataract.
  - Keratoconus.
  - Nystagmus (see ➔ p. 204).
  - Squint (see ➔ p. 204).
  - Blocked nasolacrimal duct.
  - Increased incidence of conjunctivitis, blepharitis.
  - Increased prevalence of acquired lens opacities (see ➔ p. 202).
  - Increased prevalence of refractive errors (hypermetropia is more common) (see ➔ p. 204).
- Haematology:
  - Transient abnormal myelopoiesis (TAM) (leukaemic picture in the neonatal period, secondary to *GATA1* mutation).
  - Increased risk of acute lymphoblastic leukaemia.
  - Increased risk of acute myeloblastic leukaemia.
  - Decreased risk of solid tumours.
- Endocrine:
  - Congenital hypothyroidism.
  - Hashimoto's thyroiditis (causing hypothyroidism, rarely hyperthyroidism).
  - Diabetes mellitus (insulin dependent, autoimmune).
- Dermatology:
  - Dry skin/eczema
  - Alopecia.
  - Vitiligo.
  - Folliculitis.
  - Recurrent skin infections
  - Transverse palmar crease.
- Dental:
  - Delayed dental eruption.
  - Increased incidence of dental caries (see ➔ p. 464).
  - Malformed teeth.
  - Malocclusion.
  - Hypocalcified teeth.
- Immunology:
  - Impaired humoral immunity.
  - Impaired cell-mediated immunity.
  - Increased autoimmune conditions (Hashimoto's thyroiditis, diabetes, coeliac, vitiligo).

- Reproductive:
  - Decreased fertility in both sexes.
  - Hypospadias.
  - Micropenis.
  - Undescended testicles.
- Abnormal physiological functioning:
  - Hypersensitivity to pilocarpine.
  - Hyper-reactivity to methotrexate.
  - Predisposition to hyperuricaemia.
  - Increased insulin resistance.
- Dysmorphology:
  - Round face.
  - Flat facial profile (hypoplasia of the cheek bones).
  - Upslanting palpebral fissures.
  - Bilateral epicanthic folds.
  - Flat nasal bridge.
  - Small, low-set ears.
  - Small mouth.
  - Relatively large tongue, protruding.

Investigations

- Thyroid function test (at birth, annually thereafter, one-third will develop hypothyroidism in their lifetime).
- Echocardiography (performed in all patients with DS soon after birth).
- Hearing test: soon after birth and then annually. SNHL (see ➜ p. 520) and OME (see ➜ pp. 184–5) common.
- Vision test: screen for cataracts, then 1–2-yearly for lifetime.
- Neck X-ray (for atlanto-axial instability): perform if there is suspicion of cervical cord compression.
- Coeliac screen: if growth falters.
- Immunoglobulin subclasses: to identify deficiency of IgG subclasses—if significant bacterial infections.
- Haematology: FBC. Bone marrow test if features of bone marrow dysfunction.

Medical care

- Annual health checks and follow-up: complete physical examination (for listed clinical features).
- Growth monitoring: weight faltering common in early years. Rule out hypothyroidism, coeliac, etc. Involve dietician. Obesity is a preventable secondary handicap in later years. Encourage physical activity. Explore leisure facilities. Review caloric intake.
- Developmental assessments: annually in the early years, then before secondary school, before transition to college etc. Multidisciplinary assessments involving SLT (see ➜ pp. 402–3), OT (see ➜ pp. 390–1), PT (see ➜ pp. 374–6), etc. as required, more often in early years.
- Sleep: enquire about snoring, restless sleep, etc. OSA is common (see ➜ pp. 448–9). Refer to respiratory colleagues for sleep study. ENT colleagues for airway obstruction.

- Surgical interventions/operations: for heart anomalies, adeno-tonsillectomy, other congenital anomalies, etc. Anaesthetists pay attention to atlantoaxial instability. Antibiotic prophylaxis for certain heart lesions (e.g. mitral valve prolapse), dental procedures.
- Vaccination: recommend all routine vaccinations plus annual flu vaccinations in early years, pneumococcal vaccines.
- Liaison and referral to following specialists is common:
  - Neurologist (epilepsy (see ➲ pp. 248–55), cervical cord compression, etc.).
  - Orthopaedic surgeon (hip dislocation, scoliosis (see ➲ pp. 278–9), feet anomalies (see ➲ p. 554), etc.).
  - Cardiologist (congenital heart lesions, pulmonary hypertension, etc.).
  - Psychiatry (behavioural disorders, ADHD (see ➲ pp. 126–34), ODD (see ➲ pp. 306–8), OCD, etc.).
  - Dietician (dietetic evaluation, feeding problems (see ➲ pp. 436–7 and pp. 315–16), recommend balanced diet).
  - Geneticist (genetic counselling).
  - Audiologist (annual checks).
  - Ophthalmologist (annual).
  - Dentist (annual).
  - Dermatologist.
  - Endocrinologist (for thyroid disorders, diabetes, growth faltering).

Educational habilitation
EPs advice on SEN (see ➲ pp. 656–8 and pp. 666–7). Emphasize learning about personal, social, and health education, dealing with money, self-care, employment/career counselling. Supervised employment possible for many.

Social care
Information on allowances, benefits, leisure, long-term living arrangements, respite care, (see ➲ pp. 682–3), etc.

Prognosis
- The life expectancy for DS has increased sixfold in the past 80 years.
- The average life expectancy now is into the fifth/sixth decade.
- Mortality is increased by severe ID (see ➲ pp. 136–41), institutionalization, dementia, mobility restrictions, epilepsy, cardiac disease, etc.

Edwards syndrome or trisomy 18
- Caused by the presence of three copies of chromosome 18.
- High rate of spontaneous pregnancy loss or a poor outcome in surviving infants is seen.

Clinical features
- Fetal growth restriction—a consistent feature.
- Small placenta.
- Facial features: microcephaly, microphthalmia, small pointed chin.
- Limbs: overlapping fingers, rocker-bottom feet, and short hallux.
- Chest: short sternum.
- Congenital heart disease is common (in 90%).
- Other structural abnormalities: oro-facial cleft, radial ray defects, and kidney and brain abnormalities.

- Survival rates are reported to be 45% at 1 week, 9% at 6 months, and 5% at 1 year.
- Central apnoea and cardiopulmonary arrest are the causes of death.

Inheritance

In ~94% of cases this is caused due to *de novo* meiotic non-disjunction and is hence associated with a low recurrence risk (0.5%). In the remaining, it is caused by a mosaic trisomy 18 or a partial 18q trisomy.

Patau syndrome or trisomy 13

- Caused by the presence of three copies of chromosome 13.
- Associated with a high rate of spontaneous pregnancy loss or poor outcome in surviving infants.

Clinical features

- Fetal growth restriction.
- Holoprosencephaly.
- Microphthalmia/anophthalmia.
- Scalp defects (cutis aplasia).
- Oro-facial clefts (may be midline).
- Congenital heart defects.
- Postaxial polydactyly.
- Omphalocele.
- Kidney abnormalities.
- Severe developmental delay in survivors.
- Median age of survival is 7–10 days and survival rate at 12 months is 5–10%.
- Central apnoea and cardiopulmonary arrest are the common causes of death.

Inheritance

About 90% are caused by maternal meiotic non-disjunction, which results in a complete trisomy 13; the recurrence risk is low (0.5%). In the remaining 10%, a translocation (usually unbalanced Robertsonian translocation 13;14), mosaic trisomy 13, or partial trisomy 13, may cause Patau syndrome and the recurrence risk may vary accordingly.

Further resources

Down Syndrome Association: ☎ 0845 230 0372; ♒ http://www.downs-syndrome.org.uk
Down Syndrome Education International: ☎ 02392 855330; ♒ http://www.downsed.org
Down Syndrome Medical Interest Group: ☎ 0115 883 1158; ♒ http://www.dsmig.org.uk

Common chromosomal syndromes: sex chromosome anomalies

Sex chromosome anomalies are abnormalities affecting the X or Y chromosome. Some common examples are discussed as follows:

Turner syndrome

- This is caused by the absence of one copy of the X chromosome in girls.
- It affects 1 in 2500 live female births.
- The majority of Turner syndrome pregnancies are, however, lost spontaneously.

Clinical features

- Short stature (mean adult height of 147 cm but may be increased by growth hormone treatment in childhood).
- Short webbed neck, low hairline.
- Oedema of hands and feet (in newborn).
- Heart defects: coarctation, bicuspid aortic valve, and ventricular septal defect.
- Renal anomalies: horseshoe kidneys and renal agenesis.
- Glue ears and hearing problems are common childhood problems (see ➔ pp. 184–5).
- Delayed or absent puberty and premature menopause are associated with the presence of streak ovaries and the majority of women are infertile.
- Intelligence is usually normal, but IQ may be 10–15 points lower than siblings.
- Social adjustment problems and subtle perceptual difficulties.
- Autoimmune diseases such as hypothyroidism and diabetes mellitus.
- Osteoporosis (see ➔ pp. 454–5) and obesity are more common.

Inheritance

In a study by Birkebaek et al. (2002) it was noted that 49% of Turner syndrome was caused by 45X, 9% by a structural abnormality of one X chromosome, 19% had mosaicism with 45X/46XX, and 23% had mosaicism with structural abnormality of one X. The majority of Turner syndrome karyotypes are thought to result from parental meiotic errors generating abnormal sex chromosomes.

Klinefelter syndrome

- This is caused by the presence of an extra X chromosome in males (47XXY).
- It has a prevalence of 1 in 600–800 with a significant maternal age effect.
- It is usually diagnosed prenatally as an unexpected finding on amniocentesis or CVS. In adult males, it may be diagnosed during investigations for infertility.

Clinical features

- Facial dysmorphism is not present.
- Tall stature (final adult height 187 cm).

- Transient gynaecomastia.
- Breast cancer risk (3%) is increased compared to men in the general population, but usually occurs later on in life (mean age at diagnosis 72 years).
- Boys enter puberty normally but develop low testosterone levels.
- Testes are small in adult life.
- Usually infertile due to low sperm counts.
- Decrease of 10–15 points in IQ compared to siblings and about two-thirds have additional educational needs (usually extra help in mainstream school) (see ➨ pp. 656–8).
- Passive and unassertive behaviour has been frequently noted.
- Boys should be referred to a paediatric endocrinologist before the age of 10 for monitoring of growth and hormonal levels.
- Testosterone supplementation may be needed to help with self-esteem, facial hair growth, and libido.
- Referral to a reproductive specialist is recommended in adult life to consider assisted conception or AID (artificial insemination using donor sperm). A slight increase in aneuploidy (sex chromosome abnormalities and trisomy 21) has been noted in the offspring of these men.

Recurrence risk
The risk is low (<1%) for parents of boys with 47XXY.

Triple X syndrome

- This is caused by the presence of an extra X chromosome in a female (47XXX).
- It is usually picked up as an incidental finding at amniocentesis or CVS and has an incidence of 1 in 1000 live births.
- It is also associated with a significant maternal age effect.

Clinical features
- Tall stature with relatively small head size.
- No facial dysmorphism seen.
- Frequency of urogenital abnormalities is slightly increased.
- Puberty and fertility are usually normal, although there is a slight increased risk of premature ovarian failure.
- A 10–15-point decrease in IQ compared to siblings is noted. Speech and language delay (see ➨ p. 56 and pp. 402–3) and the need for additional educational needs (see ➨ pp. 656–8 and pp. 666–7) have been seen in some individuals.

Recurrence risk
This is low for offspring and for siblings of affected females.

Further resources
Klinefelter Organisation: ☎ 01206 870430; ⌨ http://www.klinefelter.org.uk

Common chromosomal syndromes: translocations

Reciprocal translocation

- Occurs when two or more separate chromosomes exchange pieces of chromosomes between themselves. This is termed 'balanced translocation' when the translocated chromosomes have not lost or gained any chromosomal material; this is not usually associated with a phenotype.
- An 'unbalanced translocation' occurs when chromosomal material is gained (duplication) or lost (deletion) and is often associated with a phenotype which is dependent on the genes affected and the size of the deletion or duplication.
- A parent with a balanced translocation has a risk of having children with an unbalanced translocation. The risk of having a live-born affected child is dependent on the size and content of the translocation, as large deletions or duplications may result in a miscarriage.

Robertsonian translocation

- This is the result of fusion of acrocentric chromosomes (those with a very short 'p' arm), e.g. chromosomes 13, 14, 15, 21, and 22.
- Some common Robertsonian translocations are rob(13q14q) and rob(14q21q).
- The translocated chromosome may act as a single chromosome during meiosis and may be passed on together with a copy of the normal chromosome to the offspring resulting in disease, e.g. when a parent has a rob(14q21q), they may pass on this translocated chromosome along with a normal chromosome 21, resulting in DS (see ➋ pp. 496–500) in the child.

Common chromosomal syndromes: microdeletion syndromes

- These are syndromes associated with deletion of parts of chromosomes, which cannot be identified on conventional karyotype. Specific FISH tests have to be done in order to confirm a clinical suspicion of the diagnosis.
- More recently with the use of array CGH several new microdeletion syndromes have been described.
- Many microdeletion syndromes have reciprocal microduplication syndromes. Some common examples of microdeletion syndromes are discussed as follows.

DiGeorge or velocardiofacial syndrome

This is caused by a microdeletion of the long arm of one copy of chromosome 22 (22q11 deletion).

Clinical features

- Facial features: short palpebral fissures, prominent nasal bridge and root with a pinched appearance to tip of nose, rounded ears with deficient upper helices.
- Cardiac defects: in ~75%. They could be tetralogy of Fallot, ventral septal defect, interrupted aortic arch, right-sided aortic arch, ASD, etc. Conversely, ~10% of individuals with congenital heart disease have a 22q11 deletion.
- Oropharyngeal abnormalities: cleft palate, submucous cleft palate, velopharyngeal insufficiency.
- Genitourinary abnormalities: renal agenesis, multicystic dysplastic kidneys, hydronephrosis.
- Endocrine function: hypocalcaemia (due to decreased parathyroid function), hypothyroidism.
- Immune function: recurrent minor infections may occur; in 1% abnormalities of T cell numbers and function may be seen (due to effects on thymus).
- Brain abnormalities: polymicrogyria (bilateral perisylvian) and pachygyria.
- Development and learning: speech and language delay (see ➋ p. 56) is common. Learning difficulties (see ➋ pp. 136–41) are reported in 68% of individuals and are often in the mild–moderate range. They often require special educational support (see ➋ pp. 656–8 and pp. 666–7).
- Psychiatric disorders: bipolar affective disorder and schizophrenia are described in 18% of adults.

Management

- Echocardiogram.
- Renal ultrasound scan.
- Audiometry.
- Plasma calcium: check at least once during infancy, childhood, adolescence, and pregnancy.

- Immunology: T-cell, B-cell and NK (natural killer) lymphocyte subsets. Refer to immunologist if abnormal. Live vaccines (e.g. oral polio and BCG) should be avoided until immune function has been checked.
- Referral to speech therapy (see ➔ pp. 402–3) and cleft team for palatal assessment.

Inheritance

AD (see ➔ p. 486). An affected person has a 50% chance of passing on the deletion in every pregnancy. Parental chromosome tests should be offered. If both parents do not have the deletion, the recurrence risk in their off-spring is low, e.g. <1% due to gonadal mosaicism (when some cells in the gonads carry the mutation but the other cells are normal). Prenatal testing is available. Marked inter- and intrafamilial variability is seen.

Williams syndrome

This is caused by the deletion of a small piece of the long arm of one copy of chromosome 7 (7q11.23 deletion). The elastin (*ELN*) gene is deleted.

Clinical features

- Facial features: characteristic appearance with periorbital fullness, bulbous nasal tip, long philtrum, wide mouth, full lips, full cheeks, lacy or stellate iris.
- Failure to thrive with feeding difficulties (see ➔ pp. 436–7).
- Congenital heart disease: supravalvular aortic stenosis, peripheral pulmonary stenosis; other arteries may also be involved.
- Renal abnormalities: renal artery stenosis causing hypertension; nephrocalcinosis due to hypercalcaemia; renal cysts.
- Hypercalcaemia: ~15%; disappears in second year of life but may recur later. When present, it can cause constipation, failure to thrive, and nephrocalcinosis.
- Development: variable (see ➔ Chapter 2). Ranging from mild to moderate ID (see ➔ pp. 136–41); strength in language skills (but words may be used inappropriately); poor visuospatial skills (see ➔ pp. 146–9).
- Behaviour: overfriendly personality; short attention span; (see ➔ p. 126) anxiety (see ➔ pp. 338–40).

Management

- Monitoring of blood pressure in both arms annually.
- Measurement of calcium/creatine ratio in a random spot urine and urinalysis annually.
- Serum calcium levels every 2 years.
- Thyroid function and thyroid stimulating hormone level every 3 years.
- Audiological examination every 5 years (see ➔ pp. 178–80).
- Renal and bladder ultrasound every 10 years.
- Avoid multivitamins as they contain vitamin D.
- The frequency of monitoring should be increased and appropriate treatment instituted in case of abnormal results.

Inheritance

AD, although in reality few patients with Williams syndrome go on to have children. If parents do not carry the deletion, gonadal mosaicism risk of <1% applies.

Recurrent copy number variants

A number of recurrent microdeletions and microduplications have been identified using microarray CGH testing. These CNVs have been classified as neurosusceptibility loci which have variable and reduced penetrance. Hence, while these recurrent CNVs may be contributing to a child's developmental, learning, and behavioural problems they may not be the full explanation, particularly in severe cases. Family cascade testing and prenatal testing are not recommended for these CNVs. See Table 9.1.

Table 9.1 Recurrent copy number variants

Region	Phenotypic features in addition to NDD	Penetrance (according to Rosenfeld et al., 2013)	Gene
1q21.1 del prox (in patients without thrombocytopenia-absent radius syndrome)	Rosenfeld et al., 2012[a] Dysmorphism (66%), seizures (33%), skeletal anomalies (33%), brain anomalies (44%), feeding problems/failure to thrive (55%)		RBM8A
1q21.1 dup prox	Rosenfeld et al., 2012[a] Dysmorphism (56%), clinodactyly (35%), feeding problems/failure to thrive (50%), hypotonia (31%), ophthalmological abn (31%)	17.3%	RBM8A
1q21.1 del distal	Bernier et al., 2015[a] Short stature (50%), microcephaly (22%), hyper-reflexia (35%), tremor (44%)	36.9%	GJA5
1q21.1 dup distal	Bernier, 2015[a] Scoliosis (36%), macrocephaly (26%), hyporeflexia (33%), hyper-reflexia (28%), agility abn (39%)	29.1%	GJA5
15q11.2(BP1–BP2)	Butler, 2017 Dysmorphism (39% 55/141), palatal abn (46% 9/39), seizures/epilepsy (57% 57/216), behavioural problems (55% 75/136), ataxia (28% 22/78)	10.4%	NIPA1, TUBGCP5
15q13.3(BP4–BP5)	Gillentine, 2015 (191 patients) Seizures/epilepsy (37%), schizophrenia (13%), mild dysmorphism (24.5%), behaviour problems (24%)		CHRNA7

Table 9.1 (Contd.)

Region	Phenotypic features in addition to NDD	Penetrance (according to Rosenfeld et al., 2013)	Gene
16p11.2 prox del	Shinawi, 2010 Macrocephaly (69%, 11/16), seizures (31%, 5/16), behaviour problems (38%, 6/16), abn brain imaging (70%, 7/10)	46.8%	TBX6
16p11.2 prox dup	Microcephaly (60%, 6/10), behaviour problems (60%, 6/10)	27.2%	TBX6
16p11.2 distal del	Barge-Schaapveld, 2011 (review of 44 patients reported) Dysmorphism (22.7%), behaviour problems (16%), obesity (18%)	62.4%	SH2B1
16p13.11 del	Tropeano, 2013 Seizures (32%), dysmorphism (39%), behaviour problems (33%)	21.7%	MYH11
16p13.11 dup	Tropeano, 2013 Dysmorphism, behaviour problems (45%) Allach El Kattabi, 2018 Cardiac malformation (23%) increased risk of aortic aneurysm—also suggested by Kuang, 2011	5.12% (Allach El Kattabi, 2018)	MYH11

Other features may also have been reported in smaller numbers of patients.

a Reported in 4+ patients.

Further resources

22q11 Deletion Syndromes Max Appeal: ☎ 0800 389 1049; ℗ http://www.maxappeal.org.uk
Williams Syndrome Foundation: ☎ 01732 365 152; ℗ http://www.williams-syndrome.org.uk

Single gene disorders

These are caused by mutations or deletions in a single gene. Some common examples of single gene disorders seen in paediatric clinics are described.

Marfan syndrome

This is a connective tissue disorder caused by a mutation or deletion of the fibrillin 1 (*FBN1*) gene, present on chromosome 15q21.

Clinical features
- Build: tall stature, slim build, long arm span, arachnodactyly.
- Skeletal: pectus carinatum or excavatum, scoliosis (see ➲ p. 545), pes planus.
- Cardiac: aortic dilatation, regurgitation or dissection, mitral valve prolapse.
- Ophthalmological: ectopia lentis, abnormally flat cornea, increased axial length of globe.
- Pulmonary: spontaneous pneumothorax, apical blebs.
- Skin: striae atrophicae (stretch marks), recurrent or incisional hernia.
- Spine: scoliosis, lumbosacral dural ectasia.
- Clinical diagnosis is based on the *Ghent criteria*. Clinical diagnosis may be confirmed by genetic testing of the *FBN1* gene.

Management
Patients should be under the care of the specialist multidisciplinary Marfan syndrome clinic, if possible.
- Annual echocardiogram.
- Periodic ophthalmic review in childhood (see ➲ p. 183).
- Growth monitoring.
- Spine monitoring for scoliosis (see ➲ p. 545).

Inheritance
- AD with 50% risk to offspring; high new mutation rate of ~30%.
- Prenatal diagnosis is possible if mutation in family is known.

Ehlers–Danlos syndrome

- This is a connective tissue disorder caused by mutation or deletion in the collagen genes. Depending on the clinical features, EDS has been classified into several types.
- The classical forms of EDS are EDS type I and II and are caused by mutations in the *COL5A1* and *COL5A2* genes.

Clinical features
- Soft, hyperextensible skin.
- Easy bruising.
- Thin, atrophic, cigarette-paper scars.
- Joint hypermobility (see ➲ p. 379 and p. 376).
- Risk of prematurity in affected fetuses.

EDS type III
This is the hypermobility type EDS. This is a common but usually mild disorder, associated with soft skin and hypermobility of joints. Sometimes,

joint dislocations may occur. Autonomic dysfunction, generalized pain and excessive tiredness may be present. No genetic testing is available for this disorder. Referral to clinical genetics is therefore not recommended.

Vascular EDS or EDS type IV

This is an uncommon but serious type of EDS. It is caused by mutations in the *COL3A1* gene.

Clinical features

- Characteristic facial features of prominent eyes, hollow cheeks, and pinched nose caused by decreased adipose tissue.
- Thin, translucent skin with visible veins.
- Easy bruising.
- Arterial rupture.
- Rupture of bowel, bladder, or uterus.

Other types of EDS are less common and may be associated with kyphoscoliosis, rupture of optic globe, premature ageing, etc.

Inheritance

Predominantly AD with 50% risk to offspring. Some inter- and intrafamilial variability is seen. Genetic testing is recommended mainly for the 'vascular type of EDS' or those that are associated with serious life-threatening complications.

Stickler syndrome or hereditary arthro-ophthalmopathy

This is caused by mutations in the collagen genes, *COL2A1* or *COL11A1*.

Clinical features

- Facial features: flat midface with depressed nasal bridge, short nose with anteverted nares, and micrognathia. The facial gestalt is more distinctive in early childhood.
- Ophthalmological: in ~95% some involvement of eye. High myopia, cataract, retinal detachment (60%), blindness (4%) (see ➜ pp. 202–8).
- Oropharyngeal: cleft palate (including submucous cleft palate) or Pierre Robin sequence (triad of wide U-shaped cleft palate, small chin, and glossoptosis).
- Joints: hypermobility in childhood, may be associated with hip and other joint pains. In adulthood, premature osteoarthritis may occur.
- Hearing loss: may be conductive due to glue ears (see ➜ pp. 184–5) especially in those with a cleft palate; sensorineural deafness (see ➜ p. 520) is more diagnostic.

Management

- Ophthalmological assessment (see ➜ p. 204) by vitreo-retinal specialist—prophylactic retinopexy is offered to individuals at risk of detaching the retina.
- Audiometry (see ➜ pp. 178–9).
- Referral to speech therapy (see ➜ pp. 402–3) and cleft team for assessment.

Inheritance

AD with a 50% risk to each offspring. Prenatal testing is possible if mutation is known in family.

Neurofibromatosis type 1

This is caused by a mutation or deletion of the *NF1* or neurofibromin gene.

Clinical features

Having two or more of the following features is sufficient to make a diagnosis of NF1:

- Six or more café-au-lait patches. >1.5 cm in postpubertal individuals, >0.5 cm in prepubertal individuals.
- Freckling in the axilla, groin, or neck.
- Two or more neurofibromas.
- One or more plexiform neurofibroma.
- Optic glioma: more common in children <6 years.
- Two or more Lisch nodules (benign iris hamartomas).
- Distinctive bony lesion, e.g. sphenoid wing dysplasia; pseudarthrosis of long bones.
- Family history of NF1.

Additional clinical features consist of:

- Short stature.
- Macrocephaly (see ➔ p. 238).
- Scoliosis (see ➔ p. 545).
- Learning difficulties needing extra help at school (see ➔ pp. 136–41).
- Symptoms from internal neurofibromas.
- Phaeochromocytoma causing raised blood pressure.
- Renal artery stenosis also causes raised blood pressure but more common in those <20 years of age.
- Precocious puberty: related to chiasmal optic glioma.
- Malignant peripheral nerve sheath tumours or MPNST: originate in existing plexiform neurofibromas or from deep-seated nerves. They present with pain or rapid growth. Risk of MPNST is increased following radiation and hence it should be avoided whenever possible.

Investigations and management

- Skin examination: using a Wood's light to check for the presence of six or more café-au-lait patches, assessment of existing neurofibromas.
- Ophthalmological referral: to look for Lisch nodules using slit-lamp examination. Annual ophthalmic surveillance is recommended, for children <6 years of age, for optic glioma (see ➔ p. 260).
- Annual blood pressure monitoring.
- Monitoring of growth parameters
- Developmental assessment (see ➔ p. 32).
- Clinical assessment of spine (see ➔ p. 545).
- MRI brain scan: is not routinely recommended. But should be considered in those with:
  - Rapidly increasing head circumference to exclude aqueduct stenosis.
  - Epilepsy (see ➔ pp. 248–55).
  - Acute onset of headaches (see ➔ pp. 242–3), visual disturbances, or vomiting.
  - Focal neurological signs.
  - Precocious puberty.

Inheritance

AD: 50% risk to each offspring of being affected. Prenatal testing is available if the familial mutation is known. However, due to the wide inter- and intrafamilial variability, the phenotype cannot be predicted.

Segmental NF1

- This is the mosaic form of NF1 affecting only one part of the body (varying from a narrow strip to a whole quadrant of the body).
- Distribution of features may be unilateral or bilateral.
- It is caused by a postzygotic mutation in the *NF1* gene. The risk of a parent with segmental NF1 having an offspring with NF1 ranges from <1% to 50% depending on how many germline cells carry the mutation. An empiric risk figure of 5% is quoted.
- An affected offspring would have features of NF1 but not in a segmental form as all the cells would carry the mutation.

Tuberous sclerosis

This is caused by mutations in the *TSC1* or *TSC2* gene.

Clinical features

CNS: cortical tubers, subependymal nodules, subependymal giant cell astrocytomas may manifest as seizures, e.g. infantile spasms (see ➲ p. 262).
- Skin: facial angiofibromata, fibrous plaques, subungual fibromas, hypomelanotic ash-leaf macules, shagreen patch, 'confetti' skin lesions.
- Ocular: retinal nodular hamartoma (tend to be asymptomatic), retinal achromic patch.
- Cardiac: rhabdomyoma (may present antenatally).
- Renal: angiomyolipoma, multiple renal cysts.
- Respiratory: pulmonary lymphangiomyomatosis (usually presents in adult life).
- Skeletal: bone cysts.
- Oral: pits in dental enamel, gingival fibromas.
- GI: hamartomatous rectal polyps.
- LD (see ➲ pp. 136–41): ~50% of individuals with tuberous sclerosis have a normal IQ. Learning difficulties are linked to seizures and may range from mild to moderate. Children who present with infantile spasms in the first 2 years of life are more likely to have learning disability.
- Behavioural problems: autism (in 25–61%). Risk is higher if tuber in temporal lobe (see ➲ p. 223), hyperactivity, attention deficit (see ➲ pp. 126–34), sleep disturbance (see ➲ pp. 466–8).

Investigations and management

- Ophthalmological assessment (see ➲ p. 204): for retinal hamartomas.
- Cranial imaging: CT scan. To look for cortical tubers, subependymal nodules, and subependymal giant cell astrocytomas.
- Renal ultrasound scan to look for angiomyolipomas and renal cysts.
- Echocardiogram in infants to look for rhabdomyomas.
- Mutation analysis of *TSC1* and *TSC2* genes.
- Refer family to clinical genetics for examination, investigation, and counselling of at-risk relatives (see ➲ pp. 484–5).

Inheritance

AD with 50% risk to each offspring if a parent carries the mutation. About 60% of cases arise as a result of a new mutation in the family. If neither parent is affected there is a 2% risk of recurrence due to gonadal mosaicism. Prenatal testing is on offer if the mutation in the family is known.

Approach to evaluation of a child with learning difficulties and/or behavioural problems

- Cognitive difficulties occur in 2–3% of the population.
- They are often multifactorial.
- It can be difficult to differentiate the contribution of genetic susceptibility factors from that of environmental factors especially in children with mild learning difficulties without any other associated features.
- In children with moderate to severe learning difficulties (see 🔁 pp. 136–41), after a careful personal and family history and a detailed clinical examination the following baseline investigations should be carried out: chromosomes, fragile X, thyroid function tests, urine: amino acids, organic acids, and MPS (see 🔁 pp. 150–1).

Common syndromes associated with learning difficulties

Several genetic syndromes are associated with developmental delay and learning difficulties (see ⊃ pp. 136–41). Some of the more common ones likely to be seen in a paediatric clinic are discussed:

Fragile X syndrome

- This is the most common genetic cause of ID in boys, with approximately 1 in 5500 males carrying the full mutation.
- The *FMR1* gene is on the X chromosome and contains trinucleotide repeats of CGG.
- These repeats are likely to expand when passed on to their offspring, particularly when inherited from the mother. This is called *anticipation*. Box 9.1 shows the classification of different trinucleotide repeat sizes in fragile X syndrome.

Full mutation

Males with full mutation present with features of fragile X syndrome. These include:

- Physical features: long face, large prominent ears with cupping of pinnae, joint hypermobility (see ⊃ p. 379), large testes post puberty.
- Developmental delay (see ⊃ pp. 30–1 and p. 30): hypotonia, mild motor delay, speech and language problems ranging from no speech to mild delay.
- Learning difficulties (see ⊃ pp. 136–41): most boys have additional educational needs. IQ is reduced but may range from 41–88 (the latter is seen in mosaics). A degree of supported living as adults is required in most full mutation carriers.
- Behavioural problems (see ⊃ pp. 362–3): overactivity, poor concentration, impulsivity (see ⊃ p. 417), ASD (see ⊃ pp. 114–25), echolalia.

Female full mutation carriers are less affected, as they have a normal X which produces variable amounts of the protein. Up to 50% of females will show learning difficulties and behavioural problems, but are less severely affected compared to males. Those with skewed X-inactivation are more likely to show symptoms.

Premutation

- Those with premutations are less likely to present with developmental delay (see ⊃ Chapter 2), learning difficulties, and behavioural problems (see ⊃ pp. 362–3). Hence in a child with neurodevelopmental problems, in whom a premutation allele is identified, further investigations should be done to find out the cause.

Box 9.1 Allele sizes in fragile X syndrome

- Normal: <45 repeats.
- Intermediate allele: 45–54 repeats.
- Premutation carriers: 55–200 repeats.
- Full mutation: >200 repeats.

- Premutations are likely to expand into a full mutation when passed on from a premutation carrier mother to her children. Fathers that carry a premutation pass it on to all their daughters, but these are less likely to expand. They cannot pass it to their sons, as the sons will inherit the Y, not X, chromosome from them.
- Adult female premutation carriers are at risk of premature menopause and adult male premutation carriers are thought to be at a risk of FRAXTAS (fragile X tremor ataxia syndrome).

Intermediate alleles

These may represent precursors of a premutation in a successive generation. They do not have a phenotypic effect on the individuals who carry them.

Inheritance

X-linked inheritance with carrier mothers being at a 50% risk of having an affected son and a 50% risk of having a carrier daughter (who may be affected). Prenatal testing is available and consists of maternal blood sampling for fetal sexing at 9 weeks, followed by chorionic villus sampling to test the mutation (usually in case of a male pregnancy).

Angelman syndrome

This is a neurobehavioural disorder caused by a disturbance in the maternally imprinted region of chromosome 15q11.13, which includes the *UBE3A* gene.

Clinical features

- Severe developmental delay (see ➲ pp. 30–1): speech is particularly poor or even absent.
- Wide-based ataxic gait.
- Characteristic EEG (2–3Hz large amplitude slow-wave bursts) with or without seizures.
- Microcephaly (see ➲ p. 238).
- Excitable, happy personality (the syndrome was previously termed 'happy puppet syndrome' due to the happy affect with the wide-based gait).
- Love of water and fascination with reflections.
- Facial features: deep-set eyes, wide smiling mouth, and prominent chin.
- Hypopigmentation in some patients (blonde and blue-eyed).

Inheritance

The recurrence risk depends on the mechanism by which the Angelman syndrome has been caused.

- In 70% of individuals it is caused by a deletion of maternal chromosome 15q11–13; identified using a FISH test or routine karyotyping. The recurrence risk is low (<1%), if parental testing is normal.
- In 20% a mutation in the imprinted *UBE3A* gene is the cause; women carrying a *UBE3A* mutation are at a 50% risk of passing on Angelman syndrome in each pregnancy. If men carry the mutation, their children are not affected as the gene is silenced.

- In 2–5% it results from paternal uniparental disomy of chromosome 15; recurrence risks are low (0.5%)
- In 2–5% an imprinting defect is the cause; recurrence risk may be as high as 50% if due to an imprinting centre mutation.

Prader–Willi syndrome

The most common genetic syndrome associated with obesity and neurodevelopmental problems is Prader–Willi syndrome.

Clinical features
- Neonatal central hypotonia (see ➔ pp. 272–6).
- Feeding difficulties (see ➔ pp. 436–7) and failure to thrive in infancy.
- Rapid weight gain between 1 and 6 years of age.
- Facial features: almond-shaped eyes, V-shaped mouth may be present in young children.
- Truncal obesity.
- Small hands and feet.
- Small genitalia, hypogonadotropic hypogonadism, fertility is rare.
- Short stature.
- Behaviour: insatiable appetite and food-seeking behaviour, ritualistic behaviour, insensitivity to pain.
- Developmental delay and learning difficulties are present (see ➔ pp. 136–41): mean IQ of 60. Adults may be able to live independently but need some degree of support and supervision.

Inheritance
- In 75% of individuals Prader–Willi syndrome is caused by a deletion of paternal chromosome 15q11–13. The recurrence risk is low at <1% if neither parent has the deletion.
- If a father has the deletion there is a 50% risk of Prader–Willi syndrome but this is rare due to decreased fertility; if a mother has the deletion she is at a 50% risk of having a child with Angelman syndrome this too is rare but has been reported.
- In 24% of individuals it is due to maternal uniparental disomy of chromosome 15, recurrence risk is low; 1% have an imprinting centre mutation with recurrence risk of 50%.

Rett syndrome

This is a severe X-linked dominant neurodevelopmental disorder that affects females and is caused by mutations in the *MECP2* gene.

Clinical features
- Normal prenatal and perinatal development.
- Loss of acquired skills: speech, communication, and hand skills.
- Postnatal microcephaly (see ➔ p. 238).
- Stereotypic hand movements (see ➔ p. 266).
- Seizures and abnormal EEG (see ➔ p. 230).
- Episodes of hyperventilation and breath-holding.
- Bruxism.
- Cold feet.
- Scoliosis (see ➔ p. 545).

- Spontaneous outbursts of laughter/crying.
- Autistic features (see ➲ pp. 114–25).
- Severe developmental delay (see ➲ pp. 30–1 and pp. 32–4).

Inheritance

The majority have a new mutation, which is not inherited. The mutation is usually on the paternal X chromosome. There is a small risk of gonadal mosaicism. Affected girls do not reproduce due to severe mental disability and hence familial cases are rare. It is lethal in males, unless it occurs as a result of somatic mosaicism or occurs in a male with Klinefelter syndrome (47XXY) (see ➲ pp. 502–3).

X-linked intellectual disability syndromes

- This should be suspected in boys with ID (see ➲ pp. 136–41) where other common X-linked causes, e.g. fragile X syndrome, have been ruled out. A family history (see ➲ pp. 234–5) of brothers of the proband being affected and/or maternal uncles being affected strongly point to this diagnosis.
- Several genes on the X-chromosome are expressed in the brain and are important for normal neurodevelopment. Several X-linked intellectual disability syndrome genes have been identified so far, e.g. *CUL4B*, *OPHN1*, etc., but individually these are a rare cause of ID.
- Due to the significant recurrence risks involved, it is important that these individuals are referred to the genetics service (see ➲ pp. 484–5).

Further resources

Angelman Syndrome: ☎ 0300 999 0102; ☞ http://www.angelmanuk.org
Fragile X Society: ☎ 01371 875100; ☞ http://www.fragilex.org.uk
Prader–Willi Syndrome Association (UK): ☎ 01332 365676; ☞ http://www.pwsa.org.uk
Rett UK: ☎ 01582 798 911; ☞ http://www.rettuk.org

Other common genetic referrals

Congenital anomalies

- Several patients with isolated congenital anomalies are referred to the genetics service.
- The presence of more than one structural abnormality or the accompaniment of other problems such as dysmorphism (see ➔ pp. 492–4), developmental delay (see ➔ Chapter 2), or behavioural problems may indicate a syndromic diagnosis which may be associated with a significant recurrence risk.
- However, some isolated congenital anomalies may be associated with a recurrence risk, e.g. cleft lip and palate, cleft palate, spina bifida, congenital heart disease, and craniosynostosis (Table 9.2).
- This risk is in addition to the 2–3% risk in the general population of having a baby with a congenital anomaly in any pregnancy.
- Isolated congenital anomalies are often multifactorial in inheritance. Some non-syndromic isolated congenital anomalies may be inherited often in an AD manner and may show reduced penetrance, e.g. cleft lip and palate.

Sensorineural hearing loss

- Severe deafness affects 1 in 1000 children between infancy and early childhood (prelingual years).
- Approximately 60% of SNHL is genetic in origin.
- For causes of SNHL, see ➔ pp. 168–9.
- The most common gene accounting for recessive form of SNHL (in ~50%) is the connexin 26 gene. The carrier frequency of this gene in European, North American, and Mediterranean populations is 1 in 50. Pendred syndrome is another common recessive form of SNHL and accounts for 5% of severe deafness (see ➔ p. 172 and p. 183).
- For investigations of SNHL, see ➔ pp. 182–3.

Table 9.2 Recurrence risks of common isolated congenital anomalies

Anomaly	Sibling risk in %	Offspring risk in %
Cleft lip and palate	4	4.3
Cleft palate	1.8	3
Congenital heart disease	2–3	3–5
Neural tube defects	3	4
Craniosynostosis		
Coronal	5	–
Sagittal	1	–

Autism

- The cause is unknown in the majority of patients (~90%) and is multifactorial in aetiology.
- The genetic causes that should be considered are:
  - Chromosomal abnormalities.
  - Fragile X syndrome (see ➔ pp. 516–17).
  - Rett syndrome (see ➔ pp. 518–19).
  - Tuberous sclerosis (see ➔ pp. 513–14).
  - Mutations in neuroligin-3 and neuroligin-4 (X-linked autism).
- Siblings of individuals with autism are at a 3–5% risk of developing the disorder with an additional 5–7% risk of having a milder communication disorder. In those patients with a family history of autism, the risk will vary depending on the type of inheritance suspected.
- For further details on autism and ASD, see ➔ pp. 114–25.

Further resources

Bardet–Biedl syndrome: ☎ 01633 718415; ⌨ http://www.lmbbs.org.uk
Beckwith–Wiedemann syndrome: ☎ 07889 211000; ⌨ http://www.bws-support.org.uk
Child Growth Foundation: ☎ 020 8994 7625; ⌨ http://www.childgrowthfoundation.org
Cleft Lip & Palate Association (CLAPA): ☎ 020 7833 4884; ⌨ http://www.clapa.com
Contact a Family (UK): ⌨ http://www.cafamily.org.uk
Deaf Education through Listening & Talking (DELTA): ☎ 0845 108 1437; ⌨ http://www.deafeducation.org.uk
Genetic Alliance UK: ☎ 020 7704 3141; ⌨ http://www.geneticalliance.org.uk
National Deaf Children's Society (NDCS): ☎ 0808 800 8880; ⌨ http://www.ndcs.org.uk
National Organisation for Rare Disorders (US): ⌨ http://www.raredisease.org
Online Mendelian Inheritance in Man (OMIM): ⌨ http://www.ncbi.nlm.nih.gov
PubMed: ⌨ http://www.ncbi.nlm.nih.gov/PubMed
Restricted Growth Association: ☎ 0300 111 1970; ⌨ http://www.restrictedgrowth.co.uk
Royal National Institute for Deaf People (RNID): ☎ 0808 808 0123; ⌨ http://www.rnid.org.uk
Unique: ☎ 01883 330766; ⌨ http://www.rarechromo.org
Undiagnosed children (any disorder/syndrome): ⌨ http://www.makingcontact.org

Neuro-orthopaedics

Definition

- Neuro-orthopaedics is an innovative clinical specialty that combines neurology and orthopaedics and involves a systematic multidisciplinary approach to musculoskeletal issues caused by disorders affecting the central and peripheral nervous systems, neuromuscular junctions, and muscles resulting in disability.
- It is concerned with the treatment of functional and structural consequences of neurological disorders on the musculoskeletal system.
- Since the underlying disease is not completely treatable most of the time, orthopaedic treatment cannot result in a permanent cure but can improve function and limit disability.

Aetio-pathogenesis

- A wide spectrum of neuromuscular disorders that interfere with control and functioning of the muscles, can lead to functional and structural deformities of the musculoskeletal system (Table 10.1).
- Physiologically, muscles adapt to everyday needs in terms of power development and operating length. At the same time, stretching during everyday life promotes growth of the muscles and ensures that they are long enough to preserve adequate mobility of the joints. The neurological lesion can result in positive effects such as altered muscle tone due to loss of inhibition of the lower motor neurons (spasticity/clonus) resulting in muscle shortening and contractures due to the inability of the muscles to stretch during normal play. The underlying muscle activity may be spastic or flaccid.

Table 10.1 Prevalence rates for the most common neuromuscular disorders

Level	Neuromuscular disorder	Prevalence (per 100,000)
Upper motor neuron	CP	300–400
	TBI	50–250
	Spinal cord injury	2
Upper and lower motor neurons	Spina bifida	50–70
Lower motor neuron	SMA	1–3
	Post-polio syndrome	18–90
Peripheral nerve	Charcot–Marie–Tooth disease	3–80
	Friedrich's ataxia	0.5–4
Neuromuscular junction	Myasthenia gravis	5–35
Muscle	DMD	0.7–4.7
	Myotonic dystrophy	7–26
	Congenital myopathies	0.6–3.9
Others	Arthrogryposis	30

- Loss of connection to, or lesions of, the lower motor neurons can result in negative effects such as weakness, hypotonia, poor balance and coordination, and sensory deficits. A sensory disorder of varying severity may be present and loss of proprioception, can lead to loss of dynamic control over the joints and overloading of the ligamentous structures with progressive instability.
- Since the underlying neurological problems cannot usually be resolved at causal level, they act permanently on the musculoskeletal system.
- Since the growing skeleton is more plastic than the fully-grown counterpart, secondary skeletal deformities occur particularly during childhood, which can further aggravate the locomotor function. This can result in muscle contractures, lever arm deformities, and joint instability resulting in degenerative arthritis over time.
- The loss of control over part of the motor system affects everyday functions such as walking, standing, sitting, or the use of the upper extremity.
- One important diagnostic step in neuro-orthopaedics is to distinguish between *functionally beneficial* and *disruptive changes* of the musculoskeletal system. For example, spasticity sometimes can be beneficial when it compensates for muscle weakness.

Epidemiology

Each neuromuscular disease is relatively uncommon yet causes a significant burden of disease socioeconomically. Epidemiological studies in different global regions have demonstrated that certain neuromuscular diseases have increased in incidence and prevalence rates over time. The prevalence rates for the most common neuromuscular disorders based on region of involvement are outlined in Table 10.1.

Approach to diagnosis and management

- The approach to neuro-orthopaedic patients is by necessity multidisciplinary, because a variety of non-surgical and surgical options are available to treat the musculoskeletal deformities.
- The MDT involving a paediatric neurologist, physical medicine and rehabilitation physician, paediatric neurosurgeon, orthopaedic surgeon, PT, OT, and a social worker are essential to identify the patient's needs and plan treatment.
- In evaluating each patient, the team must consider the primary diagnosis, natural history of the disease, prognosis for progression, severity and direction of any deformity, potential for improvement in function, the ability to alleviate pain, and potential for improvement in hygiene and cosmesis.
- Neurological investigations to obtain an accurate diagnosis are essential in the management of each patient.
- Before the involvement of the orthopaedic and rehabilitation teams, patients will have been diagnostically investigated with routine blood tests, radiological and electrodiagnostic investigations, and in some cases invasive procedures such as muscle or nerve biopsies.
- Genetic testing is now widespread, and a positive result can eliminate the need for invasive procedures.
- The ICF is a framework from the WHO for describing and organizing information on functioning and disability. It provides a standard language and a conceptual basis for the definition and measurement of health and disability. It establishes a common language for describing health and health-related states in order to improve communication between different users, such as healthcare workers, researchers, policymakers, and the public, including people with disabilities.

Neuro-orthopaedic evaluation

A detailed history followed by a thorough neuro-orthopaedic evaluation using a systematic and comprehensive protocol is essential to identify the underlying cause of the problem or for reassuring the family. This allows for monitoring of changes over time and better communication with other members of the healthcare team.

History

This is achieved by means of a detailed interview involving the child, parents, or caregivers and should encompass the following headings: chief complaint, history of present illness, past medical and surgical history, birth and development history, family history, social history, previous subspecialty evaluations, investigations and treatment, therapy, orthotics and durable medical equipment, functional impairment with regard to activities of daily living, recreational activities, and educational activities.

Examination

This is done with appropriate exposure maintaining the patient's dignity. This involves a quick general examination, a detailed neurological examination, and a comprehensive orthopaedic examination. The orthopaedic examination is done in the following positions:

Standing
- Evaluate the 'HAT' segment (head, arm, and trunk) in relation to the locomotor segment (lower extremities) in the coronal, sagittal, and transverse planes.
- Look for any leg length discrepancy.
- Ask the patient to bend forward to look for any structural spine deformities (Adam's forward bending test).
- Ask the child to squat and then stand up with arms folded to assess the flexibility of the three major joints of the lower extremity and strength of the triceps surae, quadriceps, and gluteal muscles.
- A single leg stance test is useful to evaluate balance and also hip abductor strength (Trendelenburg test).
- A single heel rise test is useful for evaluating ankle plantar flexion strength. A double heel rise test is useful to assess flexibility of the subtalar joint and integrity of the tibialis posterior muscle.
- Ask the patient to toe walk and heel walk.

Lying down supine
- Evaluate the range of motion at each joint—hip, knee, ankle, and foot.
- Evaluate the range of motion at each joint in response to rapid and slow stretch to differentiate between spasticity (rapid passive mobilization) and contracture (slow passive mobilization).
- Evaluate stability at each joint.
- At the ankle, the Silfverskiöld test is used to assess for gastrocnemius versus gastrocnemius and soleus contracture.
- At the knee, the popliteal angle is measured to evaluate for hamstring contracture. The bilateral popliteal angle test (with opposite hip flexed) is more sensitive than the unilateral popliteal angle test (with opposite hip extended).
- At the hip, measure the hip flexion contracture using the Thomas test.
- Evaluate range of motion and stability at each upper extremity joint.

Lying down prone
- Measure the rotation profile of the lower extremities at the hip (hip internal and external rotation), the tibial torsion using the thigh foot angle and the thigh to transmalleolar axis angles, and the relation of the hindfoot to forefoot using the heel bisector.
- The Duncan–Ely test measures the rectus femoris contracture and spasticity.
- The foot is evaluated for hindfoot valgus and varus. The flexibility of the hindfoot is evaluated.

Lateral decubitus
- Evaluate hip abductor strength.
- Evaluate for iliotibial band contracture using the Ober test.

Sitting
- Assess for hypotonia using the Meryon test by lifting the child up from the armpits.

- Assess for the child's ability to sit straight. Backward bending indicates weak psoas or rectus abdominis and/or contracture of hamstrings. Use of the upper limbs to sit straight indicates weakness of trunk muscles.
- Evaluate patellofemoral joint tracking.

Functional activities
- Lower extremity: walking, running, jumping, single leg hop.
- Upper extremity: reaching, grasp and release, manipulating objects of different size.

Evaluation of orthotics and durable medical equipment
These are evaluated for appropriateness, fit, and size.

Data analysis

Gait analysis

- Gait analysis is the systematic study of human locomotion, using the knowledge and skill of the observers, augmented by instrumentation for measuring body movements, body mechanics, and the activity of the muscles.
- Gait analysis is used to assess human walking and identify gait impairments, facilitate decision-making for treating individuals with conditions affecting their ability to walk, and to evaluate the functional outcomes of different treatment modalities used to optimize gait impairments.
- Gait analysis includes incorporation of data obtained from different techniques used to evaluate human walking including a detailed history, standardized physical examination of the neuromusculoskeletal system, measurement of functional outcomes using validated outcome measures, two-dimensional video (coronal and sagittal planes), three-dimensional instrumented quantitative gait analysis, foot pressure (pedobarograph) study, diagnostic imaging, and examination under anaesthesia. This is called a diagnostic matrix.
- Instrumented three-dimensional gait analysis includes measurement of temporospatial parameters of gait, kinematics (measurement of joint angles), kinetics (measurement of forces at each joint), dynamic electromyography (measuring muscle function during gait), measurement of energy expenditure and efficiency of gait, and quantitative evaluation of lower extremity alignment, muscle tone, balance, and selective muscle control.
- A detailed gait evaluation observing any abnormalities at the pelvis, hip, knee, ankle, and foot segments in the coronal, sagittal, and transverse planes should be done with the patient walking towards and away from you. The sagittal plane is the most important plane for decision-making in gait disorders.
- A two-dimensional gait video analysis and three-dimensional instrumented gait analysis is usually performed preoperatively to facilitate surgical decision-making in ambulatory children with gait problems and 1 year postoperatively to evaluate functional outcomes.
- A diagnostic matrix incorporating data from a detailed physical therapy evaluation, gait analysis, radiographs, functional outcome measures such as the Functional Mobility Scale (FMS), Functional Assessment Questionnaire (FAQ), Pediatric Outcomes Data Collection Instrument (PODCI) and examination under anaesthesia are used for fine tuning surgical decision-making.
- Shiners Hospital Upper Extremity Evaluation (SHUEE): the SHUEE test is a two-dimensional video evaluation of upper extremity function used to facilitate surgical decision-making of upper extremity problems.

Common orthopaedic problems

- Most of the neuromuscular disorders share common musculoskeletal issues such as joint contractures, joint instability (subluxation or dislocation), and deformities (spine and extremities).
- These develop secondary to a combination of positive (spasticity/ dystonia) and negative (hypotonia, weakness, poor balance/ coordination, lack of selective muscle control) effects of the primary neurological condition.
- They result in functional disability due to decreased motor performance, mobility limitations, reduced functional range of motion, loss of function for activities of daily living, decreased quality of life, and increased pain.
- Feeding/eating disabilities, constipation, and GOR, along with obesity and malnutrition, are commonly associated GI-related complications.
- These in addition to immobility result in poor bone health and osteoporosis making these patients at risk for pathological fractures. The increased fall risk noted in these patients also contributes to the increased risk of fractures.
- Table 10.2 summarizes the common orthopaedic issues encountered in each of the neuromuscular disorders.

Management principles

Children with neuromuscular disorders are at risk of having their childhood squeezed out by treatment. The following principles are recommended to provide balance between medical interventions and preserving childhood.

- *Understand the natural history of the disease.* This allows us to prevent/ delay secondary musculoskeletal problems from developing, plan the treatment interventions, and prevent adverse outcomes. Example: hip surveillance for preventing hip dislocations in children with CP.
- *Appreciate the significance of sensation and perceptive disabilities.* A child with spina bifida has decreased sensation in the lower extremities resulting in recurrent ulcers and Charcot arthropathy.

Table 10.2 Common orthopaedic problems in neuromuscular disorders

Neuromuscular disorder	Spine (%)	Hip (%)	Knee (%)	Foot and ankle (%)	Rotational deformities (%)
CP	0–75	30	20	30	10–60
Spina bifida	20–94	1–28		20–100	
DMD	20–80	35		70–100	
SMA	70–100	11–38			
Peripheral neuropathy	10	6–8		70	
TBI				15–30	
Spinal cord injury	60–100	25–82	11	40	
Arthrogryposis	20–60	30	30	60–80	20

- *Recognize the limitations of treatment.* For most of the neuromuscular disorders we cannot cure the primary neurological lesion and hence our treatment just manages the effects.
- *Be cautious with comparisons to typically developing children.* Our aim in these children is to optimize their function, make them comfortable, and not necessarily make them 'normal'.
- *Focus on appearance, function, and comfort, not on deformity.* Management priorities are based on the severity of the condition and on individual needs, e.g. in a child with a mild disability, we aim to improve appearance to allow integration in the community. In those with moderate disabilities we aim to improve function and those with severe disabilities we improve comfort to enhance care and quality of life.
- *Focus on providing effective functional mobility not on ambulation.* This is to promote social and intellectual development. They must be practical, energy efficient, and effective.
- *Establish appropriate priorities.* Adults with severe neuromuscular disorders rate communication and socialization above self-care and mobility. Our goal is to help the family understand that independence, social integration, and mobility are more important than ambulation.
- *Focus on the child's assets, make time for creativity.* Creating time for friendship with other children is very important. These children also have talents and try to appreciate and develop these talents. This is usually more productive than time spent in overcoming the child's disability.
- *Shift priorities with age.* Focus on mobility and self-care in early childhood, on socialization and education in middle childhood, and vocational preparation in late childhood.
- *Maintain family health.* The parents of these children are under a lot of stress and it is important to protect the health and well-being of the marriage/relationship and family. Help the family find support groups to provide information, support, perspective, and friendship. Recognize that all treatments have a cost and avoid overwhelming the family.
- *Avoid management fads.* History of medical treatment includes many treatments that were either harmful or ineffective, e.g. extensive bracing, exhaustive therapies, and misguided surgeries. Steer the family away from ineffective treatment strategies.
- *Protect the child's play experience.* Play is the occupation of the child and is important for the child's physical, mental, and emotional well-being.

Treatment

- The underlying primary neurological lesion cannot be cured in most patients and hence these patients often require treatment over a protracted period, and not infrequently for life.
- Treatment is aimed at preventing the progression of contractures and deformities and for providing stability to the skeletal system.
- The primary lesion results in secondary effects such as contractures and deformities. Tertiary compensatory mechanisms develop to counter the secondary effects. Our aim is to prevent the secondary effects from developing or getting worse and treating them appropriately.
- The compensatory mechanisms usually spontaneously resolve after correction of the secondary effects.

The following treatment modalities are useful:
- Self-management—diet, exercise, home exercise programme, foot care.
- Rehabilitation—physical therapy, occupational therapy, speech therapy, orthoses.
- Durable medical equipment—orthotics, seating and mobility, standing and positioning systems.
- Non-operative treatment:
  - Medical treatment to address spasticity, dystonia, or involuntary movements. Drugs such as baclofen, benzodiazepines, trihexyphenidyl, and dantrolene sodium.
  - Botulinum toxin injection to the muscles and phenol chemodenervation to control spasticity.
  - Serial stretch casting to stretch out joint contractures.
- Orthopaedic surgery—is necessary to improve function and quality of life:
  - Soft tissue surgery to resolve myostatic contractures—aponeurotic lengthening, tendon lengthening, tendon transfers or releases. Sometimes bone shortening can be done to resolve contractures.
  - Bone surgery to correct lever arm deformities—osteotomies.
  - Combination of soft tissue and bone surgery to reconstruct joint subluxation or dislocations, hip, knee, foot, and ankle and upper extremity deformities. In severe deformities, salvage procedures like arthrodesis or bone resection may be necessary.
  - Spine deformity surgery to correct neuromuscular scoliosis.
  - To manage fractures.
- Neurosurgery—may be needed to control hypertonia and movement disorders:
  - Selective dorsal rhizotomy to control spasticity in ambulatory children with CP spastic diplegia.
  - Intrathecal baclofen pump to control hypertonia (spasticity/dystonia) in ambulatory or non-ambulatory children with CP.
  - Deep brain stimulation to control involuntary movements in patients with dystonia.
  - Peripheral neurectomies to control spasticity.

Prognosis
- Neuro-orthopaedic problems arise secondary to the positive or negative effects of the underlying neurological lesion and therefore, these cannot be cured but can be managed.
- Orthopaedic measures can correct deformities and improve the functional status, but recurrences, especially during growth, are almost unavoidable since the underlying neurological condition continues to exert its influence unchanged.

Rehabilitation

- Patients with neuromuscular disorders have sensory, autonomic nervous system, and cognitive functional deficits and other malfunctions of the nervous system, in addition to musculoskeletal issues that must be diagnosed and treated.
- Optimal rehabilitation of the patient can be ensured only through the efforts of a MDT of specialists including occupational, physical, and speech therapy, orthopaedics, orthotists, paediatrics, and rehabilitation medicine.
- Most patients require inpatient and/or outpatient rehabilitation after surgery to optimize their functional ability.

Orthopaedic management of cerebral palsy

Definition

A group of disorders of the development of movement and posture causing activity limitations that are attributed to non-progressive disturbances that occurred in the developing fetal or infant brain. The motor disorders of CP are often accompanied by disturbances of sensation, cognition, communication, perception, and/or behaviour and/or a seizure disorder.

- The CNS lesion or dysfunction may have occurred pre-, peri-, or postnatally.
- CP is not a result of a progressive or degenerative brain disorder. CP is static encephalopathy but the motor impairment and functional consequences may progress over time.

Epidemiology

Globally prevalent and pan-racial, with a prevalence rate of 2–3 per 1000 live births and possibly higher in developing countries.

Classification

Physiological classification: describes the type of movement disorder present

- Spasticity: results from damage to the pyramidal system. Increased muscle tone is proportional to velocity of stretch:
  - Loss of inhibition of reflex arcs means that muscles may contract out of phase, i.e. when it is not desirable for them to do so. This is particularly true of muscles that cross more than one joint, e.g. hip flexors, adductors, hamstrings, rectus femoris, and gastrocnemius.
  - Spastic muscles and their antagonists show varying degrees of weakness. This is the commonest form of CP and the one most amenable to orthopaedic intervention.
- Dystonia/rigidity: increased tone which is not velocity dependent.
- Athetosis: abnormal writhing movements caused by damage to the basal ganglia.
- Ataxia: disturbed balance caused by a cerebellar lesion.

Geographic classification: explains which region of the body is involved

- Hemiplegia (ipsilateral upper and lower limbs and trunk).
- Diplegia (bilateral lower limbs, minimal upper limb involvement).
- Total body involvement.

Role of the orthopaedic surgeon

As part of the MDT approach for these patients, *orthopaedic input* is important for the following:

- Spasticity management and posture control.
- Prevent or treat contractures of muscles and joints.
- Prevent or treat hip dislocations.
- Improve gait and upper limb function where possible.
- Prevent and treat neuromuscular scoliosis.

Orthopaedic assessment

Please refer to the assessment of a child with neuromuscular disorder for detailed assessment of a child with CP (see pp. 92–101).

Spasticity management

- Spasticity results from damage to the pyramidal system and is one of the main primary problems in children with CP that drives musculoskeletal pathology.
- Spasticity compass: spasticity treatment modalities can be categorized as those that act focally or in a generalized manner and those that are reversible or irreversible. Focal modalities are useful when ≤3 muscles are spastic. When spasticity is more global, modalities which act in a generalized manner are useful. Usually, multimodal spasticity management is recommended to prolong the effect (Fig. 10.1).
- Physical therapy: a stretching programme encourages muscle growth, adding sarcomeres to the muscle length.
- Orthotics: these may be used to provide passive stretching. They can also aid function, prevent deformity, and provide stability either by local control or on more proximal joints by the effect on the ground reaction force.
- Serial casting: allows stretching of myostatic contractures, reduces muscle tone by interfering with muscle spindle excitation, uses viscoelastic properties of the muscle tendon unit to produce creep, and adds sarcomeres to muscle length.
- Baclofen (generalized/reversible): baclofen may be given orally or intrathecally. The intrathecal route has the advantage that larger doses reach the target tissue—the spinal cord—thus reducing side effects seen with the high doses given orally. It is used for patients with predominant lower limb spasticity but there are no strict indications yet.
- Botulinum toxin (focal/reversible): having determined which muscles are spastic, these can be injected with botulinum toxin at the neuromuscular junction with ultrasound or nerve stimulator guidance

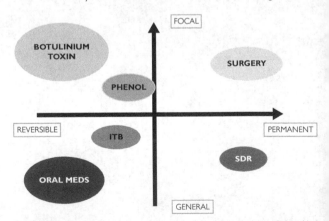

Fig. 10.1 Spasticity compass showing the different treatment modalities (reversible/irreversible) for managing spasticity depending on whether it is focal or global/generalized. ITB, intrathecal baclofen; SDR, selective dorsal rhizotomy.

for better localization. The toxin blocks the release of acetyl choline at the neuromuscular junction (synapse) thus reducing tone and relaxing the muscles until new nerve ending sprout at around 3 to 6 months (Box 10.1).

- Phenol (focal/reversible): produces chemical denervation by denaturing the nerve protein and interferes with nerve conduction. The effect lasts for about 6–12 months.
- Orthopaedic surgery: surgical lengthening of a musculotendinous unit will decrease spasticity. Muscles firing out of phase can be transferred to become an antagonist.
- Selective dorsal rhizotomy: this is a neurosurgical technique that sections a proportion of the dorsal sensory rootlets (between L1 and S1) found on electrical stimulation to be most responsible for the abnormal reflex arc that causes spasticity:
  • It produces a permanent decrease in muscle tone.
  • Ambulatory spastic diplegic patients are the most likely to benefit.
  • NICE guidelines from 2010 state that patients should be selected and treated by a MDT; however, criteria for treatment are still evolving.

Orthopaedic surgery

Surgery is performed to:
- Lengthen musculotendinous units: at the origin, at the musculotendinous portion (fractional lengthening), or within the tendon (Z lengthening or tenotomy).
- Transfer tendons: the tendon of a muscle which is firing out of phase is transferred, usually to become an antagonist to the function it originally performed. This reduces its deforming force and enhances the action of the weak antagonists.

Box 10.1 Key considerations when injecting botulinum toxin

- Botulinum toxin is useful for dynamic shortening but will not affect fixed muscle contractures.
- If weakness is a major factor, botulinum toxin may be disadvantageous as it will further weaken the muscle.
- Sedation or general anaesthetic is helpful if multiple muscles are to be injected.
- Dose is calculated according to the size of the muscle and the weight of the patient. Several preparations are available and their concentrations differ.
- Accurate placement is important and after insertion of the needle and confirmation of position with a nerve stimulator or ultrasound, the syringe plunger should be pulled back to ensure the needle is not in a blood vessel.
- Injections must be followed by a course of intensive physiotherapy plus splinting/serial casting to obtain the maximum benefit and prolong the effect of the botulinum toxin.
- Effects are temporary (3–6 months) but repeat doses can be given after 6–12 months.

- Cut and reorientate deformed bones (osteotomies).
- Relocate subluxated or dislocated joints (usually hips).
- Fuse joints (rarely).

Gait abnormalities

These are seen in ambulatory children with CP (GMFCS level I–IV). Every child is different but some of the common gait abnormalities noted are:

- *Intoeing*: in CP this usually is due to excessive femoral anteversion. It can be treated with derotational osteotomies.
- *Vaulting*: there is difficulty in clearing the foot from the ground during swing and so the foot in stance phase has an early heel raise to allow the opposite leg to swing through without hitting the ground.
- *Short leg gait*: the pelvis dips on the affected side during stance.
- *Scissoring*: spasticity in the hip adductors means the legs tend to cross over each other in the coronal plane during walking and it can be difficult to get one leg past the other.
- *Toe–toe gait*: this may be due to spasticity in the calf muscles preventing dorsiflexion at the ankles which consequently remain in equinus throughout the gait cycle and the heel does not reach the ground. Alternatively, there may be adequate dorsiflexion at the ankle but flexion of the knee throughout stance makes it impossible for the heel to reach the ground.
- *Crouch gait*: there is flexion of the knee >30° throughout the gait cycle. Excessive dorsiflexion at the ankle (which can cause a crouched gait) may allow the heel to contact the ground.
- *Stiff knee gait*: the knee has a reduced range of motion through the gait cycle. It may be due to spasticity of rectus femoris reducing the range of flexion during swing.

Typical foot deformities

- Planovalgus foot with equinus hindfoot and midfoot break (commonest in diplegics) and equinus/equinovarus foot (commonest in hemiplegics).
- Gait abnormalities are treated with non-operative options until about 8 years of age as the gait of a child matures to that of an adult. After the age of 8–10 years, a patient may be considered for *single-event multilevel surgery*.
- Single-event multilevel surgery includes a variety of procedures, often bony and soft tissue, tailored to the individual patient and aiming to address all gait abnormalities simultaneously with a single period of rehabilitation. Functional outcome measures such as the Gait Outcomes Assessment List (GOAL) questionnaire should be used to evaluate outcomes.

Hip surveillance

Hip surveillance

- Hip surveillance is the process of monitoring for hip displacement through regular clinical examinations and radiographs.
- Hip displacement occurs due to muscle imbalance that can lead to subluxation and dislocation over time. This is silent in the early phase and only detectable with radiographs.
- If left untreated, dislocations can cause pain, decreased quality of life (problems with sitting imbalance and difficulties with perineal hygiene due to restricted movement), and degenerative arthritis.
- Displacement occurs in up to 75% in those with CP spastic quadriplegia (GMFCS level IV/V) and in 33% of children with CP overall.
- If not identified and acted upon early, the need for a complex and significant surgery can result, even leading to the need to remove the hip joint (salvage surgery) in the most severe situations.
- Research has shown that careful, planned tracking, otherwise known as surveillance, together with timely orthopaedic surgery, can prevent or reduce the need for these salvage surgeries and improve the quality of life in these children.
- The exact frequency of hip surveillance varies based on assessment of risk factors—age of the child, GMFCS level, CP subtype (physiological/ geographic classification). For example, children with bilateral CP (diplegia/quadriplegia) should have a radiograph by the time they are 18 months old and then 6–12-monthly thereafter.
- Clinical evaluation includes evaluating for risk factors like age of the child, CP subtype, and GMFCS level. Examination of the hip involves measuring for hip abduction in each hip and is considered abnormal if <30°.
- Radiographic assessments are made of the Reimer's migration index and acetabular index on a standardized anteroposterior radiograph of the pelvis with both hips done in the supine position using a standardized position and radiographic technique. A horizontal reference line is drawn through the triradiate cartilage of the acetabula (Hilgenreiner's line). A line perpendicular to this is drawn at the edge of the acetabulum (Perkin's line). The Reimer's migration index is the percentage of the femoral head lying lateral to Perkin's line. The acetabular index is the angle that the roof of the socket makes with Hilgenreiner's line (Fig. 10.2).
- Many children become 'windswept', i.e. one hip lies in adduction and is at risk of posterior dislocation; the other in abduction and is at risk of anterior dislocation.
- Therapy aims at trying to retain as symmetrical a range of movement as possible although evidence that therapy and positioning of the child reduces the dislocation rate is lacking.
- Surgery is performed to prevent dislocation. If a hip is allowed to dislocate and becomes painful then this is a difficult situation to remedy.
- Preventative surgery (soft tissue releases) is indicated where the migration index is >40%, the increase in migration index is >10% between visits, and the acetabular index >27%
- Reconstructive surgery is indicated if the migration index is >50% despite soft tissue releases. Reconstructive surgery usually consists of femoral and pelvic osteotomies +/− open reduction of the hip (Fig. 10.3 and Fig. 10.4).

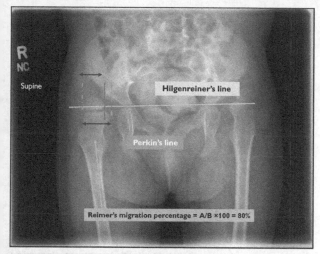

Fig. 10.2 Anteroposterior radiograph of the pelvis with both hips showing measurement of the migration percentage for hip surveillance.

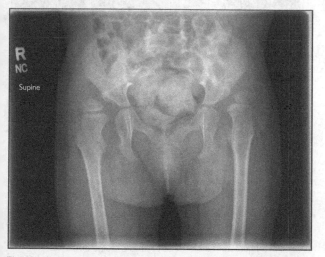

Fig. 10.3 Preoperative anteroposterior radiograph showing bilateral hip dislocation in a child with CP.

(a)

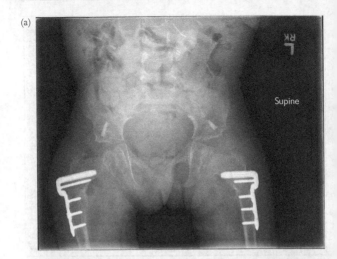

(b)

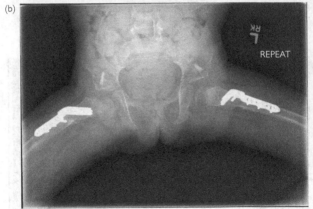

Fig. 10.4 (a) Postoperative anteroposterior radiograph showing relocated bilateral hips following a reconstructive surgery. (b) Postoperative lateral radiograph showing relocated bilateral hips following a reconstructive surgery.

- Hips must then be monitored until skeletal maturity as there is a risk of recurrent subluxation with growth. Functional outcome measures like the Caregiver Priorities and Child Health Index of Life with Disabilities (CPCHILD) questionnaire must be used to evaluate outcomes.

Spine

- The overall lifetime risk of developing scoliosis is about 0–75% depending on the GMFCS level. Those with spasticity are at highest risk.
- Scoliosis is most common in non-ambulatory patients. Unlike idiopathic scoliosis, the curves tend to be long 'C'-shaped curves down to the pelvis with an apex at the thoracolumbar junction.
- Untreated, the scoliosis can progress due to muscle imbalance and cause pain, sitting imbalance, and decreased respiratory function and quality of life.
- Bracing does not affect curve progression but may improve sitting comfort.
- Indications for surgery: progressive deformity (curves >50°), sitting imbalance, pelvic obliquity.
- Surgery usually involves posterior spine instrumentation with or without fusion depending on the age of the child. This has shown to improve sitting balance and quality of life (Fig. 10.5 and Fig. 10.6).

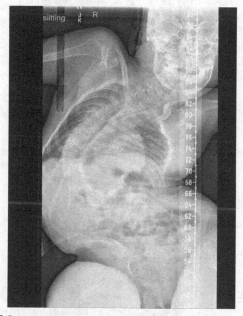

Fig. 10.5 Preoperative anteroposterior radiograph showing a C-shaped thoracolumbar scoliosis in a child with CP.

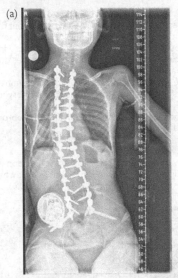

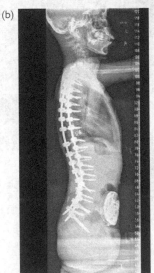

Fig. 10.6 (a) Postoperative anteroposterior radiograph showing correction of the scoliosis deformity. (b) Postoperative lateral radiograph showing correction of the scoliosis deformity.

Upper limbs

- In addition to spasticity, weakness, altered sensation, dystonia, and poor selective motor control are all a problem for the involved upper limb.
- For the hemiplegic patient, tasks are more easily performed with the 'good' hand and so the affected hand may become neglected and pattern of 'learned non-use' develops.
- Goals of treatment need to be carefully agreed with the patient and carers.
- The aims for those with total body involvement are usually to improve ease of care, including dressing and hygiene.
- Those with diplegia have little upper limb involvement.
- Hemiplegic patients are the most likely to be helped in terms of cosmesis and function.
- Assessment should focus on measuring sensation (which is predictive of spontaneous use of the limb), spasticity, selective motor control, strength, and contractures of both muscles and joints, e.g. it may be possible to fully extend the fingers with the wrist flexed but not with the wrist in neutral due to shortened length of the finger flexor musculotendinous unit.
- An idea of function and how the two hands are used together needs to be gained using functional evaluation tests (SHUEE).

Treatment

The following principles must be followed:

- The involvement of the MDT (including physiotherapist, OT, and orthopaedic surgeon) is vital for treatment planning and implementation.
- Goals must be clearly defined.
- Each patient should have a physiotherapy programme to stretch spastic muscles and strengthen weak ones in order to try and prevent contractures and maximize function.
- Constraint-Induced movement therapy(CIMT) encourages use and awareness of the affected limb by restricting the 'good' hand. This reduces the pattern of 'learnt non-use' and has been shown to maintain long-term improvements.
- Malposition of the wrist and thumb significantly impact function.

Surgery

- Surgery (musculotendinous releases and transfers, bony fusion), aims to improve positioning of the joints thereby improving function and cosmesis. It does not improve the fine dexterity of the digits.
- Because most muscles cross more than one joint, it is important to consider the limb as a whole when planning surgery.
- Just as with the lower limb, it is usual to perform several procedures in one sitting (single-event multilevel surgery-SEMLS).
- It is important to note that no amount of surgery is going to improve the function of a neglected hand, and so there must be reasonable spontaneous use of the hand before surgery is considered for functional gain.
- Validated outcome measures must be used to demonstrate efficacy of treatments.

Duchenne muscular dystrophy

- DMD is the most common dystrophinopathy and is inherited as a XLR disorder, seen in males.
- The basic defect involves cell membrane instability leading to progressive myocyte destruction.
- There is a progressive loss of muscle function and weakness.
- Typical presentation is in a young male child with complaints of the child walking awkwardly or not being able to run.
- It may present as a new-onset toe walking.
- There is history of a slight delay in motor milestones.
- Examination shows proximal muscle weakness affecting the hips and the shoulder, difficulty in taking steps, and a positive Gower sign.
- Medical management with steroids (deflazacort or prednisolone) has been found to reduce the incidence of scoliosis and prolong independent ambulation. Despite the medical treatment, orthopaedic problems are encountered in a child with DMD.
- The primary cause of orthopaedic problems is progressive muscle degeneration. Common orthopaedic problems are joint contractures, scoliosis, and osteoporosis which may cause fractures of the spine and long bones.
- The treatment principles change depending on the functional stage of the child. The stages are ambulatory stage, early non-ambulatory stage, and late non-ambulatory stage.
- Orthopaedic evaluation should commence at the time of diagnosis and at least every 6 months.
- The goals of the orthopaedic care are to preserve motor function as far as possible, improve bone health, prevent joint contractures, and maintain spine without any deformity.

The following orthopaedic problems are seen in early child with DMD.

Joint contractures

- Ankle equinus and equinovarus is developed due to gastrocnemius–soleus and posterior tibial muscle contractures and weakness of the peroneal and tibialis anterior muscles. Mild ankle equinus contracture can compensate for quadriceps weakness but more severe contractures need treatment.
- Hip flexion, external rotation occurs due to tensor fascia lata, and hip flexor contracture.
- Knee flexion contracture develops due to quadriceps weakness and hamstring contracture. It makes walking more difficult.
- Upper extremity weakness leading to loss of shoulder abduction, elbow flexion can be seen.
- In late childhood increasing contractures in the lower extremity, and decreasing muscle strength results in the inability to walk, increased falling episodes. At this point, knee–ankle–foot orthoses can be considered to provide knee stability. Soft tissue surgery (tendon lengthening) can be considered in a select group of patients.
- In adolescent patients, contractures tend to progress despite stretching and physiotherapy. It does not affect sitting. Surgical treatment for contractures can be offered to maintain ambulation or standing.

Scoliosis

- The incidence of scoliosis in DMD is 75–90% (see ➙ Table 10.1 p. 524).
- The common presentation is scoliosis of the lumbar or thoracolumbar spine in the late non-ambulatory phase of the disease.
- The pulmonary function deteriorates rapidly with curve progression.
- There is no role for spinal braces.
- Wheelchair modification can be used initially but early surgical treatment is recommended when the curve is >30° with posterior spinal instrumentation and fusion before significant deterioration of pulmonary function.
- Spine surgery has been shown to stabilize pulmonary function deterioration and improve sitting ability and quality of life.

Spinal muscular atrophy

- SMA is an AR disorder, associated with lack of survival motor neuron-1 (SMN1) protein due to loss of the *SMN* gene located on chromosome 5.
- This leads to loss of alpha motor neurons in the anterior horn cells of the spinal cord. This loss causes muscle weakness and atrophy.
- There is a 'backup gene', *SMN2*. Modulation of the low-functioning *SMN2* has been utilized in the newer treatment modalities such as risdiplam.

Classification

- Based on the time of onset of symptoms:
  - Type 1: onset of symptoms before 6 months of age, most severe form.
  - Type 2: starts manifestation at 6–12 months, may present with delayed walking.
  - Type 3: manifests in adolescence with proximal weakness.
  - Type 4: onset of symptoms in adulthood.
- Treatment and care plans should be customized to meet the specific individual needs of the patient and family.
- Physiotherapy is recommended for optimizing positioning, seating, and mobility. It also aids in the prevention of contractures and for maintaining joint range of motion.
- Newer medical therapy has emerged as a promising option.
  - Nusinersen has been used since 2016. It has been found to increase motor function in type 2 SMA. Nusinersen is an antisense oligonucleotide. It was shown to enhance exon 7 inclusion in *SMN2* messenger ribonucleic acid transcripts and production of full-length SMN protein.
  - Gene therapy using recombinant AAV9 has been used recently.
  - However, the effects of these new modalities on bone health remain unknown.

Orthopaedic issues in SMA are joint contractures, hip instability, spine deformity, and fractures.

Joint contractures

- Hip and knee flexion contractures are common in non-ambulatory children. The ankle equinus is rarely seen.
- The functional loss is due to muscle weakness and not due to contractures (in types 2 and 3), and hence, rarely surgical treatment is recommended.

Hip instability

- Hip dislocation is very common in type 2 SMA. It does not influence the function or the walking ability.
- The results of hip reconstruction are fraught with high rates of redislocation.
- Hence, in the majority of patients, surgical intervention is not recommended.
- Patients with painful hip(s), either unilateral or bilateral, should be offered surgical treatment aimed at pain relief.

Spine deformity

- A long C-shaped thoracolumbar curve is present in almost all of type 2 and about half of the patients with type 3 SMA.
- About one-third of patients have associated kyphosis.
- Curve progression is very common if not treated.
- Early treatment is recommended as the curve magnitude may affect pulmonary function and breathing.
- Bracing has a limited role in scoliosis treatment.
- Posterior spinal fusion and scoliosis correction is recommended for curves >40°. In type 3 patients, surgery should be performed while the patient is ambulatory.
- In children <10 years of age, scoliosis correction with various growth-friendly systems is recommended.

Fractures

- Fractures are common in type 2 and 3 SMA.
- Supracondylar femur and ankle fractures are common in type 2 SMA, whereas in type 3 SMA, upper extremity fractures are more frequent.
- Non-operative treatment is recommended for non-ambulatory children.
- Surgical fracture stabilization is recommended in ambulatory patients.

Myelomeningocele

- This is a common cause of long-term childhood-onset disability.
- Myelomeningocele is a neural tube defect involving protrusion of spinal cord and meninges from the spinal column. It results from failure of the neural tube to close.
- There is a cystic swelling, which includes dura and spinal nerve roots, seen as a protrusion in the spine.
- There is dysplasia of the spinal nerve roots and the spinal cord that leads to sensory and motor paralysis below the level of the lesion.
- In addition, there might be loss of bowel and bladder function.
- There could be associated lesions of the brain and spinal cord that may impact prognosis, such as hydrocephalus, Chiari malformation, syrinx, diastematomyelia, and tethered spinal cord.
- Muscle strength assessment should be done regularly.
- New-onset weakness may be due to tethered cord, syrinx, or shunt malfunction. If suspected, an MRI scan is recommended.
- Orthopaedic inputs for these children aim to maximize function and minimize disability and discomfort.

Orthopaedic issues in a child with myelomeningocele are as follows:

Spinal deformity

- It is more common in the high thoracic lesion, the incidence is <10% in sacral level myelomeningocele.
- Scoliosis and kyphosis are more severe in those with more proximal spinal cord lesions.
- Generally, the deformity is progressive and is not effectively treated by bracing.
- Surgery should be considered for curves of 50° or more and is typically required by around 8–9 years of age. This helps to maintain sitting balance, especially in the non-ambulant patient.

Hip problems

- Hips are prone to contractures (especially flexion) and dislocation in all levels of spina bifida. Contracture release may be offered.
- L2 and above lesions have bilateral hip dislocations.
- Usually, they are not treated surgically considering the high risk of complications.
- Controversy remains about undertaking surgery to relocate the hips in those with higher-level lesions, but those with lesions of L5 and below should have bony surgery to reconstruct their hips, as should any patient with a painful dislocation.
- For unilateral hip dislocations in lower lesions (ambulatory children), relocation surgery is considered.

Knee problems

- Flexion or extension/recurvatum contractures are common. May need serial casting and release of contracted muscles.
- Orthosis is used to prevent a recurrence.
- Surgery may be required to manage knee flexion or extension contractures that do not respond to stretches.

Foot and ankle deformities

- A vast majority of children with myelomeningocele develop foot and ankle deformity. The muscle imbalance causes deformity.
- A variety of foot deformities occur including club foot, vertical talus, and cavovarus feet. A progressive cavovarus deformity may be due to a tethered cord requiring referral to a neurosurgeon.
- In the non-ambulant child, it is important to have feet that rest comfortably on the footplate of the wheelchair.
- In walkers, a supple, pain-free, plantar grade foot is the aim. A plantigrade brace able foot is desired.
- Management ranges from the use of custom-made orthoses to serial casting or surgery, including soft tissue and bony procedures.
- Lack of sensation and the risk of pressure sores are important considerations.

Rotational deformities

- External tibial torsion is common. Internal tibial torsion may also be seen.
- There is limited role of non-operative modalities in treating rotational deformity.
- Usually, surgical treatment in the form of derotational osteotomy is necessary if the deformity is interfering with function.

Fractures

- Patients with spina bifida are prone to pathological fractures which tend to heal with abundant callus formation.
- The majority of the fractures are treated by non-operative means.
- With the plaster casts and splints, extra precautions need to be taken considering insensate skin.

Hereditary motor and sensory neuropathy

- This is a broad group encompassing motor and sensory polyneuropathies predominantly involving distal lower limbs.
- They may present with gait disturbance and instability, frequent ankle sprains, and foot deformities.
- Charcot–Marie–Tooth disease is one of the most common neuropathies. A duplication on chromosome 17 which codes for peripheral myelin protein 22 is the cause for the neuropathy.
- Peroneal muscles are commonly involved resulting in varus deformity of the foot and ankle. Tibialis anterior, intrinsic muscles of the foot and hand are involved.
- Orthopaedic problems that are commonly seen are pes cavovarus, claw toes, hip dysplasia, scoliosis, and weakness of the hand muscles.
- The onset is gradual, the most common presentation is in the second decade of life.
- The presenting symptoms are gait disturbance, unsteadiness, and difficulty in running. Initially, planovalgus foot is present that progresses to pes cavovarus and claw toes and to ankle equinus in some patients.
- Foot deformities are bilateral. The first ray plantarflexion is common due to peroneal longus pulling on the first metatarsal.
- Initially, the deformity is flexible, and tends to progressively become rigid.
- Coleman block test is used to differentiate between the origin of the hindfoot varus and its correctability.
- Foot drop and rigid equinus may be seen in some due to weak tibialis anterior.
- Intrinsic wasting of hands and weak grip may be noticed.

Treatment

- In initial stages, custom-made shoes to accommodate for mild deformity are used.
- Infra- and supramalleolar orthosis, Lace-up ankle brace are recommended for mild to moderate deformities but have limited success in controlling progression of the deformity.
- Surgical treatment in the form of soft tissue release with tendon transfers and bony osteotomies to realign the deformed bones and restore the muscle balance may be needed to address symptomatic cavovarus feet.

Hip dysplasia

This may be seen in some patients. It is usually diagnosed on radiographs and the patient may be symptomatic.

Scoliosis

Scoliosis may be seen in up to one-third of patients. Atypical curves are common such as a left-sided curve and kyphosis in contrast to adolescent idiopathic scoliosis. There is a limited role of bracing in the treatment. Curves >50° need surgical treatment.

Bone health in children with neuromuscular conditions

- The risk of developing osteoporosis is high in children with neurological disorders due to several reasons and it is secondary to osteopenia from decreased weight bearing (also see ➋ pp. 454–5).
- These children may have poor nutrition with decreased intake of calcium, and vitamin D.
- Swallowing and feeding disorders may enhance the problem of malnutrition.
- Decreased sunlight exposure may further contribute to vitamin D deficiency.
- In addition, medications such as glucocorticoids and antiepileptic medications may lead to vitamin D deficiency.
- Healthcare providers need to know how to improve bone health and prevent fragility fractures.

Osteoporosis is defined by two criteria: low BMD + history of fracture.
- The presence of low BMD is defined as a z-score of less than –2.0 on a DXA scan which measures bone mineral content per unit of area. Typically, it is measured at lateral distal femur or the whole body.
- The presence of a significant fracture history is defined as a long-bone fracture of the lower extremity (Fig. 10.7), vertebral compression fracture, or two or more long-bone fractures of the upper extremities.
- Osteoporotic fractures can cause significant pain and impairment.
- The child may need hospitalization and surgical treatment in the hospital. This may lead to further loss of mobility and cause additional decline in bone density. The treatment may also lead to absence from the school for the child and loss of work hours for the parents.
- Fractures are common in children with neuro-orthopaedic disorders. The frequency is variable.
- Non-ambulatory kids with CP have a 20% chance of having a fragility fracture.
- In DMD, the highest fracture incidence rate was observed in boys treated with daily deflazacort. The baseline fracture incidence was 1.2%. During a median follow-up of 4 years, incidence increased to 27.7%.
- High risk of vertebral fracture was associated with length of deflazacort use in DMD patients, regardless of the age at the start of therapy; ~20–60% of boys experience lower extremity fragility fractures and ~30% experience symptomatic vertebral fracture.
- Increased fracture risk (especially involving lower extremity) has been reported in SMA type 1.

Evaluation

- The nutritional status of the child should be evaluated. Assess for decreasing weight velocity and/or low BMI. Nutritional counselling is important to correct nutritional deficiencies, if any.
- Dietary history to estimate calcium intake should be obtained.
- Blood investigations including calcium, phosphate, parathyroid hormone, and 25-OH-vitamin D should be obtained.

- X-rays of the affected extremity should be done if a fracture is suspected clinically.
- DXA scan to assess the BMD should be done.

Treatment

- Promote weight bearing: bearing weight increases the BMD. Physiotherapy referral for a standing programme should be done and the child may need to use a standing frame.
- Prescribe adequate calcium and vitamin D. Recommended daily doses are 700 mg elemental calcium for 1–3 years of age, 1000 mg for 4–8 years of age, and 1300 mg for 9–18 years of age. It is important to provide dietary counselling to increase dietary calcium intake. It recommended to give vitamin D supplementation of 800–1000 international units per day.
- Consult with orthopaedic service for fracture management.
- Bisphosphonates can be considered after consulting with paediatric endocrinology. They suppress bone resorption and help to build bone density. However, long-term effects on a growing skeleton remain unknown. In children, typically IV administration three to four times a year is undertaken. Pamidronate and zoledronic acid are commonly used.

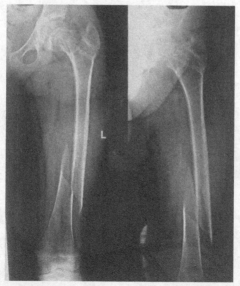

Fig. 10.7 Radiographs showing a femur fracture in a child with SMA type 2.

Child protection and safeguarding

Introduction to child protection and safeguarding

On average, one child per week dies through direct abuse in the UK, most deaths being in children <1 year of age and mainly at the hand of a family member. Other children go on to suffer physical disability and many more develop long-term mental health difficulties and have curtailed life chances.

- Child protection and safeguarding are everybody's business.
- *Safeguarding* is defined in 'Working Together' as:
  - Protecting children from maltreatment.
  - Preventing impairment of children's mental and physical health or development.
  - Ensuring that children are growing up in circumstances consistent with the provision of safe and effective care.
  - Taking action to enable all children have the best outcomes.
- *Child protection* is part of safeguarding and promoting welfare. This refers to the *activity* that is undertaken to protect specific children who are suffering, or are likely to suffer, significant harm, e.g. a referral to social care or a child protection medical assessment.
- In some countries, the term safeguarding is not used.
- Child abuse has been defined in 'Working Together' as: 'A form of maltreatment of a child. Somebody may abuse or neglect a child by inflicting harm, or by failing to act to prevent harm. Harm can include ill treatment that is not physical as well as the impact of witnessing ill treatment of others.'
- There are four main categories of abuse: neglect, emotional abuse, physical abuse, and sexual abuse. See later sections in this chapter for details of each of these.
- Children may be abused in a family or in an institutional or community setting by those known to them or, more rarely, by others.
- Abuse can take place wholly online, or technology may be used to facilitate offline abuse. Children may be abused by an adult or adults, or another child or children.
- An increasing range of childhood adversities are now considered within the remit of safeguarding: witnessing domestic violence as emotional abuse, bullying as a type of peer-on-peer abuse, and some criminal activity as a form of child exploitation.
- In 2019 in England, 52,260 children were subject to a child protection plan due to concerns about abuse.
- Approximately half were neglect, just over a third were emotional abuse, 8% physical abuse, 4% sexual abuse, and 4% had multiple categories recorded.
- The number of children at child protection level continues to rise; in 2012 when the previous edition of this handbook was published, there were ~39,100 'registrations'. Previous terminology referred to the child protection register.
- Approximately 20% of adults reported suffering abuse before they were 16 years old in a Crime Survey for England and Wales.
- Much abuse does not get reported. One in seven adults who called an adult help charity had never told anybody about their abuse before.

Further resources

Department for Education (July 2018). Working Together to Safeguard Children: A Guide to Inter-Agency Working to Safeguard and Promote the Welfare of Children. Available at: ℘ https://www.gov.uk/government/publications/working-together-to-safeguard-children--2

NSPCC Learning. Statistics briefing: child deaths due to abuse or neglect: ℘ https://learning.nspcc.org.uk/research-resources/statistics-briefings/child-deaths-abuse-neglect

Office for National Statistics. Child abuse in England and Wales: ℘ Perplexing Presentations/Fabricated and Induced Illness in children-guidance, Mar 2021, https://childprotection.rcpch.ac.uk/resources/perplexing-presentations-and-fii/

https://www.ons.gov.uk/peoplepopulationandcommunity/crimeandjustice/bulletins/childabuseinenglandandwales/march2020

Risk factors for child abuse

Any child can be subjected to any type of abuse, either within the home or elsewhere. Having a risk factor for abuse does not mean that abuse will happen and some parents with risk factors will be very good parents. Likewise, even where there are no risk factors children are also abused. Nonetheless, it can be helpful to have an awareness of risk and HVs (see ➔ pp. 676–7) plan their support to families accordingly.

Child factors

- Infants and young children are particularly vulnerable to physical abuse, due to their fragile bodies and lack of mobility.
- An infant's main form of communication, crying, is designed to get attention but its persistence can lead to high levels of stress in often already exhausted caregivers, thus increasing the likelihood that an abusive act might take place.
- A young child's rapidly developing brain and their dependence on adults make them very vulnerable to the effects of neglect and emotional abuse.
- Children of all ages are vulnerable to abuse, including teenagers. Teenagers are not only susceptible to sexual and criminal exploitation but also to parental neglect and emotional abuse during a time when their brains too are undergoing significant change.
- Children of all ages and social backgrounds are at risk of sexual abuse.
- Children with disabilities are at increased risk of abuse, both within and outside the family home.

Parental factors

- Parents who do not understand how to meet the wide range of children's physical, emotional, social, and developmental needs. Such parents may have a learning difficulty, be very young or even be children themselves, did not experience nurturing parenting themselves, or have had multiple caregivers such as in the local authority care system.
- Parents whose own needs get in the way of recognizing and addressing the child's needs. Examples include parental substance abuse and health difficulties, particularly mental health. Parental obsessions with their own social or work needs (in person or online) to the point of neglecting the child.
- The multiple, pervasive stresses associated with poverty.
- Domestic abuse (DA) was traditionally seen as a risk factor for child abuse. Now it is recognized as being abusive to the child in its own right; hence, many children are subject to a safeguarding plan under the category of emotional abuse through living in a home where DA exists. See ➔ p. 592 regarding DA.
- 'Toxic trio' has been used to describe the high incidence of DA, substance abuse, and mental health difficulties in cases of severe child abuse that have led to serious case reviews. The prevalence of these three factors remains valid but use of the term toxic trio is now advised against as it can be stigmatizing and inaccurate.

Community factors

- Factors which place additional stresses on parents include social isolation, poor housing, and lack of local amenities, including opportunities for children to play and interact safely.
- Communities with a high density of families with their own unaddressed needs, thus lessening the availability of local social support networks and resilience.
- Neighbourhoods that have been infiltrated by criminal gangs.

This chapter looks at the types of child abuse and the role of the paediatrician in its identification and multiagency response. To understand the effects of many types of abuse it is helpful to have an awareness of the work and theories related to the adverse childhood experiences (ACEs) agenda first.

Further resources

Association of Child Protection Professionals. Toxic terminology: https://www.childprotectionprofessionals.org.uk/blog/toxic-terminology

Adverse childhood experiences

(Also see ➲ Chapter 12.)

- Adversity in childhood, particularly the early years of life and adolescence, is associated with increased risk of poor physical and mental health outcomes in adulthood.
- All child abuse is adversity though not all adversity is child abuse, e.g. bereavement or severe illness.
- Vincent Feliti, an adult physician, identified a high rate of childhood adversity, particularly sexual abuse, reported by adults dropping out of an obesity clinic.
- The resulting first ACEs study in 1998[1] linked childhood experience of a range of child abuse and family dysfunction factors (as reported by the resulting adult) to an increased risk of poor adult physical and mental health outcomes, as identified through health records.
- The link was thought to be due to increased health-harming behaviours such as substance abuse; however, further work suggested that did not account for the size of the increase.
- *Chronic/toxic stress* from adversity has been suggested to result in neurobiological changes impacting endocrine and immune function in the child which can persist into adulthood, as well as epigenetic changes helping to explain intergenerational effects of adversity.
- Neurobiological changes may also affect development of cognitive function, e.g. executive function, resulting in difficulty managing impulse control and the assessment and response to perceived threats.
- Intrinsic differences between people's response to stress may be important, as well as learned behaviours. The theories are not all proven and a combination of factors are likely to exist.
- ACE/trauma scores refer to the number of types of adversity that a person experiences before the age of 18 years; those experiencing more than four having a higher risk of poor outcomes in adulthood, such as twice the risk of diabetes, three times the risk of cancer or heart disease, and seven times the risk of substance misuse or self-harming behaviours.
- The original ACEs questionnaire asked about physical, sexual, emotional abuse, and neglect, as well as family dysfunction—domestic violence, parental separation, substance misuse, mental health, and incarceration. The WHO ACEs questionnaire also covers bullying and experience of neighbourhood conflict.
- Epidemiological studies report similar proportions of the population experiencing ACEs. The Welsh ACEs study in 2015 found 53% report no ACEs, 20% one ACE, 13%, two or three ACEs, and 14% four ACEs.
- Some advocate for widespread population level ACEs screening but others are concerned that screening standards are not met. Treatment options may not be available or acceptable.
- However, it is helpful for paediatricians to have an awareness of potential adversities that a child might have experienced when undertaking a detailed and empathic assessment of concerns raised about school or behavioural functioning or during assessments undertaken for social care or education authorities.

- An *ACEs/trauma-informed* approach aims to educate the public and professionals about ACEs and their impact on the child, particularly the child's brain development.
- It seeks to avoid further trauma (e.g. detention when arriving late in school due to poor sleep due to DA incident the previous night) and to encourage both universal and targeted strategies as well as therapeutic options which promote resilience and optimum brain development.
- *Resilience*—some children who have experienced abuse or other adversity fare better than others in the long term, this is not yet fully understood.
- Resilience can be promoted through access to a consistent, attentive caregiver, community support, and social opportunities.
- Resilience can be improved by promoting optimal brain development via a nurturing and stimulating environment, including by being responsive to child interactions and modelling appropriate responses to threat.

Reference

1. Felitti VJ, Anda RF, Nordenberg D, et al. (1998). Relationship of childhood abuse and household dysfunction to many of the leading causes of death in adults. The Adverse Childhood Experiences (ACE) study. Am J Prev Med, 14, 245–58.

Further resources

Alberta Family Wellness Initiative (various resources and videos of lectures about ACEs and how to build a brain, including Robert Anda's 'The ACE Study: building self-healing communities' and Judy Cameron's 'The interplay between early brain and early behaviour development'): M https://www.albertafamilywellness.org/

Burke Harris N (2018). The Deepest Well: Healing the Long-Term Effects of Childhood Adversity. London: Bluebird. [Not a self-care book, rather an easy read paediatrician's review of the ACEs literature and how it affects her approach to clinical practice.]

Public Health Wales. Welsh ACEs reports, epidemiology, and helpful infographics: ℜ https://phw.nhs.wales/files/aces/

Neglect

- Neglect is the most common reason for children being on a safeguarding plan—~50% of plans.
- Definitions refer to *persistent or ongoing* failure to meet the child's basic physical or psychological needs.
- Neglect is often chronic and fluctuates, due to difficulties in maintaining improvements without addressing adults' reasons for neglectful behaviours.
- Focus on the lived experience/outcomes for the child and consider how other parents in similar situations of poverty or disability are able to meet the child's needs.
- Can begin *in utero* through poor self-care of mother/not accessing available antenatal care.
- Increased risk if parents under additional stress, DA, poor mental health, substance misuse, child with disability and/or complex health needs, and/or adult with health or learning needs.
- No parent is perfect. Neglect, however, is the persistence of neglectful behaviours.

Various categories of neglect are recognized which can overlap:

Physical neglect

- Inappropriate clothing; bedding/inadequate home conditions including unsafe appliances, windows, etc.; poor hygiene in a young child; poor supervision; not addressing social development or promoting behavioural boundaries; abandonment; inadequate food or inadequate diet.
- Leading to malnutrition or obesity (neglect if failure to engage in remedial measures); reports of scavenging food; poor growth with catch-up growth in hospital or foster care, faltering again when back with parents; hypothermia, can have red swollen hands or feet from cold injury. Poor hygiene, dirty or ill-fitting clothes, inappropriate for weather conditions, malodourous. Ostracized by peers and poor mental well-being. Frequent injuries including burns; accidental ingestion of toxic substances including parental medication or illegal drugs.

Educational neglect

- Inadequate developmental stimulation from infancy onwards; not accessing education (in school or otherwise) through actions of the carer, e.g. not enrolled; frequent absences for no justifiable reason such as child acting as a young carer without support; frequent avoidable school moves; frequently arriving late for school.
- Leading to developmental delay, particularly speech and language delay/missing sensitive phase for language and interaction development; starting school at developmental disadvantage leading to increased risk of ongoing literacy and numeracy difficulties; poor self-help skills such as toileting, dressing, or use of cutlery; not achieving potential in education and missing out on life chances which itself can lead to poorer physical and mental well-being.

Emotional neglect

- Unresponsive to child's emotional and social interaction needs/ignoring. Emotional abuse implies a more intentional act—emotional neglect is more about omission, e.g. due to parental mental health, substance misuse, preoccupation with own needs including social media.
- Leading to an increased risk of poor mental and physical health, poor interaction and social skills, and worse educational outcomes.

Medical neglect

- Not addressing medical or developmental concerns; delay in seeking medical help for injuries or illnesses; not attending medical assessments including dental assessment; not providing recommended medication or engaging in therapies.
- Leading to illness not being treated—can lead to death, e.g. diabetes, asthma. Untreated squint—irreversible amblyopia; hearing loss— impaired speech and language development; not taking thyroxine or PKU diet—avoidable mental disability; physiotherapy—secondary disability and pain; dental caries—avoidable dental pain/infections/ extractions/anaesthetic.

Role of a paediatrician in neglect

- In all clinical encounters identify and document any signs and symptoms of neglect, discuss with the carer in an empathic but clear way to help them to be addressed. Document conversations and outcomes in an objective way including offers of support and whether they are taken up or not.
- Be clear, both verbally and in the clinic letter copied to parents, what is expected of parents to adequately address a child's health or developmental needs.
- Explore and rule out medical causes of any growth or neurodevelopmental concerns.
- Check for iron deficiency if nutritional concerns. Rare cases of vitamin C deficiency/scurvy in neglect.
- Work in a multidisciplinary way to piece together objective evidence of neglect if such is suspected.
- Use 'child not brought' approach, not 'did not attend'.
- Have knowledge of and contribute to your local neglect assessment tool, such as the Graded Care Profile.
- Consider if threshold is met for referral to social care.
- Facilitate identification of neglect through advocating for and using joined-up clinical records and IT systems across and between health organizations.

Emotional abuse

- Emotional abuse is the second most common reason for a child being subject to a safeguarding plan, affecting more than one in three children.
- 'Working Together' tells us that it is the persistent emotional maltreatment of a child such as to cause severe and persistent adverse effects on the child's emotional development.
- Sometimes called psychological abuse, can overlap with emotional neglect if extreme unavailability of parent to child's emotional and social needs. Often occurs with other forms of abuse, particularly neglect.
- Conveying to a child that they are worthless or unloved, inadequate, or valued only insofar as they meet the needs of another person.
- Not giving the child opportunities to express their views, deliberately silencing them, or 'making fun' of what they say or how they communicate.
- Age or developmentally inappropriate expectations being imposed on children/interactions that are beyond a child's developmental capability, including treating the child as their friend rather than their child.
- Overprotection and limitation of exploration and learning, or preventing the child participating in normal social interaction.
- Seeing or hearing the ill-treatment of another, e.g. DA (frequent reason for a child protection plan).
- Serious bullying (including cyberbullying), causing children frequently to feel frightened or in danger, or the exploitation or corruption of children.
- Some level of emotional abuse is involved in all types of maltreatment of a child, though it may occur alone.

Signs and symptoms of emotional abuse

- Lack of attachment to parent or excessive clinginess to parent, aggression to peers or animals. Emotionally labile, poor social skills, lack of friends, inappropriate language and actions, attention seeking, continence difficulties, not forming relationships, risk-taking behaviours, lack of care for own safety, mental health problems.
- Observation of faltering growth (with catch-up growth when living in different circumstances), apathetic look; frozen watchfulness; withdrawn; excess clinginess or opposite, i.e. indiscriminate attachment to strangers; parent openly overly critical of child or name calling in front of professionals.
- Not responding to child's emotional or interaction needs.
- Hypervigilance—child always on guard for the next threat, could be emotional insult or physical abuse.
- Lack of playfulness or bruises normally associated with normal play accidents—sits too still/seems too good, too aware of threat of extreme punishment, verbal or physical.

Role of paediatrician

- Consider the possibility of emotional abuse in children brought in with behaviour difficulties, observe and record parent–child interactions.
- Consider if parental risk factors are present such as DA, substance misuse, etc.
- Alert the parent in an empathic though clear way to your concerns, may or may not be appropriate on first meeting. May be helpful to take a 'wondering' approach to the enquiry with parents.
- May need to discuss concerns with colleagues or other professionals working with the family. Offer to explore help in a multidisciplinary way.
- Rule out medical cause of growth concerns.
- Consider if threshold met for referral to social care.

Further resources

For all types of abuse:

NSPCC Learning. Statistics briefing: child deaths due to abuse or neglect: ℘ https://learning.nspcc. org.uk/research-resources/statistics-briefings/child-deaths-abuse-neglect

Royal College of Paediatrics and Child Health (RCPCH) Child Protection Evidence and RCPCH Child Protection Companion found at the RCPCH Child Protection Portal: ℘ https://childprotection. rcpch.ac.uk/

Physical abuse

- Physical abuse is the third most common reason for a child being subject to a child protection plan, accounting for ~8–9% of cases.
- Physical abuse, sometimes referred to as non-accidental injury, has been defined as may involve hitting, shaking, throwing, poisoning, burning or scalding, drowning, suffocating or otherwise causing physical harm to a child. Physical harm may also be caused when a parent or carer fabricates the symptoms of, or deliberately induces, illness in a child.
- Babies are most at risk of physical abuse.
- Babies' bodies, especially their brains, are particularly vulnerable to the effects of physical abuse.
- Bruising and other injuries in non-mobile babies is rare with normal handling, 'Those who don't cruise rarely bruise.'
- Accidental injuries to babies who are not yet mobile can happen, but with normal supervision the cause is likely to be known to the baby's carer.
- All potential or actual injuries in non-mobile babies should be assessed by an experienced paediatrician who should give an opinion as to whether or not there are likely to be safeguarding concerns. Part of that assessment should involve establishing whether or not there are social concerns relating to that family.
- Small bruises in non-mobile babies have been termed sentinel bruises as they can be highly significant, leading to the discovery of occult injuries such as multiple fractures. In retrospect, some babies presenting with severe abusive injuries had previously been seen with a small bruise, particularly on the face.
- A baby's main form of communication, crying, is designed to gain immediate attention. Public health campaigns and support are designed to help carers cope with crying babies.
- Hitting a child is illegal in Scotland and a ban comes into force in Wales in 2022. It is still legal in England and Northern Ireland as 'reasonable punishment'—as long as no mark is left and no implement used.

> For all forms of injuries, it is essential to bear in mind the developmental abilities of the child when considering whether a proposed mechanism of injury is plausible or not.

Bruising

- Bruising is the most common examination finding in physical abuse.
- It is not possible to reliably age bruises—do not give an opinion on the likely age of a bruise.
- As children become more mobile, they are likely to have more bruises through normal mobility and play.
- Bruises incurred *accidentally* tend to be on bony prominences such as knees and lower legs, back of the head, lower spine, and the T zone of the face—forehead, nose, upper lip, and chin.

- The pattern of accidental bruising in wheelchair users is different, with more bruising to the hands, abdomen, thighs, knees, and feet.
- Blunt injury to the forehead can track downward giving bilateral 'black eyes'. Circumstances of the forehead injury still need to be explained.

Consider or suspect abuse if

- Bruising in non-mobile babies.
- Bruising away from bony prominences.
- Bruises on ears, around the eye, cheeks, mouth, neck, upper arms, abdomen, buttocks.
- If bruising to the suprapubic area, thighs, or genital areas, consider child sexual abuse (CSA).
- Bruising in the pattern of a handprint from a slap, or an implement, e.g. belt, wire such as phone charger wire used as a whip, stick, sole or heel of a shoe, etc.
- Clusters of bruises may represent fingertip bruising in a grip pattern. Try putting your fingers over to see if pattern fits; if so, it can be helpful to photograph the bruises with and without fingers overlying in order to demonstrate your point in the context of a medical assessment.
- Bruising to arms and outer thighs may be defensive injuries.
- The suggested mechanism doesn't seem likely; there are very large bruises or clusters of bruises; bruises of similar shape or frequent bruising.
- Petechial bruising is more common in abuse, in the absence of a medical cause.
- Petechia in the area of the superior vena cava can occur in suffocation (but also in superior vena cava obstruction or violent coughing or vomiting).
- Note that severe abusive head trauma (AHT) and fractures can occur without bruising.

Medical causes to be considered

- Children with permanent inborn coagulation disorders or transient (e.g. viral-related) coagulation disturbances can have more and larger bruises (need less force to produce a bruise/bruise more easily) but the *distribution of those bruises is still likely to be in keeping with normal patterns*.
- Platelet levels need to be very low (20×10^9/L) for spontaneous bruising; at $20–50 \times 10^9$/L there is a mild bleeding diathesis.
- Vasculitis should not be confused with bruising.
- Birth marks including subcutaneous cavernous haemangiomas can be mistaken for bruising and may occasionally need repeat examination at a later date to be sure.
- Mongolian blue spot birthmarks can cover extensive areas of the body.
- Take blood for a coagulation screen if extensive bruising, subdural haematoma, or concerns about a coagulation disorder.
- Be aware that some viral infections can produce transient inhibitors which result in a temporary coagulation disorder, hence if blood tests are indicated, take them as soon as possible in order to establish the child's coagulation status as close to the alleged incident as possible.

Burns

- About 5–14% of children admitted to burns units are thought to have burns due to abuse.
- Burns are the second most common cause of death in physical abuse.
- Children 0–1 year of age have the highest prevalence of abusive burn injury.
- Scalds are the most common type of abusive burn injury.
- Young children are most at risk of abusive hot water scald injury.
- Children are at risk of other types of abusive burn injury throughout childhood.
- Burns due to neglect are nine times more common than those intentionally inflicted.
- Children who have a burn before 3 years of age are seven times more likely to be identified as being abused or neglected by 6 years of age, hence such burns have been described as sentinel.[1]
- Children <1 year get a full-thickness scald burn after 1 second in a liquid of 60°C.

Accidental scalds

- Usually from hot drinks, affecting the face, neck, and upper body.
- Asymmetrical distribution, usually anterior body and unilateral.
- The border is irregular, often with splash marks and uneven burn thickness.
- Difficult to reliably age burns, effectiveness of first aid can alter healing.

Abusive scald injuries

- Usually from tap water, such as forced immersion in hot bath water (Fig. 11.1a).
- Affecting the lower body, mainly the legs, perineum, and buttocks.
- Symmetrical distribution and even upper border.
- Splash marks less likely but sparing of creases.
- Sparing of areas of skin in firm contact with the bath, e.g. buttocks or soles of feet.
- Can have 'glove and stocking' distribution—see Fig. 11.1b.
- May have fingertip bruising/grip marks where the child was forcibly held.

Non-scald burn injuries

- Abusive contact burns, often affect posterior of body.
- Outline of implement seen, e.g. iron.
- Accidental contact burns, e.g. the palm of the hand.
- Cigarette burns—stubbing on skin gives circular outline, 1 cm diameter or less if roll ups. If accidental brushing past then likely to be less defined edge and have a tapering tail.
- Other burn mechanisms—flames, hairdryer, caustic fluids. or powder and microwave.

Differential diagnosis

Infections, including impetigo; drug reactions; photodermatitis; skin disorder, such as eczema; traditional heat therapies, such as moxibustion; accidental friction burns.

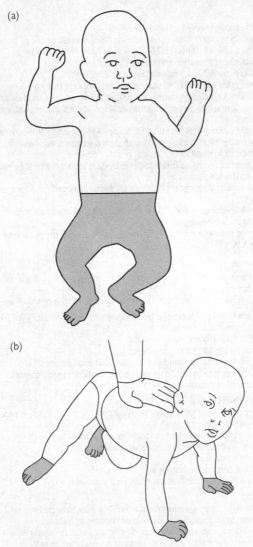

Fig. 11.1 (a) Abusive scald immersion pattern. (b) Abusive scald 'glove and stocking' pattern.

Bites

- Children commonly bite other children.
- Human bites form one or two annular/oval bruises or set of puncture wounds, overall diameter 2.5–5 cm, may have central bruising.
- Individual tooth marks may be seen.
- Bites are painful and likely to be remembered.
- Animal bites are more 'V' shaped and may include tearing injury.
- It is difficult to clearly identify if a bite was inflicted by a child or an adult due to dental bite pattern differences. Note dental maturity at aged 12 years.
- Forensic dentist may be asked for an opinion regarding the possible perpetrator by excluding those with dental patterns incompatible with the imprint in question.
- Very limited access to forensic dentists, operate on regional or national basis in the UK.
- Good-quality photographic documentation is needed for a forensic opinion.
- If DNA evidence is likely, then arrange for forensic samples via multiagency working.
- Forensic sampling is beyond the remit of most child protection services in the UK.

Fractures

- In children <1 year of age, 25–56% of fractures are thought to be from abuse.
- About 80% of abusive fractures are in children <18 months of age.

In the absence of metabolic bone disease or clear history of relevant trauma, *suspect* possible abuse in:

- Any fracture in a pre-mobile child.
- Rib fractures, particularly posterior.
- Metaphyseal (bucket handle) fractures of the long bones.
- Femoral fracture in a child who is not yet walking/trying to walk.
- Fracture of humerus in a child <18 months.

Also *consider* abuse in:

- Any fracture where the given mechanism is not consistent with the child's developmental age.
- Fractures where the given mechanism is not consistent with the type of fracture—consider an orthopaedic opinion.
- Multiple fractures.
- Spiral fracture of the humerus.
- Inconsistencies in the history or delayed presentation.

Note that:

- Non-weight-bearing children with disability may have pathological fractures from osteopenia, often a distal femoral fracture.
- Birth trauma, especially shoulder dystocia, can cause fractures.
- Supracondylar fracture of the humerus is usually accidental.
- Premature infants can have metabolic bone disease of prematurity.

- Rickets/symptomatic vitamin D deficiency can cause fractures but the bone disease should be demonstrated as being active at the time, i.e. radiological changes or increased parathyroid hormone levels. Hence the need for *parathyroid hormone measurement to be taken at the time of the fracture*, not just vitamin D and bone profile.
- Skull fractures—linear fracture is the most common type and could be either abusive or non-abusive. Needs assessment in context of history. Can't date skull fractures.
- Skull fractures thought to have been from abuse are more likely to be multiple or to cross suture lines.
- It is difficult to date fractures radiologically; estimates are in weeks not days.
- Occult fractures such as rib, metaphyseal, hand, or pelvic fractures may be revealed on radiological investigation of suspected physical abuse, e.g. skeletal survey.
- Rib fractures are more likely to be identified when healing/callous is visible radiologically, hence the importance of follow-up radiology in 10–14 days.
- Squeezing the thorax is the proposed mechanism causing rib fractures, such as in shaking.
- Rib fractures have been described in cardiopulmonary resuscitation but not posterior rib fractures.
- Consider advice from orthopaedic surgeon regarding forces required for the fracture in question.
- Consider advice from a metabolic bone consultant if metabolic bone disease is suspected.
- Children with osteogenesis imperfecta will continue to have fractures when in foster care.

Abusive and non-abusive head trauma (AHT and nAHT)

- AHT is the most common cause of death from physical abuse.
- Mortality rate up to 30%, ~50% of survivors have some form of disability.
- AHT mainly affects infants, especially those <6 months.
- Subdural haemorrhages are statistically associated with AHT.
- Subarachnoid haemorrhages are found evenly in both AHT and nAHT.
- Extradural haemorrhages are statistically associated with nAHT.
- Cerebral oedema, hypoxic ischaemia, diffuse axonal injury, and closed head injury are statistically associated with AHT rather than nAHT.
- Presentation can be through subtle signs such as irritability or isolated vomiting. May present with breathing abnormalities or seizures.
- Subdural haemorrhage may present less acutely with increasing head circumference.
- AHT can be difficult to identify—have a low threshold to suspect it.
- Many babies present more than once before AHT is diagnosed.
- Also found on investigation of suspected physical abuse, including rib fractures.
- Trilogy of encephalopathy, retinal haemorrhages, and subdural haemorrhage thought to be related to shaking.
- Confessions of perpetrators—shaking main mechanism in infants, with or without direct blow/s.

- Statistically associated with retinal haemorrhages and apnoea.
- Investigate with CT. MRI can find parenchymal brain injuries when CT normal.
- Look at cervical spine for associated injuries.
- Ultrasound not good at picking up subdural haemorrhage.
- Subgaleal and cephalohaematomas associated with birth trauma.
- Subgaleal haematomas can be large, cross suture lines; associated with hair pulling in older children—abusive and non-abusive.

Differential diagnosis
- Birth trauma, coagulopathy, and metabolic disorders, particularly glutaric aciduria.
- Note subdural haemorrhage from birth trauma usually resolves within 4 weeks.

Eye and retinal injuries
- Retinal haemorrhages are strongly associated with abuse.
- Proposed mechanism from shearing forces due to rapid and forceful head movement.
- The presence or absence of retinal haemorrhages should be confirmed by an ophthalmologist.
- Children can have direct eye injuries associated with abuse.

Ear, nose, and throat
- Epistaxis is associated with suffocation in children <2 years, whether intentional or unintentional.
- Bruising to the ear is associated with abuse.
- Direct trauma to the oropharynx can occur in abuse, including forceful feeding.

Torn labial frenum
- Historically a torn labial (lip) frenum (or frenulum) was said to be pathognomonic of abuse; however, research does not support this statement, though abuse does need to be considered.
- It is possible to injure the labial frenum accidentally; however, such events are likely to be recalled by carers due to bleeding.
- A congenital anomaly may also need to be considered.

Visceral injuries
- High mortality rate.
- Hepatic, splenic, pancreatic, or small bowel injuries.
- Liver and spleen in young children less protected by ribs.
- Have low threshold to investigate when abdominal bruising.
- Suspect abuse in children with intra-abdominal injuries in the absence of a clear trauma history such as a road traffic accident.
- May be occult, often with no overlying bruising; need to be actively searched for, especially in an unconscious child.

Poisoning
- Consider accidental or deliberate poisoning in a stuporous or unconscious child at any age.

- Potential substances accidentally ingested by young child may not be readily admitted by carers, such as GHB.
- Keep an open mind and take samples at an early stage if no clear medical cause is evident for clinical presentation.
- Consider neglect or FII/physical abuse if poisoning identified.

Anogenital bleeding

- May present acutely as an emergency or non-acutely in clinic.
- Needs careful history and examination to rule in or out a range of medical causes; examine the whole child.
- Consider any accidental cause offered regarding its plausibility.
- Most accidental causes are witnessed.
- Injury to the posterior fourchette, particularly if severe, raises concern of CSA, unless a clear witnessed accidental cause can be provided.
- If no cause can be established, or if there are concerns of CSA, then refer to social services for a strategy meeting and possible forensic examination.
- Can be helpful to discuss with the on-call forensic doctor regarding a need to referral to social care but if a referral for forensic examination is needed then this needs to be via a multiagency approach with social care and police.
- If emergency surgery is clinically indicated, then liaise with the forensic clinician regarding forensic samples if there is any concern about CSA.

Causes of anogenital bleeding

- Lichen sclerosis et atrophicus, sexually transmitted infections (STI), foreign body, urethral prolapse, midline fusion anomalies, endocrine causes, tumour, including haemangioma.
- GI conditions including anal tear from constipation, gastroenteritis, intussusception.
- Trauma, either accidental such as a straddle injury, or sexual trauma.
- Vulvovaginitis does not usually cause bleeding. See ℘ https://brits pag.org/wp-content/uploads/2018/10/Leaflet-Vulvovaginitis.pdf for helpful parent leaflet.

Genital infections

- Any sexually transmitted infection in a child under 13 years—referral to social care for strategy discussion with clinician with specialist skills in CSA who will guide assessment and treatment. See ➔ p. 457.
- Genital warts—CSA should be considered, particularly if the warts first appear in a child aged 4 years or older. See flow chart: ℘ https://www. stmaryscentre.org/application/files/4514/7793/0541/2013-anogeni tal-warts-flow-chart-final-version-4-September-2013-St-Marys-SARC. pdf.

Female genital mutilation (FGM)

- FGM involves the partial or total removal of, or injury to, external female genitalia for non-medical reasons.
- Usually performed without anaesthetic or clean knives; the child is often forcibly held.

- Results in a range of morbidity and death from infection or blood loss at the time or due to late complications, including during child birth. Is a cause of neonatal harm. Urinary complications also occur.
- Known by many names, including cutting and sunna.
- Four types described. *Type 1*, clitoridectomy, removing the outer part of the clitoris; *type 2*, excision, removing part or all of the clitoris and cutting the inner and/or outer labia; *type 3*, infibulation, narrowing the vaginal opening (deinfibulation refers to reopening of the vaginal opening to allow intercourse or childbirth); *type 4*, other harmful procedures to the female genitals, including pricking, piercing, cutting, scraping, or burning.
- Most FGM is carried out on young girls, often infants. Sometimes used on women to exert sexual control.
- Culturally rooted in north African and sub-Saharan countries, also Yemen, Malaysia, and Indonesia.
- No religion mandates FGM.
- It is illegal to carry out FGM in the UK and in many other countries.
- FGM is currently the only type of child abuse in the UK where it is *mandatory* to report it to police—Serious Crime Act 2015.
- Any 'regulated professional' such as health and social care, or education staff must inform the police if a girl <18 years:
  - Is seen (on examination) to have had FGM.
  - Says that she has had FGM.
- It is not mandatory to refer to the police if you think a girl is at risk of having FGM. You should though discuss with safeguarding colleagues and social care regarding a referral for assessment of risk.
- If you think the girl is at imminent risk of FGM then call the police on 999 (as per any other imminent serious risk to a child). Otherwise, if informing the police, this can be done in a non-urgent way, e.g. via telephoning 101.
- Courts have a range of powers including FGM or travel banning orders—these might need to be put in place urgently.
- It is not mandatory to refer to the police if a woman >18 years has had FGM but it is illegal to perform it. See Royal College of Obstetrics and Gynaecology guidance if needed regarding medical reasons for genital surgery and the law.
- Alerting signs to a girl being at risk of or having had FGM include her mother having had the procedure, the family being from a country where FGM is often practised, the girl saying that she is going on a long or special holiday away from school, new or frequent pain or urinary difficulties, walking or standing difficulties, reluctance for medical examination, and/or psychological or behavioural difficulties.
- The incidence of FGM is unclear in the UK. The WHO states that >200 million girls/women have had FGM.
- Local pathways for medical confirmation of FGM involve clinicians who have expertise in CSA-type examinations or gynaecologists.
- Find out about local support options, both medical and via specialist voluntary organizations.
- Be aware that some adult women have appeared in the media saying they consent to FGM; however, this is by far the exception.

Reference

1. Pawlik MC, Kemp A, Maguire S, et al. (2016). Children with burns referred for child abuse evaluation: burn characteristics and co-existent injuries. Child Abuse Negl, 55, 52–61.

Further resources

e-Learning for Healthcare, including communication skills videos. Available at: ℘ https://portal.e-lfh.org.uk/

Government FGM resources. Available at: ℘ https://www.gov.uk/government/publications/female-genital-mutilation-resource-pack/female-genital-mutilation-resource-packgov

Fabricated and induced illness

- ∋Fabricated and induced illness' (FII) and 'Perplexing Presentations' (PP) are diagnostic terms introduced by the RCPCH in 2002, and updated in 2013
- In the UK it replaced Munchausen syndrome by proxy which largely focuses on the adult, though other countries still use that and other terms.
- RCPCH 2009 guidance states that 'Fabricated or Induced Illness by Carers (FII) can cause significant harm to children. FII involves a well child being presented by a carer as ill or disabled, or an ill or disabled child being presented with a more significant problem than he or she has in reality, and suffering harm as a consequence.'
- FII is an area of child protection that is complex and may be stressful to all concerned when trying hard to achieve the best outcome for the child. New RCPCH guidance was published in March 2021 and the following points are in line with this guidance.
- RCPCH introduced the term 'Perplexing Presentations' (PP) in 2013 and the new guidance describes PP as "a situation, when there are alerting signs of possible FII (not yet amounting to likely or actual significant harm), when the actual state of the child's physical, mental health and neurodevelopment is not yet clear, but there is no perceived risk of immediate serious harm to the child's physical health or life".
- The new RCPCH guidance states that 'FII is a clinical situation in which a child is, or is very likely to be, harmed due to parent(s) behaviour and action, carried out in order to convince doctors that the child's state of physical and/or mental health and neurodevelopment is impaired (or more impaired than is actually the case)'.
- FII can (rarely) involve active illness induction (e.g. suffocation, poisoning, etc.) with the aim of then presenting that child as ill.
- Fabrication is more common, may falsify specimens (e.g. adding blood or sugar to urine) or charts/records.
- Providing a false history, either of symptoms or of reported diagnoses made elsewhere, is the most frequent.
- FII is not a category of abuse; it is a medical diagnosis in a child that describes a mechanism leading to abuse.
- Outcome for the child is one of the four abuse categories, usually emotional abuse, neglect, or physical abuse.
- Can result in significant morbidity or death through the illness induction itself or via medical treatment including unnecessary medication or surgery.
- Harm is caused through adversities associated with medical investigations and medical/surgical treatments, including altered feeding and/or elimination routes, endured unnecessarily.
- Psychological harm through being presented as ill, or more ill than they are, loss of education, and socializing opportunities.
- Perpetrator usually the mother but can be the father, can be intergenerational.
- Child may, and often does, have a genuine illness but the child is presented as more ill, or less functionally or developmentally able, than they actually are.

- Common alleged illnesses tend to be those which rely on history to diagnose and where the child could appear well in clinic, e.g. seizures; apparent life-threatening events/brief resolved unexplained events; allergy; feeding difficulties; bowel difficulties; asthma; blood loss; mobility difficulties, particularly musculoskeletal; neurodevelopmental, including autism; false allegations of abuse or accidental overdose.

Perplexing presentations

- In 2013, the RCPCH suggested the additional term of perplexing presentation, to be used when there are alerting signs that make FII a possibility but significant harm is not thought to have been inflicted.
- FII in its full form is thought to be relatively rare, particularly illness induction.
- Perplexing presentations, however, are more common.

Medically unexplained symptoms

FII and perplexing presentations are diagnostic concepts that differ from medically unexplained symptoms in that in medically unexplained symptoms the child's parents agree with medical staff that the symptoms do not have a medical origin and they engage in a rehabilitation plan to support the child.

When to consider FII

- Symptoms not seen in clinic or by other observers, including school (beware genuine situation-specific symptoms).
- Symptoms or signs not found when the parent is absent.
- Symptoms don't match known clinical conditions.
- Investigation results that don't fit with signs or symptoms.
- Unexpectedly poor response to treatment.
- Parental insistence on repeated assessments or invasive investigations or treatments that are not warranted (note: parents do have a reasonable right to a second opinion).
- New symptoms as soon as old ones resolved.
- Parent not consenting to sharing of information with other health professionals, education, or social care.
- Recurrent formal complaints from parents.
- Education staff, relatives, or other carers expressing concern.

Investigation and referral to social care

- Investigation of significant harm should be led by children's social care (CSC), including chairing of strategy meetings; hence, refer to social care when concerned about significant harm/the child is in imminent danger.
- If significant harm is found via a case conference or in court then the category of abuse will be physical, emotional, neglect, or sexual, depending on the circumstances of the case.
- As with other concerns it is possible to refer to CSC without informing parents if it is thought that informing them would endanger the child. In FII there can be circumstances when that would be the case, but not necessarily.

- If significant harm is not thought to have taken place, particularly if the diagnostic situation is not clear, then it may or may not be helpful to refer to social care.
- It can be helpful to refer to social care requesting their help to verify or exclude diagnoses, e.g. when parents do not consent to the doctor obtaining information from other sources such as other relatives or school. The parent's behaviour can therefore be seen as neglectful as it impedes the child's health needs being addressed.

Both FII and perplexing presentations are predominantly health-related conditions, hence the investigation should have a large health component—to investigate and manage the health component. This may need the support of CSC.

It is important to

- Establish how ill the child actually is; what diagnoses, if any, are verifiable, including the diagnosis of FII.
- Establish the current functional level of the child and what the expected functional level of the child would likely be given the verified diagnoses.
- To communicate that information to parents (not a lone clinician—helpful to have a witness).
- Establish and support a rehabilitation plan.
- To monitor and review the rehabilitation plan—possibly long term.

In order to investigate and manage the health component there should be:
- One consultant who is the clinical lead for the clinical components of management.
- Support and input from the named or designated doctor regarding the safeguarding decisions to be made, including deciding if or when to refer to CSC.
- Diagnoses, symptoms, and signs to be verified or refuted based on evidence, such as clinic letters from all health professionals, review of laboratory results, and information from carers and other involved adults including school.
- A chronology may well be helpful as part of this investigation, though is not necessarily needed. CSC may ask for one but this should not delay a referral if such is needed. The referral needs to be detailed and clear.
- A professionals meeting should be held to come to a consensus view among clinicians regarding which diagnoses are verified and the nature of a rehabilitation plan.
- Unless there is reasonable cause not to, then parents are kept informed about the doctor's need to be clear about the facts and diagnoses which are currently causing concern (either at the level of perplexing presentations or FII).
- The outcome of the investigation into the child's diagnoses, developmental level, and level of daily functioning could be that all, some, or none of these as currently presented are verified.

- The level of further support, including the need for CSC support, will depend on the parent's reaction to this consensus opinion and ultimately on the underlying motivation for parental actions, such as:
  - Parental anxiety combined with lack of understanding.
  - Pecuniary motives such as disability/mobility funding or other benefits, either governmental or through social media.
  - Parental mental health difficulties, including personality disorder or somatization.
  - Fixed parental beliefs.
- Factors which may contribute to the complexity and time-consuming nature of investigating perplexing presentations and FII include poor healthcare communication arrangements such as lack of copy letters and separate healthcare records systems.

Child sexual abuse

- CSA is the fourth most common reason for a child being subject to a safeguarding plan, ~4% or 5%.
- Of adults aged 18–24 years when asked, 11% considered themselves as having been sexually abused as children.
- CSA can be either contact or non-contact.
- *Contact CSA* includes assault by penetration (e.g. rape or oral sex) or non-penetrative acts such as masturbation, kissing, rubbing, and touching outside of clothing.
- Penetration may be with the penis, digital, or with an object.
- May or may not involve a high level of violence.
- In the UK any sexual activity with a child <13 years is unlawful as they are deemed unable to consent.
- In the UK, sexual activity in 13–17-year-olds may be CSA or child sexual exploitation (CSE) and may warrant referral to social care, depending on circumstances. Discussion with a senior colleague is advised.
- *Non-contact CSA* includes looking at or being involved in the production of sexual images, watching sexual activities, encouraging children to behave in sexually inappropriate ways, or grooming a child in preparation for abuse.
- Sexual abuse can take place online, plus technology can be used to facilitate offline abuse.
- All children, both girls and boys, are at risk of CSA.
- Children with disabilities are at increased risk.
- Perpetrators can be men, women, or other children.
- Child perpetrators should also be seen as victims of CSA.
- Most CSA goes unreported.
- Most CSA is carried out by somebody known to the child or family.
- There is a close link between CSA and long-term physical and mental health issues (see ⊃ p. 326).

Alerting features of CSA

- Disclosure by the child or young person.
- Unexplained anogenital bleeding or discharge, trauma to posterior fourchette.
- Sexually transmitted infection, especially in a child <13 years.
- Behavioural change, including increased anxiety or aggression.
- Displaying sexually inappropriate behaviours or knowledge inappropriate for age.
- Soiling or incontinence without another obvious cause.
- Change in school attendance or academic performance.
- Maladaptive stress relief activities, including self-harm and substance misuse.

Response to concerns of CSA

- Keep careful notes of history and examination, particularly of any disclosure by the child and of the referral to social care.
- If concerned about CSA but unsure then discuss with senior safeguarding colleagues +/– local CSA clinicians regarding next steps.

- Both acute and non-acute/historical CSA concerns should have a multiagency approach including a strategy discussion.
- Medical assessment of CSA should be by clinicians who have specific skills and competencies which include taking forensic samples and who are working within a recognized CSA service, may be a Sexual Assault Referral Centre.
- Most paediatricians will not have such skills, though both community- and acute-based paediatricians are encouraged to gain expertise through additional training; see ℛ https://www.rcpch.ac.uk/resources/facu lty-forensic-legal-medicine-fflm-guidance.

Acute CSA examination

- Timing of examination in acute CSA should be within 24 hours as rapid healing can mask physical signs and forensic evidence can be lost.
- Retain clothing for forensic evidence.
- Advise not to wash if possible before examination.
- Sexually transmitted infections, blood-borne virus screening, and relevant treatment/s should be addressed, may involve genitourinary medicine clinic.
- Post-exposure prophylaxis to HIV (72 hours maximum) and pregnancy prevention should be addressed.
- If urgent surgery required in context of possible CSA, then liaise with CSA/forensic clinician on call regarding preservation of evidence if at all possible.

Non-acute/historical CSA

- An assessment and examination can still be helpful.
- The timing is not urgent but should be reasonable.

CSA examination

- Will only be carried out with appropriate consent.
- Will only be carried out with assent of the child.
- Genital examination does not always take place.
- Holistic paediatric history and examination, not just of the alleged CSA.
- Should have access to colposcopy/photographic documentation.
- If forensic samples are indicated, these should be managed in line with Faculty of Forensic and Legal Medicine guidance and chain of evidence.
- Holistic nature includes reassurance of normal anatomy, general health as appropriate.
- Includes access to or signposting to psychological support.

Further resources

See 'Physical signs of child sexual abuse' for details of examination where there are concerns about CSA. Available at: ℛ https://childprotection.rcpch.ac.uk/resources/physical-signs-of-child-sexual-abuse/

Child exploitation

Includes child sexual exploitation (CSE) and child criminal exploitation (CCE); associated activities include county lines and child trafficking. Linked to modern slavery.

- Exploitation of the child or young person is facilitated though their vulnerability, be that due to intrinsic child factors, family factors, contextual environmental factors, or a combination.
- There is an imbalance of power in the relationship which is exploited by the abuser in order to control the young person.
- Can be difficult to escape CSE and CCE due to threats and blackmail.
- Online child and parent voluntary sector advice and support may be helpful in addition to statutory services.

Vulnerability factors for all forms of exploitation

- Direct childhood adversity factors including emotionally abusive relationship with parent figure, neglect, physical abuse, CSA, and poor mental health in the C&YP.
- Family adversity such as parental separation, bereavement, parental mental health difficulties, parental substance misuse, and parental incarceration.
- Learning or social interaction difficulties in child (or parent).
- Lack of school access through exclusion, part time timetable, or educational neglect.
- Living in a neighbourhood where there is gang or CSE activity.
- Friendship group involved in exploitative activities.

Grooming

- Grooming is associated with exploitation, whereby C&YP are manipulated into forming a trusting relationship with another person who then exploits and abuses them, often sexually but can be for criminal activity.
- Grooming can be in person or online.
- Someone they know or a stranger.
- Takes the form of a romantic relationship, mentor, or dominant figure.
- Can involve gifts, outings, and positive attention.
- May increasingly isolate C&YP from friends and family.
- Increasing control over C&YP's thoughts and actions.
- C&YP usually unaware they have been groomed and may vehemently deny such.

Signs of grooming and exploitation

- Increasingly secretive.
- Unexplained gifts and outings.
- Much older boyfriend or girlfriend.
- Alcohol or substance misuse, may be new or increased.
- Missing from home or school episodes.
- Sexualized behaviours, out of keeping with age.
- Signs of distress including self-harm or emotional distress.
- Sexually transmitted diseases or urinary infections.

- Traumatic injuries from physical or sexual violence.
- Can result in long-term poor mental health and substance misuse.

Child sexual exploitation

- CSE is a form of CSA. It occurs where an individual or group takes advantage of an imbalance of power to coerce, manipulate, or deceive a child or young person under the age of 18 into sexual activity (a) in exchange for something the victim needs or wants, and/or (b) for the financial advantage or increased status of the perpetrator or facilitator (UK Department for Education, CSA definition[1]).
- Can be online or in person.
- 17-year-olds can be victims of CSE as consent is coerced.
- Four types have been described, peer on peer, older boyfriend or girlfriend, via an organized network, or via a person in a position of responsibility such as a sports coach etc.
- Can be linked to gang activity, either with CSE being the main activity of the gang or as form of power and control within a gang whose main focus is other forms of criminal activity.
- Perpetrators not always older than victim, can be the same sex and may have originally been victims who are then encouraged to find other victims.
- Can involve trafficking either between countries, counties, or neighbourhoods of a city.

Child criminal exploitation

- Child is pressured or manipulated into cooperating with criminal activity, some comparisons with grooming in CSE.
- Activities include carrying drugs/weapons, carrying out violent acts.
- Often involves gangs ranging from informal peer groups to named street gangs or organized criminal gangs.
- Threats and criminal convictions make it difficult to escape that way of life.
- *County lines*—supply chain using children as young as 11 years to transport drugs from large urban areas to small towns, run by (very) organized criminals.
- *Cuckooing*—coercing (vulnerable) adults into allowing their accommodation to be used to store drugs or to accommodate children or other members of the county lines operation.

Child trafficking

- The illegal movement of a child from one country to another or from one part of a country to another.
- Purpose—various types of exploitation, e.g. CSE, CCE, modern slavery, child marriage, forced marriage, and illegal adoption.
- All child trafficking is child abuse, along with a multitude of abusive acts they are also likely to suffer including neglect in all its forms.

Modern slavery

- Affects adults and children, often linked to human/child trafficking.

- Main types: labour exploitation, sexual exploitation, domestic servitude, criminal exploitation, and organ harvesting.
- Some statistics suggest ~50% is labour exploitation—likely adult figures.
- *National Referral Mechanism (NRM)*—government-run system for support and protection.[2]
- In 2018, 23% of referrals to the NRM were UK nationals.
- Always needs a multiagency response.
- Difficult to leave due to threats to self, friends, or family. May not see self as victim.
- Children involved in criminal activities including moving drugs, cannabis cultivation, and benefit fraud.
- C&YP often hidden, rarely leave the accommodation, and reluctant to give family history or education details.
- Visits to health and dental care can be opportunities to establish basic details, hence reluctance or inability to provide such can be *alerting signs*. May sense abnormal relationship between C&YP and accompanying adult.
- Beware that adults may not be the child's parents.
- Don't directly challenge adults—seek advice from police or social care—may need to be urgent.

Radicalization

Radicalization can also be a form of child exploitation, with similar risk factors and methods. Can involve being persuaded to hold violent extremist views.

Contextual safeguarding

- Looks at factors outside the family that increase young people's risk of abuse such as CSE, CCE, etc.
- Risks from peers, within schools, online, and in neighbourhoods.
- Systemic factors including building and open spaces design, and school and transport systems.

Cultural and sex-linked abuse

Respect for cultural backgrounds is important but should never prevent child abuse being identified or acted upon. Examples of culturally related abuse include the following.

- 'Honour-based' killing: ~12 per year in UK; often women or teenage girls (can be boys) murdered by family member for supposedly bringing dishonour to family or religion; take concerns seriously.
- Child marriage: consider absence from school, change in behaviours, pregnancy.
- Breast ironing/flattening: practised by some African cultures. Female family members binding or pounding breast tissue with heavy and/or hot objects to damage breast tissue in order to delay or prevent its development. Allegedly to protect the pubescent girl from attracting sexual advances.
- Witchcraft beliefs: being accused of being possessed by demons and/or being beaten for such (emotional abuse and/or physical abuse).

- Persecution for severe learning difficulties or other disabilities in some societies.
- Persecution of people with albinism: in some African countries people with Albinism are mutilated (dead or alive) for their body parts which are used in witchcraft or illegal medicinal practices. Some live in protected communities for safety. Also linked to infanticide.
- FGM: see ➲ pp. 577–9.

References

1. Department for Education (2017). Child Sexual Exploitation: Definition and a Guide for Practitioners, Local Leaders and Decision Makers Working to Protect Children from Child Sexual Exploitation. Available at: ℘ https://assets.publishing.service.gov.uk/government/uploads/system/uploads/attachment_data/file/591903/CSE_Guidance_Core_Document_13.02.2017.pdf
2. GOV.UK. National Referral Mechanism statistics: ℘ https://www.gov.uk/government/collections/national-referral-mechanism-statistics

Further resources

NSPCC (various topics including child exploitation): ℘ https://www.nspcc.org.uk/
Office for National Statistics. Child abuse in England and Wales: ℘ https://www.ons.gov.uk/peoplepopulationandcommunity/crimeandjustice/bulletins/childabuseinenglandandwales/march2020

Disability and child abuse

- C&YP with SEND are at increased risk of being abused.
- Data from the England and Wales Crime Survey year ending March 2019 found that adults who had a disability were much more likely to have experienced abuse before 16 years of age (32%) compared to those who did not have a disability (19%).
- C&YP (and adults) with learning difficulties are more vulnerable to all forms of exploitation, particularly CSE.
- Adults with learning difficulties are also more at risk of exploitation including modern slavery and of their homes being exploited (see → pp. 587–8). Note these adults might also be parents.
- Can be difficult to get a clear history from a child with learning difficulties or developmental language disorder, or for such to be taken seriously. Children with SEND more likely to say things without understanding the meaning or consequences, making parents and the child more vulnerable. This doesn't mean abuse didn't happen—can be very complex.
- Some children with autism have related sensory processing difficulties and may experience pain differently, not displaying as much distress as a typically developing child for a given injury. Such a possibility would need careful assessment.
- C&YP with some forms of disability are in need of intimate care and are very dependent on adults—may have a range of carers from within and outside of the family.
- See → pp. 570–1 for bruising pattern in wheelchair users.
- Behavioural change might be part of the underlying disability, diagnosis, or pain, but the possibility that they may be distressed behaviours in response to some form abuse needs to be borne in mind.
- Updated neglect assessment tools may not yet be validated for families where there is a child with a disability, e.g. Graded Care Profile; historically, a version for such children was produced.
- Parenting can be difficult anyway, but can be harder for parents of children with additional needs, especially where support from agencies and extended family is limited.
- Evidencing neglect in such circumstances is difficult, but practitioners should keep the child's lived experience in mind and how other families in similar circumstances are able to make reasonable adjustments in order to adequately support their child.
- Work in a multiagency way to support families but also to identify neglect. Put action plans into place to support the child and family and review their success or otherwise.
- Work with parents and professionals, including teachers, to help to hear the child's voice/understand and document their lived experience, particularly if concerns regarding *unaddressed health or developmental needs* such as:
  - Pain from various causes including spasticity or dental caries.
  - Hunger and failure to thrive.
  - Distressed behaviours from some form of abuse.

- Not promoting independence in activities of daily living—including feeding and toileting when the child is capable of achieving these.
- Drowsiness from inadequate sleep.
- Obesity associated with failure to engage in remedial measures.
- Many conditions vary in how much they respond to treatment but safeguarding should be considered when reasonable treatments, interventions, compliance with therapies, etc. are not being engaged with by parents or other carers and failure to do so is significantly impacting the child's well-being.
- Be as objective as possible regarding evidencing nutritional neglect. This is harder when condition-specific growth charts are not readily available or accepted locally, e.g. CP. Access to appropriate growth measuring equipment is also important.
- Be aware of children acting as *young carers* for parents or siblings with significant health needs; refer for local support.
- Remember that the best interest of the child is of primary importance, whether that be for a healthy, typically developing child, a child with disability or complex health needs, or a child receiving palliative care.
- The situation can be complex if parental wishes do not align with the best interests of the child as seen by health professionals. Identify if there are any safeguarding issues or areas of conflict; seek advice and support.

Further resources

Linney M, Hain RDW, Wilkinson D, et al. (2019). Achieving consensus advice for paediatricians and other health professionals: on prevention, recognition and management of conflict in paediatric practice. Arch Dis Child, 104, 413–16. Available at: ℜ https://adc.bmj.com/content/104/5/413

Domestic abuse

- Sometimes termed domestic violence, but *domestic abuse* (DA) more accurately allows for the range of abusive acts, including physical and sexual violence, emotional, social, or financial control.
- Witnessing DA is child abuse and is the reason for many children being on a safeguarding plan for emotional abuse.
- Children are affected not only by seeing or hearing DA but by seeing the effects on a parent's physical and mental well-being.
- Effects for children include a wide range of emotional and behavioural problems such as aggression, withdrawal, sleeping, eating and toileting difficulties, distressed behaviours, and even suicide.
- DA is common. In a Crime Survey for England and Wales year ending March 2019, 5.7% of 16–74-year-olds reported experiencing DA, 4.2% of those by current or former intimate partners and 2% by other family members.
- In 2019, 8.4% of women and 4.2% men aged 16–59 years reported DA in the UK. Higher rates are reported in other countries.
- Both men and women can be perpetrators, either in heterosexual or same-sex couples. However, most DA victims are women with men as the perpetrator. Both partners of a couple can be perpetrators.
- DA affects all social, professional, and religious groups.
- Calls to the national DA helpline in the UK increased 65% during the Spring 2020 Covid-19 lockdown, particularly as that lockdown eased and victims were more able to seek help. Escaping DA became a stated reason to leave the house during subsequent lockdowns.
- Christmas and other holidays are times when support mechanisms outside of the family are limited, leading to increased risk of DA.
- Sometimes children are perpetrators of DA towards parents. *Adolescent to parent violence and abuse* includes children <16 years of age.

Professional response to child protection and safeguarding

This chapter has so far mainly focused on the clinical aspects of child protection. In order to contribute effectively to safeguarding children, however, paediatricians need more than clinical knowledge and acumen; they also need appropriate skills and behaviours to work in services that deliver high levels of communication and team and interagency working. Paediatricians engage in safeguarding children both in day-to-day clinical work where safeguarding concerns may arise, as well as in services specifically set up to assess child protection concerns.

Further resources

Royal College of Nursing (2019). Safeguarding Children and Young People: Roles and Competencies for Healthcare Staff (4th edn) [known as the Intercollegiate Document]. Available at: ℘ https://www.rcn.org.uk/professional-development/publications/pub-007366

Child protection medical assessment

- A specific medical assessment undertaken at the request of social care or police to aid their investigation, usually due to concerns about a possible physical injury or severe, acute neglect. In England sometimes called a Section 47 assessment. CSA assessments might also be seen as a child protection medical assessment.
- RCPCH/Child Protection Special Interest Group (CPSIG) standards and good practice guidance for child protection medical assessment services can be found at ℜ https://childprotection.rcpch.ac.uk/resources/serv ice-delivery-standards/.
- The medical assessment is holistic, though primarily aims to provide an *opinion* regarding the nature of symptoms and signs, particularly regarding visible examination findings, e.g. whether they represent an injury and if so, how that injury might have been incurred.
- The child's safety is paramount and any necessary medical treatment should be provided first.
- A paediatrician or other senior clinician should attend a *strategy meeting* (often virtually or joining by phone) to establish the need or otherwise for a child protection medical assessment, social care concerns, expectations, and background information.
- Consent is needed for a child protection medical assessment and should be a topic discussed at the strategy meeting. If there is no parental consent but concerns are very high then social care may apply for an Emergency Protection Order (EPO).
- The paediatrician should engage with the strategy discussion to help establish the level of safeguarding concern in that particular situation.
- May need further information such as photographs of furniture, toys, etc. related to an alleged set of circumstances; ideally these can be brought to the planned child protection medical assessment if identified at the strategy meeting.
- Child protection medical assessment should be conducted within 24 hours of referral to health from CSC/police.
- Take a history from parent/carers or other relevant adults. Cover current concerns, also birth, past medical, and developmental history (see ➋ p. 234).
- Endeavour to hear the voice of the child, talk to them without parent present.
- Need a chaperone for history and examination (health staff for examination).
- Examination should be a top-to-toe physical examination (including oral and ENT), or as much as there is consent and assent for. Measure, plot, and interpret height, weight, and BMI.
- Record the child's demeanour and interaction with parents.
- Look for and record signs of neglect, including dental neglect—consider obtaining a dental assessment.
- Document all visible findings.

- Investigations may include blood tests or radiology (if non-accidental injury is suspected—skeletal survey in a child <2 years, CT head for <1-year-olds) (see ℘ https://www.rcr.ac.uk/publication/radiological-invest igation-suspected-physical-abuse-children).
- Review health records for potential concerning history, including evidence of medical neglect.
- Documentation, reports, and opinion—see following sections.
- If significant concerns for a child, it may be appropriate to see their *siblings*, particularly younger siblings, for a child protection medical assessment as well.
- All clinicians involved with child protection medical assessments should attend regular *peer review* meetings where their practice can be reviewed on a regular basis by colleagues in a challenging but supportive manner, including the phrasing of opinions in reports.

CSA examinations details are not covered in this chapter. Paediatricians wishing to undertake this work are directed to specific training courses, e.g. those provided by RCPCH and Faculty of Forensic and Legal Medicine, and to specialist texts such as 'Physical Signs of Child Sexual Abuse' (also known as the 'Purple Book') published by the RCPCH (see ℘ https:// childprotection.rcpch.ac.uk/resources/physical-signs-of-child-sexual-abuse/).

Documentation

For all documentation:
- Contemporaneous documentation is important in all contexts, whether obviously safeguarding at the time or not. When/who made an entry should be clear—don't use generic logins on digital systems.
- Retain email if clinical information/decisions (including date/who sent/received it) in health records.
- Routinely identify and record who accompanies a child to scheduled/unscheduled care and which school is attended.
- Benefits include identifying vulnerable children out of education, illegal private fostering arrangements; young people accompanied by non-family members may be linked to exploitation.
- Evidence of concerning interactions or presentation of child/family/accompanying adult should be documented, just as much as that of history, clinical concern, and injuries if present.

For a child protection medical assessment, in addition:
- Use a standard proforma—likely to be completed by hand. Store in health record.
- Drawings and photographs are important evidence to support you later when explaining why you did or did not think the significant visible findings were a safeguarding concern.
- Record visible findings/injuries via body map drawings, annotated with dimensions and numbered corresponding to the subsequent report. May need more detail on a freehand diagram—photographs may not reflect all you see so drawings are still important.
- Record interpreter's ID and language used.

Photographic documentation—for child protection medical assessments

- Aim to photograph all significant visible findings—ideally use a clinical photographer for a child protection medical assessment service but can be a clinician.
- If a clinician takes photographs in a child protection medical assessment service then they should link with a clinical photography department in the same or another trust for governance and image processing. RAW files preferable to JPEG—maintenance of image detail when magnified. Ensure secure storage.
- Take specific consent for photography, including that it will be part of the child's health record, will be made available to peer review, and that social care or the courts may ask for a copy in the future.
- Photography sequence—identification of child as first and last image in sequence (consent form or possibly facial image), anatomical image (so you can see which part of the body it is), detailed image of visible finding with L-shaped ruler—not pressing on skin as that distorts skin contours, ruler not hiding any of the visible finding.
- Consider if an image of the injury with the alleged implement or an overlying hand would help to record size/shape match.
- Don't leave images on the camera—upload to a secure system then delete off camera.

- Don't delete images from a sequence—may raise questions in court regarding missing evidence.
- Never include the face in an image of intimate parts (breast, anogenital).
- If appropriate facilities not currently available, can use NHS Digital approved Pando app as images not held on device.
- Colposcope used in CSA photographic documentation, including video.

Reports and opinions

- Clinic letters and discharge summaries are all reports which could become or contain evidence.
- *Professional opinion*—that of the examining clinician.
- *Expert opinion*—that of an expert commissioned by a legal team or the court.

Provisional/interim/initial findings report from child protection medical assessments

- The child protection medical assessment opinion conveyed verbally to the social worker/police *at the time of the assessment* should be *backed up in writing* and a copy given to the attending professional/s.
- Can be handwritten, needs identifiers of child/clinician/organization.
- Sufficiently detailed to allow safeguarding measures to be taken that day.
- Keep a copy in the notes.
- There may be email conversations too which contain medical opinions in the form of answers to social workers' questions. Copies should be kept in the child's health record.

Child protection medical assessment full typed report

- Deliver to social care within 10 working days or sooner if needed, e.g. EPO court proceedings. CSC will have already had your written provisional report.
- This is a report for social care, primarily to describe your assessment and to state your opinion on the questions posed by social care who are enquiring into whether or not the child has suffered or is likely to suffer significant harm through some form of abuse.
- Be professional, objective, fair, and respectful. Remember that this report is likely to be given to the parents by social care, particularly if going to case conference.
- If quoting the child or parent then use quotation marks, and make sure you repeat the statements accurately. Clearly distinguish between what was said to you (what you heard) and what you were told was said.

Contains

- Your details (name, General Medical Council number, qualifications, role, experience, supervising consultant name, health provider organization name).
- Circumstances of child protection medical assessment (date, time, location, people present and roles, consent taken, how referral came about).
- History from social care.
- History from parent or carer regarding the injury/incident in question.
- History from child.

- Birth and past medical/developmental history—from parental report and notes review.
  - Brief, though sufficient to set context for assessment, e.g. significant diagnoses, including neurodevelopmental diagnoses or ongoing assessments such as autism.
  - State if history of coagulopathy or frequent fractures in child or family is present or not and of previous child deaths.
  - Expand if relevant issues, e.g. evidence of frequent injuries or ingestions or inappropriate health-seeking behaviours, either excessive or suggestive of medical neglect. Previous child protection medicals.
  - If there is evidence suggestive of inappropriate health-seeking behaviour then say so—don't assume those who read your report will make the same interpretation that you do or will read between the lines—they often won't. You will have come to your opinion through your medical experience and expertise that the main readership of your report won't have.
  - State where information is from—parents told you or medical records. Do they match?
- Family and social history—consider how much family and social history is needed in order to set the context. Much of this is likely to have been given to you by social care so you don't need to report it all back to them.
- Examination/observation findings (positive and negative):
  - Parent–child interaction/child's demeanour and behaviour/ presentation of child, e.g. clothing/hygiene/growth parameters and centile—interpret them, is child's growth normal or not?
  - Remember who your readership is and if detail of general systems examination needed then say why and what it means, otherwise no need to put this detail in report—'general examination normal' will suffice. If baby or injury to head then more specifics such as ENT examination or frenula important.
  - You do need all the detail of the top-to-toe examination in your records though—on the proforma.
- Injuries/visible findings list with descriptions and dimensions—numbered corresponding to your line drawing annotations. Can sometimes add in brief opinions here such as 'Injury 4: there was a brown bruise, approximately 1 cm diameter to left shin—likely to have been incurred accidentally during normal play as stated by parent and child'. This then leaves the opinion section free to concentrate on the more significant findings. Don't do this for the concerning injuries though, just use the opinion section, or if you do comment elsewhere in the report, make sure they are all consistent.
- Investigation details, what was carried out, results to date, and what is still outstanding. Interpretation of results. An addendum may be needed for later results, parents should have this information too as much as possible.
- State if photographic documentation carried out.
- Summary—briefly pull together significant positive or negative/ concerning aspects of history and examination.
- Opinion—see following section.

- Any onward referrals or treatment given.
- Discharge details, e.g. home with parent (which), or another family member on a Section 20, or Police Protection Order (PPO), etc.

Opinion

- Provide an opinion, not just a summary of events and examination.
- State what your opinion is regarding the likelihood of how an injury has been incurred or whether the child has suffered some form of abuse or not, based on your history and examination.
- Likelihood—is it more likely than not that an event or abuse has taken place?
- Likelihood is similar to probability which is a mathematical concept. In family courts, the test for abuse having taken place is 'on the balance of probability' hence your opinion also needs to be considered in those terms. So, if in your mind you are 51% or more sure that an event has taken place (such as a particular mechanism for an injury, or that medical neglect is present), then you can say that in your opinion it is more likely than not that ... has happened.
- Alternatively, you could say that on the balance of probability that ... has happened; however, note some teachings are that we should not use the words 'balance of probability', yet many clinicians find no issue with using this phrase in the courts.
- You may want to say 'very likely' or 'highly probable', depending on how sure you are.
- The standard of proof in family law (e.g. whether the child needs to be subject to an order/go to foster care etc.) is 'on the balance of probabilities'.
- Criminal courts (e.g. whether a person is guilty or assault) use a much higher level of test—'beyond all reasonable doubt'.
- State how you arrived at your opinion—as a judge said in a teaching session, 'Show your workings out', i.e. your reasoning. For example, you may have already described injury 2 as consisting of linear red marks with pale areas of skin between and given the dimensions. In the opinion you may say 'The pattern of injury 2, is the shape and size of an open adult hand and is likely to be a slap mark'.
- See section on physical abuse regarding aspects to consider when opining on an injury (see ➋ pp. 570–9).
- You were not there (usually) at the time of the injury, so in general you are giving an opinion on the likely mechanism of an injury, not who did it or with what intent. You should though state whether any alleged mechanism is likely to have caused the injury.
- State if your opinion relates to aspects of the history or the examination or both, e.g. there may not be any injuries to see but there might be concerning aspects of the history that you wish to comment on, or concerning parent–child interactions observed.
- Lack of visible signs of an injury might be due to the possibility of healing during the time lapse from the alleged incident; if that is a possibility or is likely, then say so/which.

- Beware that something being a 'possibility' is different from it being 'likely'. A possibility could mean a 10% chance, being likely or probable is taken to mean a >50% chance.
- Be as clear as possible and try to be helpful (social workers have a difficult job to do and we are all trying to get the best for the child and family) but don't stray beyond your area of expertise or the facts!
- If it really isn't possible to state whether or not a visible finding is of concern or not, then say so.
- Try to avoid words like 'inconclusive' or 'unascertained' as these may be interpreted in a different way by your reader than how you meant them. Better to say in some form of sentence such as 'There are no specific features regarding the history or examination of injury 3 so unfortunately I am unable to say if it represents a safeguarding concern or not'.
- Interpret investigation findings in relation to your opinion. A normal skeletal survey may make no difference to your opinion that the baby has suffered physical abuse—if that is the case then say so, don't leave social workers or lawyers to read between the lines.
- Similarly, if the pattern of bruising or behavioural history is suggestive of CSA then say so and recommend further assessment as appropriate.
- While the report to social care is not intended as a court report, they are often provided to court by social care. The more detailed and clear you are in your opinion, and the reasoning for that opinion, then in general the less likely it is that you will be asked to answer further questions in a court report or to attend court.
- It is sometimes appropriate to refer to the evidence base, particularly systematic reviews such as RCPCH Child Protection Evidence (formerly Core Info) or the RCPCH Physical Signs of Child Sexual Abuse. This can be particularly helpful regarding the likelihood of abuse associated with bruising to particular body sites.

Court report

- Make sure you get a letter (or email) of instruction; this should tell you what they are asking for and may take the form of specific questions.
- If related to a child you have seen in clinic or for unscheduled care, then a chronology of your involvement is likely to be needed (who referred, when you saw the child, key points of what you were told, what you found, what you did, etc.), including the reasoning for your actions at key points.
- If this relates to a child who you saw for a child protection medical assessment, then the court may well have seen your initial report addressed to the social worker. The further information the court requires may therefore be clarification on specific points.
- Stick to answering the questions and don't stray off the point.
- Don't get caught out—it's not possible to age bruises when a lawyer asks you any more than it was when the social worker asked.
- Don't include third-party or hearsay information, only what you heard, you saw, or you did. This might include you seeing a letter from another clinician and what that stated.
- Try to avoid medical language but if it is needed, then explain it.

- It may be that the court wants a specific report regarding a child protection medical assessment rather than using the social care one. In which case, the structure is similar to the report for social care but without the additional detail of birth, past history, family and social history, etc. Important points like relevant underlying diagnoses should be included, e.g. the child has CP and is a wheelchair user. Limit the history to what you were told by whom and the key aspects of the examination. As always, take care to be clear in your opinion, and to show your reasoning for your opinion (see previous 'Opinion' section).
- As with the report for social care, start with your standard paragraph about you, e.g.:
  - My name is Dr … MB ChB, MRCPCH. I have worked at St Elsewhere Hospital as a consultant community paediatrician for 3 years and have 8 years' experience of seeing children for child protection medical assessments. I am on the child protection rota once a week and I attend monthly peer review. My General Medical Council number is … .
- Format the document in numbered paragraphs and pages. Each page needs three identifiers.
- State your involvement with the child—e.g. seen in community paediatric clinic due to referral from the GP because of [xxx] concern. Or you were on call for child protection and the referral was from social care with [xxx] concern.
- If you are answering specific questions, then it is best to quote the question and answer, e.g.:
  - Question: 'In your opinion, could injury 3 in your report to social care dated dd/mm/yyyy have been incurred by bumping into the sofa and if not why not?'
  - Answer: No, it is very unlikely that injury 3 was incurred by bumping into the sofa. Injury 3 is extensive bruising around the right eye which is likely to have been incurred through blunt force applied to an area that is normally well protected from injury. Photographs of the sofa shown to me by …, the social worker, show the sofa to be soft with no hard edges visible. Billy was non-mobile at the time so would only have bumped into anything when being carried. No history of injury was given at the time of my assessment.'
- Finish with the statement 'The information in this report is true to the best of my knowledge'.

Police/witness statements

Police often obtain your report from social care; however, they may ask for a statement. This will be on specific numbered paper or a digital file that they will forward to you. Similar to the court report, confine yourself to your involvement, not hearsay or the family or medical history unless absolutely necessary in order to address the issue at hand.

Going to court

Sometimes you will be called to court, despite having provided a good, clear report. You are there purely to assist the court in terms of your medical evidence. You are not there to advocate for the child or to win the case.

In advance prepare by
- Going on a court skills course. You can also ask to visit the court to familiarize yourself.
- Check if this is a family court or a criminal court—the test for evidence is very different. The family courts use balance of probability and the criminal courts use beyond reasonable doubt (see ➋ pp. 599–600).
- Respond promptly regarding availability, though there may not be a choice.
- Work out where the court is at least the day before and how you are going to get there in good time. Factor in time to settle once arrived, though also be prepared for long waits.
- May need to take an anatomical model for demonstration in CSA case.
- Read all your reports, look at the images and line drawings in advance to remind yourself—the lawyers will have gone over it all in detail and picked up on any discrepancy either within or between documents, including handwritten notes and may use these to discredit your testimony. Avoid these in the first place.
- Consider practising answering questions on the case with a colleague.

On the day
- Dress respectfully and professionally, turn off your phone when in the courtroom.
- Tell the clerk that you have arrived.
- Take copies of your reports—to further remind yourself while waiting to be called.
- The court will have copies of all reports in a paginated bundle (big folder with numbered pages and paragraphs) and you may be asked to look at a specific page and paragraph and to comment on it.
- You will be asked to take an oath—choose from a religious oath or to affirm/non-religious.
- You need to confirm who you are and your qualifications.
- You will be asked questions from the prosecution (local authority usually), defence (parents usually), and the guardian ad litem team who represent the child.
- Address answers to the judge—you should be told how to do this, e.g. 'Your Honour' or in higher courts 'My Lord' or 'My Lady'.
- Take care over your answer, be as clear as possible, and beware an adversarial style of questioning from barristers. You may ask for a question to be repeated if necessary.
- As per your report, don't stray outside your expertise and if you don't know then say so. Remember you are there as a professional witness, not an expert witness.
- You will be told when you may leave the court—bow your head briefly to the judge on leaving.

Expert witnesses are commissioned by the court to address specific issues such as further opinion on a bruise, X-ray, or metabolic bone disease. Their report will draw on their experience but also a review and interpretation of the research literature.

Legal framework and children's social care processes

The laws, governmental guidance, terminology, and timescales vary between the four nations of the UK and beyond, though the principles and process are largely similar. NSPCC Learning provides a helpful summary of child protection systems for the four nations of the UK (see ℜ https://learning.nspcc.org.uk/child-protection-system).

The current safeguarding framework in England is described here:

Children Act 1989

The Children Act 1989 provides the key principle that children are best looked after within their families, with their parents playing a full part in their lives, unless compulsory intervention in family life is necessary. It provides the legal basis of CSC assessments and orders:

- *Section 17*. The local authority has a duty to safeguard and promote the welfare of children in their area. *Children in need* are children who need 'local authority services to achieve or maintain a reasonable standard of health or development. Need local authority services to prevent significant or further harm to health or development.'
- *Section 20*. The local authority has a duty to find accommodation for a child, this can be done without a court order but parents must be agreeable. In child protection circumstances, parents may sign a Section 20 agreement regarding the placement of a child, often with a relative. Parents retain full *parental responsibility*—i.e. the local authority does not have any parental responsibility.
- *Section 47*. A Section 47 enquiry means that CSC must carry out an investigation when they have 'reasonable cause to suspect that a child who lives, or is found, in their area is suffering, or is likely to suffer, significant harm'. Needs to be completed within 15 working days. A child protection medical assessment might be requested as part of that assessment.
- *Police Protection Order (PPO)*. In extreme/urgent circumstances, a police officer can remove a child from their home/enforce stay in hospital if at imminent risk. Lasts up to 72 hours, parental responsibility is not shared.

> Note that your child protection typed report may be needed urgently for CSC to apply for an EPO before the 72 hours of the PPO expires!

- *Emergency Protection Order (EPO)*. CSC can apply to court for an EPO, lasts up to 8 days, can be extended for another 7 days. Gives LA shared parental responsibility with parents so the local authority can remove the child and can give consent for a child protection medical assessment.
- *Interim care order and full care orders*. The local authority can apply for a range of care orders relating to the Children Act 1989, such as an interim care order, full care order, or a supervision order which are longer lasting and allow the local authority to share parental responsibility.

Children's social care assessment and processes

- Anybody can make a referral to CSC (or NSPCC) if they are worried about significant harm to a child. Members of the public may remain anonymous but professionals may not.
- Information about local referral pathways, phone numbers, etc. should be available on the local authority website and ideally your health provider website.
- Telephone referrals should be backed up in writing, stating specifically what you are worried about, your actions to support the child and family and what you are requesting from CSC. Keep details in health record.
- It is good practice to seek consent before sharing information or making a referral to CSC unless to do so puts the child at risk.
- Information can though be shared without consent; information governance laws do not prevent sharing of information when there are concerns for a child's welfare.
- *Multiagency Safeguarding Hub (MASH)*—is the one 'front door' for safeguarding referrals to be received and triaged by social care. Supported by health and police regarding information gathering and strategy meetings. One working day for decision and action.
- The *triage decision* might be that an *assessment* is needed to establish whether or not the child is suffering or is likely to suffer from significant harm. That might be under Section 17—at child in need(CIN) or a Section 47 assessment.
- A medical assessment such as a child protection medical assessment may be requested to inform that assessment.
- *Interim safeguarding measures* may need to be put in place to protect the child while the assessment is being conducted, e.g. the alleged abuser agreeing to leave the house; parents voluntarily agree to allow the child to live with other relatives; for another relative to move in as a protective factor while the assessment is undertaken; an *EPO* to be applied for from the court or a *PPO* is put in place by the police while awaiting an EPO.
- The referrer to MASH is informed of the triage decision and actions which can range from no further action, referral to Early Help, Child and Family Assessment, and Section 47 assessment, to immediate removal of child. See Fig. 11.2.
- As a result of the assessment, the child may need a different level of support than they were originally receiving—see following section.

Thresholds of need and response

- Children with different levels of need for social support and intervention in family life are said to be at levels 1–4 of need; that level may change depending on amount of concern at the time (Fig. 11.2).
- Higher levels are governed by statutory assessments and even compulsory intervention in family life (court orders) if evidence is deemed to have met that threshold by the courts.
- *Level 1 /universal*: children with no additional needs, most children are at level 1.

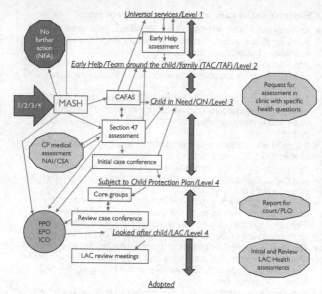

Fig. 11.2 Multiagency Safeguarding Hub (MASH) triage. CP, child protection; NAI, non-accidental injury.

- *Level 2/Early Help*: the child and family are supported by multiagency working, often led by a HV or school safeguarding lead. Team aims to help the family resolve any difficulties including housing etc. Social workers are not involved but *family support workers*, employed by the local authority, might be.
- *Level 3/CIN*: often child protection concerns just below the level of needing a child protection plan. To become a CIN there needs to have been a referral to social care that has been accepted and is allocated to a named social worker who undertakes a holistic child and family assessment.
- *Disabled children, young carers, etc.*: can also be CIN despite no child protection concerns—all CIN should have a social worker as lead professional.
- *Child and Family Assessment (CAFAS)*: looks at the developmental needs of the child, parent's ability to meet those needs, and wider factors that might impact ability to parent, including domestic violence, parental substance misuse, housing, etc. See Fig. 11.3.
- The CAFAS is led by a social worker and may lead to Section 47 assessment being opened if concern about significant harm is identified. If no concern found the outcome might be no further action.

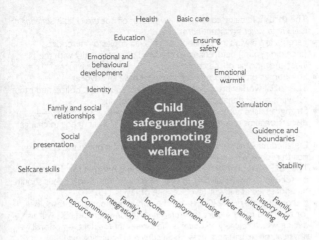

Fig. 11.3 Assessment framework.
Reprinted from Working Together to Safeguard Children (2018) The Department for Education under a Open Government Licence v3.0.

- *Level 4/subject to a safeguarding plan/LAC*: a child who is subject to a safeguarding plan will have been discussed at an initial case conference (ICC) where the outcome was that the child is placed on a safeguarding plan.
- A child who is a *looked after child* may have been discussed at an ICC and as part of the safeguarding plan a court order was obtained to remove the child from the family due to lack of positive progress with their care.
- Some looked after children have never been to an ICC as the situation was so concerning that the court order was sought early on, e.g. baby with rib fractures taken into foster care (on an EPO or interim care order) from hospital.
- Note that if abused by a known perpetrator who is no longer in contact, then the child may not go on a safeguarding plan or become a looked after child as they are now deemed safe. This is one of the reasons why statistics regarding children on plans do not equate to the number of children who we know have experienced abuse, let alone the many who professionals never hear about.
- *Pre-birth assessments and conferences*: the CSC assessment takes place prior to birth and may lead to a legal order hence the child could become a looked after child at birth.

Initial case conference

- The ICC is a multiagency meeting which decides if the safeguarding concerns meet the threshold for the child/children to be subject to a safeguarding plan.

- The threshold being considered is whether or not the child *is suffering or is likely to suffer significant harm*.
- Parents are always invited and will be given copies of all reports (including yours) beforehand to read and discuss, usually with the *independent chair* of the conference.
- Sometimes older children may attend or have an advocate.
- The social worker attends as well as health, education, police, and other relevant professionals which could include housing.
- Strength-based approaches are often used, e.g. 'Signs of Safety'— discussion aims to identify what is working well/what needs to change and how.
- Detailed minutes are produced; a copy should be put in the child's health record.
- The ICC decision may be that the threshold is not met for the child to be subject to a safeguarding plan, in which case the child's needs should be addressed at a lower level, i.e. one of levels 1–3.
- If the outcome of the ICC is that the concerns meet the threshold for the child to be *subject to a safeguarding plan*, then the ICC will also decide which *category of abuse* is most relevant (neglect, emotional, physical, or sexual) and draw up an *outline safeguarding plan*.
- A *core group* will be formed which should meet within 10 working days, thereafter 6-weekly, to review and refine the safeguarding plan/actions.
- Within 3 months a *review case conference* will be held and if significant progress is found then the child may move to a lower level of need. If deterioration or no progress, then legal advice may be sought to escalate.
- *Public law outline* sets timescales for court reports etc. to speed up the process when the local authority seeks a court order to remove a child from parents (private law relates to private disputes between parents, e.g. custody in divorce).

Safeguarding arrangements: management and governance aspects

- UK nations have similar practice but different laws, terminology, and process details—see NSPCC website for detail by country.
- In England, the *Children and Social Work Act of 2017* led to LSCBs (Local Safeguarding Children's Boards) being replaced by *Multiagency Safeguarding Partnerships* an executive body, where the local authority, health (clinical commissioning group (CCG)), and police have equal responsibility for a local geographical area.
- They set out thresholds to be met for children at different levels of care, often described as levels 1–4.
- Arrange multiagency training and audit of safeguarding procedures.
- When a child who is thought to have suffered abuse dies or is seriously injured, then the local authority's safeguarding partnership should, within 5 working days of being aware of the incident, notify the *Child Safeguarding Practice Review Panel*, a *national* independent panel that works with the Department for Education.
- The local safeguarding partnership should also undertake a *rapid review* of the case (each service involved with the child will submit a report) to be completed within 15 working days *and* forward the report and conclusion to the national panel.
- The conclusion might be that no further review is needed, that a *local review* (more in-depth) is needed, or that there are factors which warrant a *national review*, particularly if learning is likely to relate to systemic/process issues that need to be addressed. It may be that professional practice was good—not all harm can be prevented.
- The Child Safeguarding Practice Reviews replace Serious Case Reviews in England. The new arrangements aim to ensure greater consistency, wider overview, and learning from reviews.
- Statistical data resulting from these notifications can be found at ℅ https://explore-education-statistics.service.gov.uk/find-statistics/serious-incident-notifications.
- The NSPCC maintains a national repository of Child Safeguarding Practice Reviews/Serious Case Reviews, available online at NSPCC Learning.
- *Designated doctors and nurses* are employed by the CCG to provide clinical advice on safeguarding matters and oversight of all health providers in the geographical area covered by the Safeguarding Partnership. They support named staff.
- *Named doctors, named nurses, and named midwives*, where appropriate, are employed by each health provider organization to provide advice to colleagues in that organization and to ensure that safeguarding processes are set up and followed. Some departments, particularly emergency departments, have a *safeguarding lead* who is supported by the named doctor.
- Each CCG employs a *named GP* who undertakes a similar role and supports the *safeguarding leads* for each GP surgery.

- *Local Authority Designated Officer*—an experienced social worker who undertakes an investigation/assessment when there are safeguarding concerns involving a person who is in contact with children through work or volunteering, e.g. teachers/sports coaches.
- *Disclosure and Barring Service*—pre-employment/volunteering checks, plus maintains a list of people barred from working with children (or vulnerable adults) sourced from certain criminal convictions or referrals by employers or Local Authority Designated Officers.

Further resources

Department for Education (July 2018). Working Together to Safeguard Children: A Guide to Inter-Agency Working to Safeguard and Promote the Welfare of Children. Available at: ℅ https://www.gov.uk/government/publications/working-together-to-safeguard-children--2
NSPCC Learning: ℅ https://learning.nspcc.org.uk/
tri.x. Proceduresonline.com. Safeguarding partnership arrangements: ℅ https://www.proceduresonline.com/resources/sgp/p_child_sg_review.html

United Nations Convention on the Rights of the Child

- All UN states have ratified this convention apart from the US; the Convention came into force in the UK in 1992. For more information, see ♪ https://www.unicef.org.uk/what-we-do/un-convention-child-rights/.
- Of the 54 Articles, many have relevance to safeguarding and child protection including Article 3, best interests of the child; Article 19, protection from violence, abuse, and neglect; Article 24, the right to the best possible health; Article 28, the right to an education.
- Articles 32–35 cover topics of exploitation and trafficking.
- Article 39 refers to children who have experienced neglect, abuse, exploitation, or torture, or who are victims of war, who must receive special support to help them recover their health, dignity, self-respect, and social life. This could be interpreted as a therapeutic response to trauma.

Child deaths

- Approximately 6000 children die in the UK every year.
- Compared to European countries with lower rates, it is estimated that the UK has ~2000 excess child deaths per year.
- Over half of child deaths occur in the first year of life, often related to prematurity.
- The next most common age group in which children die is the late teenage years.
- Accidents are a major cause of child death after infancy.
- Suicide is a major cause of child death.
- The UK has a higher child death rate than many similarly developed countries.
- See RCPCH 'Why Children Die' report from 2014 for more details (℞ https://www.rcpch.ac.uk/resources/why-children-die-research-recommendations).

Sudden infant death syndrome (SIDS)

The sudden and unexpected death of an infant <12 months of age, with onset of the lethal episode apparently occurring during normal sleep, which remains unexplained after a thorough investigation, including performance of a complete postmortem examination and review of the circumstances of death and the clinical history.

- In the 1980s, epidemiological research established that babies put to sleep on their tummies (prone) had a much higher rate of SIDS than those sleeping on their backs.
- The resulting 'Back to sleep' public health campaign, led by The Lullaby Trust, started in the 1990s and led to an 81% decrease in SIDS over the following 25 years.
- SIDS rates have been stable since 2014. In 2018, the incidence was 0.30 per 1000 live births (℞ https://www.ons.gov.uk/).
- Approximately 200 babies per year currently die through SIDS, in the 1980s it was 2000 per year.
- Babies are most at risk during the 2nd, 3rd, and 4th months of life, boys have a slightly higher risk.
- Low birth weight and premature babies are also more at risk.

Modifiable risk factors include sleeping position—place baby on his/her back to sleep, position baby in the cot so as not to slide down under blankets—feet to foot (foot of the cot), avoid overheating, keep head uncovered, sleep in the same room as parent for first 6 months, do not co-sleep in bed or on a sofa, do not use alcohol/drugs, use a firm and flat mattress, avoid smoking during pregnancy and exposing baby to second hand cigarette smoke, and breast feed if possible.

Sudden unexpected death in infancy/childhood (SUDI/SUDC)

The death of an infant or child whose death *was not anticipated as a significant possibility 24 hours before the death*, or where there was *a similarly unexpected collapse* leading to or precipitating the events which led to the death.

A thorough investigation may lead to a diagnosis or explanation for the death (*explained SUDI/SUDC*). If no clear diagnosis or explanation, then for an infant the death will be described as *SIDS* and for children >12 months of age it will be a *SUDC*.

Child Death Review (CDR) process

It is important to disseminate learning gained from reviewing child deaths. What follows is a brief review of the new system being rolled out across England, as recommended in 'Working Together'; other nations will have their own systems. The CDR is a separate process from child safeguarding. The CDR process in England is currently acquiring more resources and structure, becoming a distinct field of expertise in its own right.

The new CDR guidance for England states that all child deaths should be reviewed. Detailed guidance can be found at: ℜ https://www.gov.uk/gov ernment/publications/child-death-review-statutory-and-operational-guida nce-england.

CDR partners (CCG and the local authority) should employ a senior paediatrician as a *designated doctor for child deaths*, who is often a senior paediatrician involved in a *Joint Agency Response* (JAR) to a child death—also known as the SUDC paediatrician on call.

Immediate actions after a child's death include:
- Supporting the child's family—this should be continued by a named 'key worker' throughout the process.
- Decide whether a death certificate can be issued.
- Decide whether a JAR is needed.
- Does the death meet criteria for an *NHS Serious Incident* (STEIS or similar)?
- Begin *notifications*, including the GP, child health computer systems, stop routine appointments being generated, etc.
- A *medical lead* should also be identified to support the family, may be known to them already and will aim to answer their medical questions, at times through the key worker.

Joint Agency Response

CDR guidance states that the following circumstances mandate that a JAR is needed as the death:
1. Is or could be due to external causes.
2. Is sudden and there is no immediately apparent cause (including SUDI/SUDC).
3. Occurs in custody, or where the child was detained under the Mental Health Act.
4. Where the initial circumstances raise any suspicions that the death may not have been natural.
5. In the case of a stillbirth where no healthcare professional was in attendance.

- In practice, regarding item (2), you will need to call the SUDC paediatrician when *the child's death, or the collapse leading to the death could not have been reasonably predicted 24 hours beforehand*. See earlier section on SUDI/SUDC.

- If a JAR is needed, then the on-call health professional, police officer, and social worker need to be contacted immediately. Be aware of your local referral route.
- It may be that a *coronial* investigation is needed.
- A *postmortem examination* may be needed, either a standard *hospital postmortem* or a highly detailed *forensic postmortem*.
- In a JAR, an initial *information sharing meeting* is likely to take place in the first 24–48 hours.
- Investigations include a joint home/scene of collapse visit by the senior health professional and police.

Child Death Review Meeting (CDRM)

- The CDRM is a multiagency meeting of professionals directly involved with the child *and* those investigating the death. Findings of investigations, including postmortem results, will be reviewed at this meeting.
- The CDRM may take several forms depending on the circumstances of the death. After a JAR, it is likely to be an individual case discussion held within the first 3 months; however, if a neonatal death or other hospital death, the discussion might take place as part of a regularly programmed mortality review meeting.
- The CDRM reviews the background and investigations with the aim of establishing contributing or modifiable factors regarding the child, social and physical environment, and service delivery.
- Parents are not invited to the CDRM but may put questions via their key worker.
- The CDRM drafts the *analysis form* and sends this to the Child Death Overview Panel (CDOP).

Child Death Overview Panel

- The CDOP is an independent multiagency review panel that scrutinizes all aspects of the child's death.
- The local CDOP reviews all child deaths, i.e. all deaths of all persons <18 years of age, including any live born baby. Still births are not included.
- Two or more local areas may join to form a CDOP such that it reviews at least 60 child deaths per year in order to be of sufficient size to identify thematic modifiable factors that could be acted upon.
- Resulting local and national reports regarding data and thematic learning are produced.
- *Notification Form (previously Form A)*—initial notification of death to CDR partners, completed by professional involved with the child.
- *Reporting Form (previously Form B)*—completed by responsible officers during the investigation and sent to the CDOP.
- *Analysis Form (previously Form C)*—initial draft created at the CDRM and sent to the CDOP for completion. Completed analysis form to be shared with National Child Mortality Database.
- *eCDOP*—a digital version of the statutory forms which facilitates standardization of approach, more rapid data collection and therefore more timely analysis and learning at the National Child Mortality Database.

National Child Mortality Database

Commenced in 2019, this database receives reports from CDOPs regarding all child deaths in England; analysis and learning is disseminated (🔗 https://www.ncmd.info/).

Learning Disabilities Mortality Review (LeDeR) programme

If the child is >4 years old and had a LD, the CDR partners will notify the LeDeR mortality review process. This is a programme commissioned from Bristol University and reviews all deaths of people with a LD.

Adoption, fostering, and looked after children

Reasons for children entering care

The UN Convention on the Rights of the Child is the most widely ratified UN convention. It sets out important rights on issues relevant to the lives of children who enter public care. The full expression of these rights would reduce the need for children to enter care and is an advocacy issue.

- Article 3: the best interests of the child must be a top priority in all decisions and actions that affect children.
- Article 9: children must not be separated from their parents against their will unless it is in their best interests (e.g. if a parent is hurting or neglecting a child). Children whose parents have separated have the right to stay in contact with both parents, unless this could cause them harm.
- Article 19: governments must do all they can to ensure that children are protected from all forms of violence, abuse, neglect, and bad treatment by their parents or anyone else who looks after them.
- Article 20: if a child cannot be looked after by their immediate family, the government must give them special protection and assistance. This includes making sure the child is provided with alternative care that is continuous and respects the child's culture, language, and religion.
- Article 21: governments must oversee the process of adoption to make sure it is safe, lawful, and that it prioritizes children's best interests. Children should only be adopted outside of their country if they cannot be placed with a family in their own country.
- Article 22: if a child is seeking refuge or has refugee status, governments must provide them with appropriate protection and assistance to help them enjoy all the rights in the Convention. Governments must help refugee children who are separated from their parents to be reunited with them.
- Article 25: if a child has been placed away from home for the purpose of care or protection (e.g. with a foster family or in hospital), they have the right to a regular review of their treatment, the way they are cared for, and their wider circumstances.
- Article 33: governments must protect children from the illegal use of drugs and from being involved in the production or distribution of drugs.
- Article 34: governments must protect children from all forms of sexual abuse and exploitation.
- Article 35: governments must protect children from being abducted, sold, or moved illegally to a different place in or outside their country for the purpose of exploitation.
- Article 39: children who have experienced neglect, abuse, exploitation, torture, or who are victims of war must receive special support to help them recover their health, dignity, self-respect, and social life.

Placing a child away from their parents is a major decision (Article 9) and requires a judgement that remaining at home puts the child at significant risk of harm. The following data are for children who entered care in England in the year April 2018 to March 2019 (Fig. 12.1):

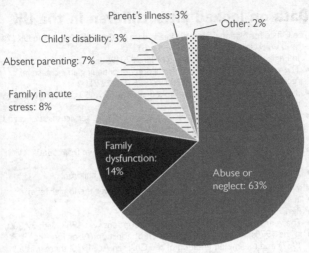

Fig. 12.1 Main reasons for children entering public care.

Reprinted from 'Children looked after in England including adoption: 2018 to 2019' *Office of National Statistics* available at https://www.gov.uk/government/statistics/children-looked-after-in-england-including-adoption-2018-to-2019, under the Open Government Licence v3.0.

There are a range of reasons why a child is looked after including:
• As a result of or because they were at risk of abuse or neglect—49,570 children, the most common reason identified.
• Primarily due to living in a family where the parenting capacity is chronically inadequate (family dysfunction)—11,310.
• Due to living in a family that is going through a temporary crisis that diminishes the parental capacity to adequately meet some of the children's needs (family being in acute stress)—6050.
• Due to there being no parents available to provide for the child—5410.
• Due to the child's or parent's disability or illness—4580.
• Due to low income or socially unacceptable behaviour—1230.

Data on looked after children in the UK

The Office for National Statistics keeps data on these children in the UK (℘ http://www.statistics.gov.uk/default.asp).

In England, for the year ending 31 March 2019:

- There were 78,150 looked after children—continuing an increase in recent years and up from 50,700 in 1996 (Fig. 12.2).
- 31,680 children started to be looked after and 29,460 children ceased to be looked after during the year.
- Maltreatment was the main reason why social care services first engaged with children who became looked after during the year.
- 72% of children were in a foster placement.
- There were 3570 children placed for adoption, down from 5360 in 2015.
- There were 5070 unaccompanied asylum-seeking children.

The following data show the trends in adoption over the longer term:

- In 1930, there were 4000 adoptions.
- By 1950, there were 14,500 adoptions.
- The year with the greatest number of adoptions was 1968, with 27,000.
- In the 1970s, following the legalization of abortion (Abortion Act 1967) and the implementation of the Children Act 1975, there was a rapid decline in the number of adoptions from 22,502 in 1974 falling to 10,870 in 1979.
- The number of adoptions continued to fall steadily over the 1980s and 1990s; there were 1800 in 1997.
- Adoptions have increased since then with 3800 in 2004 and 2005 and 3200 in 2010.

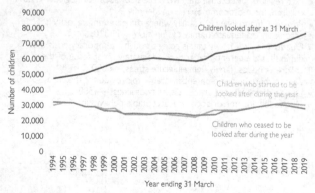

Fig. 12.2 Number of children in England looked after on 31 March each year from 1994 to 2019.

In Scotland, 14,015 children were in the care of local authorities on 31 July 2019 and 263 adoptions took place in the year to 31 July 2019. In Wales 6845 children were in the care of local authorities on 31 March 2019 and 310 children were adopted from care during the year ending 31 March 2019. In Northern Ireland, 3281 children were looked after on 31 March 2019 and 61 looked after children were adopted in the year ending 31 March 2019.

Legislative framework for looked after children and adoption

Adoption is the process that permanently transfers parental responsibility for a child from birth parents (who cease to have any parental responsibility when the adoption order is granted) to adoptive parents. It is a legal term.

Legal adoption was first introduced into the UK under the terms of the Adoption of Children Act 1926. The initial emphasis was on the needs of adults—adoption provided relief for unmarried mothers and met the desire to parent for couples unable to conceive themselves.

The Adoption Act 1976 is the main legislation governing the process of adoption in the UK but it has been updated with the Adoption and Children Act 2002 and more recently in England with the Children and Families Act 2014. Key features of the law in relation to adoption are:

- Paramountcy of the child's welfare over other issues.
- Preventing delay.
- Widening access to adoption by allowing unmarried couples, single people, and same-sex couples to adopt.
- Improving support for long-term impact of adoption by requiring adoption agencies to assess the support needs of those who are affected by adoption and setting out a more consistent approach to the release of sensitive and identifying information held in adoption records.
- Contact between prescribed persons and adopted person's relatives.
- Placement of looked after children with prospective adopters.
- Recruitment, assessment, and approval of prospective adopters.
- Adoption support services: personal budgets and the duty to provide information.
- The Adoption and Children Act Register.
- Post-adoption contact.

In Scotland, the Adoption and Children (Scotland) Act 2007 replaced the Adoption (Scotland) Act 1978 in 2008. The current legislation in Northern Ireland is the Adoption (Northern Ireland) Order 1987. Wales is governed by the Adoption and Children Act 2002.

In England, Wales, and Scotland there are national standards for the level of service adoption agencies must provide for all involved in the adoption process, including birth parents.

Adoption is solely administered through adoption services and agencies approved by the secretary of state. Therefore, private adoption is prohibited in the UK.

Further resources

Adoption Act 1976: http://www.legislation.gov.uk/ukpga/1976/36/contents
Adoption and Children Act 2002: http://www.legislation.gov.uk/ukpga/2002/38/contents
Children and Families Act 2014: https://www.legislation.gov.uk/ukpga/2014/6/contents
Adoption (Scotland) Act 1978: http://www.legislation.gov.uk/ukpga/1978/28/contents
Adoption and Children (Scotland) Act 2007: http://www.legislation.gov.uk/asp/2007/4/contents
The Adoption Agencies Regulations (Northern Ireland) 1989: http://www.legislation.gov.uk/nisr/1989/253/contents/made

Role of named and designated doctors for looked after children

The named doctor for looked after children has a trust lead for this vulnerable group. This is an operational role and functions include the following:
- Support all activities necessary to ensure that the organization meets its responsibilities for looked after children and young people.
- Be responsible to and accountable within the managerial framework of the employing organization.
- At all times and in relation to the roles and responsibilities listed, work as a member of the organization's looked after children's health team.
- There are interagency responsibilities, leadership and advisory roles, clinical roles, coordination and communication, oversight of policies and procedures, training, monitoring, and supervisory elements.

The designated doctor for looked after children has a clinical commissioning group lead for this vulnerable group. This is a strategic role and functions include:
- At all times and in relation to the roles and responsibilities listed, lead and support all activities necessary to ensure that organizations within the health community meet their responsibilities for looked after children.
- Advise and support all specialist professionals working with looked after children across the health community.
- Be responsible to and accountable within the managerial framework of the employing clinical commissioning group.
- There are interagency responsibilities, leadership and advisory roles, clinical roles, coordination, communication and liaison, oversight of policies and procedures, training, monitoring and information governance and supervisory elements including appraisal.

Further resources

Royal College of Nursing on behalf of the Royal College of Paediatrics and Child Health (2020). Looked After Children: Roles and Competencies of Healthcare Staff. Available at: https://www.rcn.org.uk/professional-development/publications/rcn-looked-after-children-roles-and-competencies-of-healthcare-staff-uk-pub-009486

The adoption process in the UK

Adoption provides a new legal family to children who cannot be brought up by birth parents. Deciding to become an adoptive parent is a major decision and there are a series of processes before a child can join a new family.

- *Register with an adoption agency*: local authorities have adoption agencies within Children's Services (England and Wales) or Social Services (Scotland) or there are independent adoption agencies run by charities. A full list of adoption agencies is available from Adoption UK.
- Prospective adopters are invited to an information meeting and can then complete a formal application. Once accepted by the agency, a social worker is allocated and from this point the agency has a maximum of 8 months to make a decision on the application.
- Training is offered to groups of prospective adopters. The challenges of parenting any child are discussed as well as the additional complexities that children for adoption may present (e.g. because of experiences of maltreatment and attachment difficulties). Many other issues such as contact with birth families are considered.
- The assessment involves the social worker visiting the prospective adopters at home over a period of time and completing a Prospective Adopters Report. This comprehensive report explores the applicants' ability to adopt. It includes information on motivation to adopt, family background, childhood experiences, current relationships, financial circumstances, and the safety and suitability of the home and neighbourhood for a child. A health assessment, local authority, and police checks are required and at least three referees are interviewed face to face.
- The assessment allows prospective adopters to understand the challenges to adopting a child and the social worker to make an informed assessment of the adopter's strengths and weaknesses. The adopters have 10 days to review the completed Prospective Adopters Report and comment.
- The application is then considered by the agency's adoption panel. Prospective adopters are invited to part of the panel meeting to answer questions. The panel makes a recommendation to the agency's decision maker. If approved, the process of finding a suitable child begins. If not approved in England or Wales, the prospective adopters can involve the Independent Review Mechanism.
- When approved, a suitable child may come from the approving agency or elsewhere. Prospective adopters can use resources such as those available through *Be My Parent* or *Adoption UK*.
- When a suitable child is found, his/her agency arranges a meeting with the agency of the prospective adopters to look at the child's needs and the ability of the prospective adopters to meet these needs. If the match meets the child's needs, an Adoption Placement Report is written and presented to the child's adoption panel to recommend, and the agency decision maker to approve, the match.

- If approved, an adoption placement plan is written detailing how introductions of the child to the family and vice versa will take place, what the contact plan will be, and what post-adoption support is needed and how this will be provided.
- Providing introductions go well, the child moves to the adopters' home. The adopters, at this point, share parental responsibility with the local authority; the child is only legally adopted after an adoption order is granted by court. This order can be applied for after a minimum of 10 weeks. When it is granted, the child is legally part of the new family and can take their surname.

Further resources

Adoption UK: ℘ https://www.adoptionuk.org/
Be My Parent: ℘ http://www.bemyparent.org.uk/
Prospective Adopter's Report (PAR) England. Guidance Notes and Additional Resource: ℘ https://corambaaf.org.uk/sites/default/files/Form%20PAR.pdf

Assessment of prospective adoptive parents or foster carers

- Prospective adoptive parents and foster carers go through an assessment process. Such an assessment has a number of functions:
  - Describe the needs of looked after children.
  - Explore the impact of maltreatment before entering public care.
  - Discuss strategies for dealing with vulnerable children.
  - Reflect on their formal and informal support networks.
  - Consider the impact on the child of separation from birth family.
  - Look at contact with birth family.
  - Explain the legal framework of accommodation, care orders, special guardianship, and adoption orders.
- Social services provide formal support mechanisms with social workers for the adoptive parents and foster carers. In addition, there is often support available from other families attending the same training course and local foster care organizations or post-adoption support groups.
- Medical issues in adoptive parents are rarely an absolute contra-indication to adopting but there are important issues that do need debate and discussion at the adoption panel. Examples include:
  - Life-limiting condition.
  - Disability.
  - Significant mental illness.
  - Smoking.
- Medical issues in foster carers are similar.
- The medical group in CoramBAAF provides a source of advice in particular health dilemmas. CoramBAAF publishes the Adoption & Fostering journal and 'Practice notes' on specific issues.

Further resources

Adoption UK: http://www.adoptionuk.org/
CoramBAAF. Health group: https://corambaaf.org.uk/corambaaf-health-group
CoramBAAF. Practice notes: https://corambaaf.org.uk/resources/practice-notes
CoramBAAF. Thinking about adoption?: https://corambaaf.org.uk/fostering-adoption/adoption

Health needs of looked after children

Looked after C&YP have higher levels of physical, mental, and health promotion needs than other children of the same age.

The evidence for looked after young people's significant mental health needs and risk-taking behaviours is described in the topic on adolescents in public care (see ➔ pp. 636–8).

There are patterns to the health needs of looked after children, though individual children may have none of these issues:

- Intrauterine exposure to *alcohol*—consider fetal alcohol syndrome or fetal alcohol effects.
- Intrauterine exposure to *drugs*—can lead to neonatal drug withdrawal symptoms and the need for morphine in the neonatal period. There can also be a longer-term impact on behaviour and neurological development.
- There is a risk of exposure to *vertically transmitted infections* such as syphilis, gonorrhoea, hepatitis B, hepatitis C, and HIV. Mothers of looked after children are more likely not to have been tested in pregnancy.
- *Neglect* of children's healthcare is a common pre-public care experience and so common problems such as squint, undescended testes, asthma, or chronic secretory otitis media may not have been addressed satisfactorily (see ➔ p. 567).
- *Immunizations* are commonly not up to date at entry to public care.
- *Developmental delay*, particularly in speech and language, is common in children entering public care (see ➔ pp. 30–1).
- Some children enter public care because their parents have learning difficulties that impact their parenting capacity. Sometimes the learning difficulties can have a genetic aetiology (e.g. fragile X syndrome or microdeletion/microduplication syndromes) and genetic testing may be warranted (see ➔ pp. 484–5).
- See ➔ pp. 324–5 for *attachment difficulties*.

Further resources

Simkiss D (2020). Meeting with prospective adoptive parents. Paediatr Child Health, 30, 186–90.

Looked after child health assessments and adoption medical assessments

- Consultations for children in care are almost unique as they are often seen by doctors without their birth parents.
- This is a disadvantage as birth parents often have important and detailed health information and many parents want to communicate this face to face with the doctor. Therefore, provided it is appropriate, social workers should encourage the birth parents to attend health assessments.
- Children in care are a vulnerable group. The *Healthy Child Programme* identifies these children as a group for targeted health visiting and school nursing.
- The Strengths and Difficulties Questionnaire must be completed to provide information on the emotional and behavioural well-being of children in care for children over the age of 4 years. This questionnaire should be completed by the child/young person's carer and discussed and validated at the health assessment appointment. Young people should be encouraged and supported to complete their own version of this questionnaire.
- The key output from a health assessment is a Health Care Plan and information from the Health Care Plan should be incorporated into the statutory review minutes and the Care Plan which are social work processes and address Article 25 in the UN Convention on the Rights of the Child. Independent reviewing officers should ask specifically for the Health Care Plan and clarify that all actions have been completed. If these have not been followed, they should be identified as recommendations from the statutory review and stated as specified in the minutes.
- It is the social worker's responsibility to provide information for an effective health assessment including:
  - Care Plan.
  - CoramBAAF Form PH (parental health).
  - CoramBAAF consent to share information forms.
  - 'Red book' (parent/carer-held child record) to be brought by carers, if available.
  - Strengths and Difficulties Questionnaire completed by carer.
- Looked after C&YP are required to have health assessments, every 6 months for children under the age of 5 and every year over that age. The current guidance on the service looked after children should receive is 'Promoting the Health and Wellbeing of Looked after Children' published by the Department of Health and the Department for Education in 2015.

Looked after children health assessment case vignettes

Two siblings placed out of the area for 3 years in a short-term foster care placement were invited to health assessment because the social worker was concerned that they were 'ruminating on their food'.

The head teacher of their school wrote a letter saying 'I am concerned that their emotional and psychological needs are not being met. They have many physical and medical problems, but the outstanding problem is their obsessive need for food (and drink). They steal, lie, and manipulate to obtain food and have to be constantly supervised.'

On examination, both siblings were stunted with a height velocity of <1 cm in the previous 12 months. After extensive investigations in hospital, a diagnosis of hyperphagic psychosocial short stature was made and the children moved to a different foster placement. In the next 12 months both children demonstrated catch-up growth, one growing 17 cm in that year!

A looked after child living with an extended family member was brought to her health assessment by the family and a social worker. The social worker reported that 'There is something wrong with her eyes, something wrong with her ears and she isn't doing very well at school'.

On examination there was hypertelorism and her nose was of an unusual shape. Audiology testing revealed a 50 dB HL. On direct questioning there was a family history of premature greying of hair in the mother and a grandfather. The grandfather also had anisochromia. A diagnosis of Waardenburg syndrome was made.

Children under the age of 5 years need to see a doctor every 6 months to ensure the medical information for the adoption process is current. Children over the age of 5 years with an adoption plan are seen at least every 12 months.

It is important that social care information is sent to the doctor to enable a comprehensive Adoption Health Report to be written. In many areas, the information forms developed by the Health Group at CoramBAAF are used to ensure that the required information as follows is obtained:
- The initial or review health assessment form (child or young person) signed by whoever has parental responsibility.
- The Care Plan and Statutory Review Minutes.
- Child's Permanence Report.
- CoramBAAF Forms M and B, which contain useful information on the obstetric and neonatal histories respectively.
- CoramBAAF Form PH (parental health) for both parents. These are an opportunity for parents to explain any health issues they have and sometimes these are directly relevant to the ongoing health of the child.
- CoramBAAF Consent Forms which address the issues of consent for treatment and for access to medical information on the child and also has a section to allow the parents to give consent for the doctor to access information on the birth parent.

- CoramBAAF Carer Report which provides detailed information on the behaviour of the child.
- School/nursery/child development centre/other relevant reports.

A comprehensive Adoption Health Report is required for the purposes of Adoption Panel, adoption court reports, and for the child's new GP when adopted.

It needs to include:
- Name, date of birth, sex, weight, and height.
- Neonatal history including:
  - Details of the birth and any complications.
  - The results of a physical examination and screening tests including blood-borne infections (hepatitis B and C, HIV, and syphilis).
  - Details of any problems in management and feeding.
- A full health history including:
  - Details of any serious illness, disability, accident, hospital admission or attendance at an outpatient department, and in each case any treatment given.
  - Details and dates of immunizations.
  - A physical and developmental assessment according to age, including an assessment of vision and hearing and of neurological, speech, and language development and any evidence of emotional disorder.
  - For a child >5 years of age, the school health history (if available).
  - How the child's physical and mental health and medical history have affected his/her physical, intellectual, emotional, social, or behavioural development.
- A full examination including height, weight, and head circumference. Comments on any dysmorphology if noted and a full systems examination including cardiovascular, respiratory, abdominal, and neurological systems.

Adoption health assessment case vignette

A 27-month-old infant presented for an adoption health assessment. She was well but presented with some speech and language delay. She was in foster care because her mother had learning difficulties. There was a family history of significant learning difficulties with maternal uncle and maternal great uncle both attending special school.

The mother was invited to the health assessment where it was explained about the possible genetic causes of LD. With her permission, genetic testing of her daughter was arranged. The results revealed that she was a carrier of fragile X syndrome. Further testing in the birth family confirmed that this was the cause of the significant LDs seen in the male members of the family.

Further resources

CoramBAAF. Health forms (UK-wide): ℛ https://corambaaf.org.uk/bookshop/corambaaf-electronic-forms/health-forms-uk-wide

Department of Health, Department for Education (2015). Promoting the Health and Wellbeing of Looked After Children. London: Department of Health. Available at: ℛ https://www.gov.uk/government/publications/promoting-the-health-and-wellbeing-of-looked-after-children--2

Contributing to an adoption panel

Purpose

An adoption panel makes recommendations on three issues:
- Should a child have a plan for adoption?
- Should prospective adopters be approved to adopt?
- Should a potential link between a child and approved adopters progress?

Membership

- An adoption panel requires a medical advisor by law. In most cases this is a community paediatrician, but other doctors such as GPs can also provide good advice to panels.
- Other members include an independent chair, a panel advisor from the adoption service, and members with experience of the care system such as foster carers or people who were adopted as children or have adopted children.

Medical role

- The medical advisor is a full member of the panel, reading all the papers for the panel meeting and contributes equally in the general panel discussion.
- In addition, the medical advisor provides specialist advice to the panel on:
  - The health and development needs of the child.
  - The health of the adopters.
- The medical advice forms part of the child's permanence report.

Medical issues in adoption

- The medical advisor is responsible for identifying health issues in the birth family that could be significant for the child.
- Potential adopters should have this information as they decide about whether to adopt a child. Important issues include:
  - Risk of vertical infections from an infected mother (hepatitis B, hepatitis C, HIV, syphilis, gonorrhoea, chlamydia).
  - Investigation of LDs in the birth family. Some of these causes can be inherited (e.g. fragile X).
  - Family history of inheritable conditions. An example is a birth grandparent with Huntington's chorea whose child (the parent of the child for adoption) has refused to be tested. In this situation, the child with a plan for adoption has a 1:4 risk of developing Huntington's chorea. The ethical advice in this scenario is not to test the child until they have reached the age of majority and can make the decision themselves, but potential adoptive parents need the opportunity to discuss this dilemma.
  - Family history of mental illness. There is an inheritable component to a number of mental illnesses. This is highest in schizophrenia and so clarity on the specific diagnosis is important in order to counsel the potential adopters on the level of risk to the child.

- The medical advisor also guides the adoption panel on health issues in the prospective adoptive parents that may be relevant to caring for a child.
- These are rarely absolute, but debates arise on the impact of mental illness, chronic disease, life-limiting conditions, and disabilities.
- The key issue to focus the discussion is what is in the best interests of the child.

Further resources

CoramBAAF provides extensive information on all aspects of adoption, including adoption panels. It has a specific text called 'Effective Adoption Panels', available at: ℞ https://corambaaf.org.uk/ books/effective-adoption-panels

CoramBAAF runs a medical group for doctors working in this field and holds an annual conference. See: ℞ https://corambaaf.org.uk/

CoramBAAF also publishes Adoption & Fostering, a journal that has articles on the medical issues in adoption. There are also relevant 'Practice notes' published by CoramBAAF including 'Reducing the risks of environmental tobacco smoke for looked after children and their carers', 'Guidelines for the testing of looked after children who are at risk of a blood-borne infection' and 'Genetic testing and adoption', available at: ℞ https://corambaaf.org.uk/resources/practice-notes

Adolescents in public care

Adolescents are the most common group of looked after children. These young people have the same issues that all adolescents face. But mental health issues and risk-taking behaviours are more common in looked after young people than other adolescents. The last survey of the Mental Health of Children Looked After (MHCLA) was carried out in 2002 so the findings, which inform policy and commissioning decisions for this group at local and national levels, are now considerably out of date. NHS Digital is currently updating the previous survey using the same methodology but the results are not yet available. Figs. 12.3–12.5 are taken from two surveys of mental health in the general population of young people and looked after young people and published by the Office of National Statistics survey[1] in 2003.

Mental health issues

Fig. 12.3 shows that looked after young people commonly experience mental health problems, particularly conduct disorders, and that the prevalence rates are considerably higher than in children not looked after.[1] Young people in public care are more commonly involved in risk-taking behaviours such as smoking (Fig. 12.4)[1,2], alcohol (Fig. 12.5)[1,2], drug use, and early sexual activity than their peers:

- In Sweden, 15–20% of girls who were involved with social services as teenagers became teenage mothers compared with <3% of the general population.[3]
- Every third girl placed in a secure residential unit and every fourth girl placed in other residential homes because of behavioural problems became mothers as teenagers.

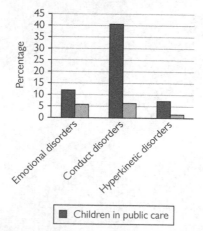

Fig. 12.3 Prevalence of mental disorders among 480 children in public care and 4609 private household children aged 11–15 years.

Source: data from Meltzer H, Corbin T, Gatward R, Goodman R, Ford T. The mental health of young people looked after by local authorities in England. London: The Stationery Office, 2003.

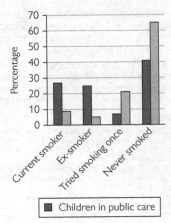

Fig. 12.4 Smoking behaviour of looked after and private household children aged 11–15 years.

Source: data from Meltzer H, Corbin T, Gatward R, Goodman R, Ford T. The mental health of young people looked after by local authorities in England. London: The Stationery Office, 2003 and Meltzer H, Gatward R, Goodman R, Ford T. Mental health of children and adolescents in Great Britain. London: The Stationery Office, 2000.

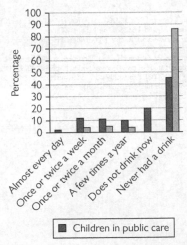

Fig. 12.5 Drinking behaviour of looked after and private household children aged 11–15 years.

Source: data from Meltzer H, Corbin T, Gatward R, Goodman R, Ford T. The mental health of young people looked after by local authorities in England. London: The Stationery Office, 2003 and Meltzer H, Gatward R, Goodman R, Ford T. Mental health of children and adolescents in Great Britain. London: The Stationery Office, 2000.

- Of boys involved with social services as teenagers, 5–6% became teenage fathers compared to 0.7% of the general population.[4]
- Almost one in five of all Swedish teenage parents in the cohort had been involved with social services.

These issues are present in many looked after young people at entry to public care and the prevalence only drops slowly over time in public care. There are a wide range of sources of useful information available on line or from NICE, but further research is needed on effective strategies.

Further resources

Department of Health, Department for Education (2015). Promoting the Health and Wellbeing of Looked After Children. London: Department of Health. Available at: ℅ https://www.gov.uk/government/publications/promoting-the-health-and-wellbeing-of-looked-after-children—2

FRANK: ℅ http://www.talktofrank.com/

House of Commons Education Committee (2016). Mental Health and Wellbeing of Looked After Children. London: UK Parliament. Available at: ℅ https://publications.parliament.uk/pa/cm201516/cmselect/cmeduc/481/48102.htm

National Institute for Health and Care Excellence (2010). Alcohol use disorders: prevention. NICE Public Health Guidance 24. Available at: ℅ https://www.nice.org.uk/guidance/ph24

National Institute for Health and Care Excellence (2017). Drug misuse prevention: targeted interventions. NICE Guidance 64. Available at: ℅ https://www.nice.org.uk/guidance/ng64

National Institute for Health and Care Excellence/Social Care Institute for Excellence (2010). SCIE Guide 40. Promoting quality of life for looked after children and young people. Available at: ℅ https://www.scie.org.uk/publications/guides/guide40/

Social Care Institute for Excellence (2017). Improving mental health support for our children and young people. Available at: ℅ https://www.scie.org.uk/children/care/mental-health/report#downloads

References

1. Meltzer H, Corbin T, Gatward R, et al. (2003). The Mental Health of Young People Looked After by Local Authorities in England. London: The Stationery Office.
2. Meltzer H, Gatward R, Goodman R, et al. (2000). Mental Health of Children and Adolescents in Great Britain. London: The Stationery Office.
3. Vinnerljung B, Franzén E, Danielsson M (2007). Teenage parenthood among child welfare clients: a Swedish national cohort study of prevalence and odds. J Adolesc, 30, 97–116.
4. Vinnerljung B, Sallnäs M (2008). Into adulthood: a follow-up study of 718 young people who were placed in out-of-home care during their teens. Child Fam Soc Work, 13, 144–55.

Unaccompanied asylum-seeking children

Introduction

Unaccompanied asylum-seeking children

Introduction

The UN Convention on the Rights of the Child Article 22 says 'children who come into a country as refugees should have the same rights as children born in that country'.

Definitions

'Refugee' is a legal term used to describe a person who fulfils the definition set out in the Geneva Convention of 1951. To be recognized as a refugee, the Convention says that a person has to show that:

> Owing to a well-founded fear of being persecuted for reasons of race, religion, nationality, membership of a particular social group or political opinion, is outside his country of nationality and is unable or, owing to such fear, is unwilling to avail himself of the protection of that country; or who, not having a nationality and being outside the country of his former habitual residence as a result of such events, is unable or, owing to such fear, is unwilling to return to it.

An asylum seeker is a person who has lodged an asylum claim with the Home Office and is waiting for a decision on the claim. The person is not allowed to work, but is entitled to basic healthcare.

If this definition applies to a child's circumstances, then the Immigration and Nationality Directorate should be notified and an application for asylum made. The Home Office can make one of the following decisions:

• To allow the asylum application and recognize the child as a refugee.
• To refuse the asylum application, but allow the child to remain in the UK on human rights grounds.
• To refuse the application and refuse any other kind of permission to remain in the UK.

The National Asylum Support Service (NASS) will support persons above the age of 18. Unaccompanied minors do not receive any support from NASS. They become responsibility of the Local Authority Children Services. If the asylum claim is refused for an unaccompanied child under the age of 18 years, discretionary leave may be granted until the child reaches 18 years of age.

Unaccompanied asylum-seeking C&YP, irrespective of immigration status, are entitled to all public health services, including medical and dental treatment, vision testing, family planning, and mental health services.

This special group of looked after C&YP should receive health assessments tailored to their particular needs. These needs include:

• Physical health including dental health.
• Previous physical trauma (e.g. fractured bones incorrectly set, perforated tympanic membranes following bomb blasts).
• Previous mental trauma including post-traumatic stress disorder or other mental illness.
• Evidence of infectious disease (e.g. cutaneous leishmaniasis, tuberculosis, hepatitis B).

- Health promotion needs (e.g. a basic understanding of puberty can be missing).
- Immunization—Health Protection Agency advice is to assume that these C&YP are unimmunized and to follow a catch-up schedule.

Further resources

Simmonds J, Merredew F (2010). The health needs of unaccompanied asylum seeking children and young people. Available at: ℘ https://www.nice.org.uk/guidance/ph28/evidence/looked-after-children-ep23-unaccompanied-asylum-seeking-children-john-simmonds-and-florence-merredew2

UASC Health: ℘ https://www.uaschealth.org/

Wade J, Mitchell F, Baylis G (eds) (2005). Unaccompanied Asylum Seeking Children: The Response of Social Work Services. London: British Agencies for Adoption and Fostering.

Leaving care and adult outcomes

- Young people leaving care need accurate information about their medical history and health needs in order to take responsibility for their own health.
- The 2010 NICE/Social Care Institute for Excellence guidance on 'Promoting quality of care for looked after children and young people' recommends that young people leaving care are given this information in a letter.
- At the medical review, the young person should be informed that he/ she would be receiving a letter with this information.
- The aim is to outline the discussion held at the last medical review, any medical advice given, and as complete a summary as possible of all health information to the young person.
- It is good practice to inform the young person about the information that would be in the letter so that he/she does not discover this information for the first time via the exit letter. This would allow any queries to be answered during the last medical review.
- The letter should be copied to the GP and social worker with the young person's consent.
- The following information should be included in the letter:
  - Birth history.
  - Past medical history: any illnesses, hospital attendances/admissions, information from reviews of looked after children.
  - Immunization history.
  - Developmental history.
  - Medication history.
  - History of allergies if any.
  - Relevant family medical history.
  - Ongoing health issues if any.
- There may be some leavers with complex medical needs where it may be more appropriate to provide a formal medical report. In these young people, the format used for medical advice to schools at transition could be adopted.

An example of a leaving care letter

Dear xxx,
When we met in September, I said I would try to get together some of the health information on you in order to write you a summary. I am sorry it has taken so long to get the information together but I hope that you find this letter useful.

You were born at xxx Hospital by a forceps delivery at 3.51 in the morning. You were born a week earlier than your mother was expecting and you weighed 2.96 kg with a head circumference of 35 cm. You were a healthy newborn baby and did not require any special care and you had a normal neonatal examination.

As far as I can tell you have no family history of illness. You have in the past had a couple of admissions to the Accident & Emergency (A&E) Department at xxx Hospital. The first was on 3 August 2005 when your left foot was caught in the wheel of a bike the day before and X-ray showed you had an avulsion fracture at the base of your fifth metatarsal, that is a small bone in your foot, and that will have healed up without any long-term effects. You then injured your left ankle in May 2007 and again was seen in the A&E Department but no significant injury was found.

You told me that you had been bitten by a dog and required sutures to your chest but I can't find any record of that in the notes that have been available to me.

You have seen Dr xxx, Consultant Child and Adolescent Psychiatrist, in recent years and a diagnosis of attention deficit hyperactivity disorder (ADHD) has been made. You are receiving treatment with methylphenidate and Equasym® XL (this is another methylphenidate preparation).

I have uncovered the details of most of your immunizations. You had diphtheria, tetanus, whooping cough, polio, and haemophilus influenzae type B immunizations on 16/11/92, 1/01/93, and 12/04/93. You had a preschool booster on 02/05/96. You had two doses of measles, mumps, and rubella vaccine on 23/12/93 and 05/04/97. I informed you when we met about the need to arrange your school leaving booster vaccines and you gave me permission to write to your GP about whether you have had the meningitis C vaccine.

You need to organize a dental appointment to ensure that your teeth are healthy.

You had a normal Guthrie test in the newborn period that ensured that you didn't have neonatal hypothyroidism or a condition called phenylketonuria.

When we met on xxx you were 15 years 9 months old and you presented as a physically healthy boy. Your growth is normal with a height of 172 cm between 25th and 50th centile, that means just below average for a boy of your age. Your weight of 68 kg was on 75th to 91st centile which is above average for a boy of your age. Examination of your heart, lungs, and abdomen was normal.

You and your carer completed the Strengths and Difficulties Questionnaire for me and those both produced relatively low scores; 6 from your carer and 9 from yourself.

To summarize, you are a physically healthy 15-year-old boy. You are up to date with your immunizations other than school leaving booster and meningitis C. You have had no significant past medical history other than a diagnosis of ADHD and a fracture of a bone in your foot in 2005. You take methylphenidate as treatment for ADHD.

With kind regards.

Yours sincerely,

xxx xxxx

Community Paediatrician

Young people leaving care face multiple transitions; accommodation from foster placement or children's home to independent living, from a legal status as a looked after child to a care leaver, from school to further or higher education, employment, training, or none of these, as well as medical transfers of care from paediatric services to adult services. These transitions are difficult to navigate.

Further resources

Munro E R, Simkiss D (2020). Transitions from care to adulthood: messages to inform practice. Paediatr Child Health, 30, 175–9.

Intercountry adoption

Intercountry adoption

Intercountry adoption is governed (in those countries that are signatories) by the 1993 Hague Convention on Protection of Children and Co-operation in Respect of Intercountry Adoption. The Hague Convention aims to:

- Eliminate abuses associated with intercountry adoption such as profiteering and bribery, coercion of birth parents, and the sale and abduction of children.
- Develop a child-centred approach with the process being more about finding a suitable family for a child than a suitable child for a childless couple.
- Improve regulation and procedures to protect prospective adopters.
- Bring about automatic recognition of adoptions in all contracting states.

Intercountry adoption may mean:
- Placing a British child for adoption outside of the UK.
- A child from abroad being placed in the UK.

Around 300 children a year are adopted into the UK. Information on the background of children in this situation can be very limited indeed; they may have been abandoned or taken to institutions by parents who provide little or no medical information on themselves or the child.

In this situation, prospective adopters need to know that there is considerable uncertainty about health issues:

- Genetic factors: a family history of learning difficulties, mental illness, or genetic disease will not be clear.
- Exposure to abuse and neglect: information on the early life experiences of children can be very limited and it is difficult to assess impact. The strongest predictor of continuing psychological deficits and impairments is overall duration of institutional privation.
- Developmental progress: at the point of assessment, the developmental status will be clear but without a trajectory it can be problematic predicting the likelihood of developmental catch up. Encouragingly, in the English and Romanian Adoptees Study there was considerable developmental catch up so that all the children were functioning in the normal range by 4 years of age when half had profound developmental delay at entry to the UK.
- Risk of exposure to infectious diseases: such as tuberculosis, hepatitis B, hepatitis C, or HIV.
- Immunization: schedules vary by country and details of vaccinations received are lost. In this situation the Health Protection Agency advice is to treat the child as unimmunized and follow a catch-up immunization schedule.

Overall, the findings from the English and Romanian Adoptees Study give a complicated picture of real success and worrying sequelae and prospective intercountry adopters need to understand this complexity. For a child from another country to be legally adopted in the UK, the prospective adoptive parents have to be assessed in a similar way to other prospective adoptive parents and so training is an opportunity to discuss these issues.

Further resources

CoramBAAF produces a practice note on 'Health screening of children adopted from abroad'. Available at: ℬ https://corambaaf.org.uk/books/practice-note-46-health-screening-children-adopted-abroad

Gov.uk. Adopting a child. Available at: ℬ https://www.gov.uk/child-adoption/adopting-a-child-from-overseas

Selman P (ed) (2000). Intercountry Adoption: Developmental, Trends and Perspectives. London: British Agencies for Adoption and Fostering.

Post-adoption support

- Between 1926 and 1990 there were 876,601 recorded adoptions in England and Wales, so being adopted is a relatively common experience.
- Post-adoption support has slowly developed to meet the needs of this population and others affected by adoption. Every local authority has an Adoption Support Service Advisor who is the first point of contact for all post-adoption queries.
- Adoption agencies have a duty to consider requests for post-adoption support, to assess what is needed, and if they are in a position to meet that need, e.g.:
  - Adopted people over the age of 18 years who are seeking information about their origins through access to their birth records or adoption records.
  - Adopted people who are seeking or have made contact with their birth parents and other relatives and are seeking advice and support.
  - Birth parents and birth relatives seeking information or counselling service.
  - Financial support (means tested).
  - Support with parenting children.
- Post-adoption support includes:
  - Statutory Adoption Leave for up to 52 weeks.
  - Adoption Allowance, regular financial support to eligible adoptive parents before and after the adoption order is granted.
  - Adoption Support Fund pays for services and training for adoptive parents.

Chapter 13

Special educational needs and disability

Academic failure at school

Introduction

Poor academic performance has implications that play out across life stages and at multiple levels:

- At the individual level, academic underachievement predicts short-term problem behaviour and dropout, and can derail educational and occupational trajectories well into adulthood. It leads to loss of confidence and poor self-esteem.
- At the institutional level, academic problems among students can create disorder and undermine the general mission of schools.
- Widespread academic failure impacts communities by influencing rates of fertility, mortality, marriage, and unemployment through its relation to educational attainment and the development of human capital.

Causes of academic failure

- Familial and social factors: poverty, parental separation, domestic violence, maltreatment, parental learning difficulties, drug abuse, mental health problems.
- Child's intrinsic factors: chronic physical or mental health problems, visible (e.g. CP) or hidden (e.g. ASD) disability, medications (e.g. antiepileptics), sensory (vision or hearing) impairment, emotional and behavioural difficulties, ADHD, conduct disorder, oppositional defiant disorder, substance or alcohol misuse.
- Environmental factors: poor-quality teaching, scarcely resourced educational environment, bullying, absenteeism.

Paediatrician's approach and assessment

- History: presenting concerns, family history of special schooling (or learning difficulties), detailed history of pregnancy (including drugs or alcohol exposure), prematurity, past medical history, enquiry about hearing or vision (low threshold for testing), general health, medications, emotional or behavioural difficulties, early development particularly speech and language, family situation/caring responsibility, sleep difficulties, school attendance, bullying, additional support at school, attentional or coordination difficulties.
- Examination: general presentation, engagement, impulsivity, mood, social interaction, dysmorphism, growth, coordination, and neurological examination, neurocutaneous stigmata, hearing and vision assessment, simple quick assessment of reading and drawing age.
- Further information and assessments: information from SEN coordinator/class teacher, OT/PT/SLT assessment as relevant, educational psychology assessment if appropriate, consider standardized questionnaires or CAMHS referral (for possible ADHD/mood disorders) if indicated.

Preventative strategies
- Primary: reducing alcohol/drugs consumption in pregnancy, improved neonatal care, reducing alcohol and drug misuse in adolescents, prevention programmes against bullying in schools.
- Secondary: early diagnosis and optimal management of chronic health, developmental and emotional problems; vision and hearing checks.
- Tertiary: specific educational and rehabilitation programmes for sensory impairments and SEN.

School absence and truancy

Introduction

- Regular school attendance:
  - Positively relates to full potential and best health outcomes.
  - During adolescence, protects from dangerous behaviours, such as substance or alcohol abuse, smoking, suicidality, violence, high-risk sexual behaviour, teenage pregnancy, and exploitation.
- In the UK, children must get an education between the school term after their fifth birthday and the last Friday in June in the school year they become 16 years old.
- School refusal:
  - Is a child-motivated refusal to attend school and/or difficulties remaining in classes for an entire day.
  - Children with school refusal feel anxiety or emotional distress towards school.
  - Is more likely to occur at transition points, i.e. between 5–6 years and 10–11 years.
- The most reported physical symptoms are headache, abdominal pain, muscle pain, dizziness, and tiredness. Nearly half of those children without a defined organic disease had been diagnosed with a psychiatric condition such as depression, anxiety, or OCD. In younger children, consider possibility of FII.
- In the US, the term 'school refusal behaviour' is used to include various forms of absenteeism, such as truancy, school phobia, and separation anxiety.
- The Department for Education regulates strict school attendance laws in the UK.
- Latest figures for pupil absence in England:
  - Overall absence rate 4.9%.
  - Persistent absentees make up 13.1% of all enrolments.
- A persistently absent child is one who misses school for at least 10% of the time.
- Secondary schools had a higher rate of persistent absence than primary schools.
- In Britain, local councils and schools can use various legal powers if child is missing school without a good reason. They can issue:
  - A Parenting Order.
  - An Education Supervision Order.
  - A School Attendance Order.
  - A fine (sometimes known as a 'penalty notice').

Contributing/risk factors for school absence

- Familial/social: parental sickness, work absence, related to unemployment, sick leave or disability, lack of parental involvement and supervision, and parental dysfunctional behaviour increase the risk of school absenteeism in children.
- School/learning environment: bullying, violence and gang culture, feeling isolated, poor relation with peers or teachers, inadequate support for SEN children.

- Individual: anxiety (separation anxiety disorder), depression and ODD, adverse childhood experiences (such as death or incarceration of a parent or financial hardship, familial substance use, or neighbourhood violence increase the risk), academic difficulties.

Truancy

- Truancy is intentional unauthorized absence from school by the pupil. Truants are children who decide not to attend school, generally without the knowledge of their parents.
- Truants have a significantly higher incidence of illegal drug use, underage drinking and smoking, antisocial behaviours, conduct disorder, and/or sexual and drug exploitation compared to non-truanting pupils.
- Schools and local authorities can issue penalty notices to parents (Education Act 1996), where pupils fail to attend school regularly.
- Local authorities play an important role in supporting schools to tackle high levels of absence. Schools are expected to collect absence data every term, enabling progress to be monitored closely, so that intervention and support can be deployed speedily for those schools which require it.
- Statistics for unauthorized school absences are also influenced by parents taking children out of school during term time for family holidays.

Community paediatrics assessment

- Background history: onset, family circumstances, parental view/attitude, academic progress, bullying at school, social services involvement, family history of learning difficulties or mental health problems.
- Medical history: pregnancy, birth, early developmental progress, chronic illness, medications, anxiety.
- Examination: complete physical examination, growth, dysmorphism, impulsivity, interaction, engagement during consultation, speech and communication.
- Investigations: try to avoid unnecessary investigations. Specific investigations if indicated such as blood counts if clinically pale or genetic testing if dysmorphic. Behaviour checklist and rating scales such as Conner's for suspected ADHD if appropriate. Educational psychology assessment is particularly helpful. Feedback from SEN coordinator may provide further insight.

Approach/support

- Collaborative approach between school, child, and parents is required.
- School and local authority can help. The school can discuss attendance problems with parents and agree a plan to improve child's attendance. A lot of local councils have teams that help parents improve their child's attendance at school including:
  - Support to reduce the burden on children where families are in difficulty (e.g. if a child is spending a lot of time caring for someone).
  - Working with families and schools to overcome bullying and other serious problems.
  - A parenting contract.

- Psychological intervention such as CBT may be helpful if anxiety is the main contributor.
- Graduated reintegration with educational and emotional support.
- Appropriate treatment of developmental/mental health problems such as depression, and ADHD.

Further resources

Department for Education. School and college behaviour and attendance: detailed information: https://www.gov.uk/topic/schools-colleges-childrens-services/school-behaviour-attendance

SEN and educational support for children with additional needs

- Section 312 of the UK Education Act 1996 states that: 'Children have special educational needs if they have a learning difficulty which calls for special educational provision to be made for them'.
- A child has a learning difficulty if they:
  - Have a significantly greater difficulty in learning than the majority of children of the same age, or
  - Have a disability which prevents or hinders the child from making use of educational facilities.
- Disability: the Equality Act 2010 defines disability as when a person has a 'physical or mental impairment which has a substantial and long-term adverse effect on that person's ability to carry out normal day-to-day activities'.
- Paediatricians have a pivotal role in providing information and strategies to support the school and their professional counterparts in education. Collaborative working requires effective management and transfer of information between agencies.
- The Equality Act 2010 requires schools to:
  - Promote equality of opportunity.
  - Promote positive attitudes towards disabled people.
  - Assess and monitor the impact of their activities on disabled people.
  - Make reasonable adjustments to ensure disabled children are not disadvantaged.
  - Improve outcomes for disabled people.

Education, Health and Care (EHC) needs assessment

The Children and Families Act 2014 transformed legislative changes relating to C&YP with special educational needs and disabilities (SEND).

The SEND Code of Practice provides statutory guidance and sets out duties, policies and procedures relating to Part 3 of the Children and Families Act 2014 in England.

SEND Code of Practice 2014

- Covers the 0–25 years age range.
- Mandates participation of C&YP and parents in decision-making at individual and strategic levels.
- Has a stronger focus on high aspirations and on improving outcomes for C&YP.
- Requires a coordinated assessment process and the new 0–25 EHC plan replaces statements and learning difficulty assessments.

EHC plan

- An EHC plan is a legal document which describes the SEN of a child or young person aged up to 25 years, the support they need, and the outcomes they would like to achieve. There were ~354,000 C&YP with EHC plans in 2019. The total number of C&YP with a statement or EHC plan has increased each year since 2010.

- The purpose of an EHC plan is to make special educational provisions to meet the SEN of the child or young person, to secure the best possible outcomes for them across education, health, and social care, and, as they get older, prepare them for adulthood.
- An EHC plan can only be issued after a child or young person has gone through the process of an EHC needs assessment. An EHC needs assessment is a detailed look at a child's SEN and the support he or she may need in order to learn.
- The special educational provisions described in an EHC plan must be provided by the child or young person's local authority. This means an EHC plan can give a child or young person extra educational support. It can also give parents and young people more choice about which school or other setting the child or young person can attend.
- Young people and parents have a right to request a personal budget when a local authority has confirmed it will prepare an EHC plan or during a review of an existing plan and a local authority is under a duty to prepare one when requested.
- In order to ensure the EHC plan is up to date and reflects the needs of the child or young person, a local authority must review it at least annually. Reviews must focus on:
  - How well the child or young person is progressing towards achieving the outcomes.
  - Reviewing whether the support offered is effective.
  - Considering if a plan is still needed.
  - Setting new targets (and potentially new outcomes).
- A plan ceases if any of the following apply:
  - The education and training outcomes have been achieved.
  - A young person aged 16 or over takes up paid employment.
  - The young person enters higher education (such as university).
  - A young person aged over 18 leaves education and doesn't want to do further learning.

Inclusion

- Inclusive education—also called inclusion—is education that includes everyone, with non-disabled and disabled people (including those with 'SEN') learning together in mainstream schools, colleges, and universities.
- Inclusive Early Years settings provide opportunities for children with and without special needs to learn, play, and socialize together. The environment, curriculum, and resources should reflect the ethos that children with special needs are welcomed, cared for, respected, and valued equally with other children.
- C&YP with SEN have a right to mainstream education.
- The majority of children with SEN complete their education in mainstream schools.
- For children with an EHC plan, arrangements are made for the child's education to continue in a mainstream school of the parents' choice.
- For some children with multiple and complex SEN, the facilities, specialist teaching, expertise, and adapted environment of a special school may be of greater benefit.

Further resources

Department for Education, Department of Health and Social Care (2015). Special educational needs and disability code of practice: 0 to 25 years. Statutory guidance for organisations which work with and support children and young people who have special educational needs or disabilities. Available at: ℘ https://www.gov.uk/government/publications/send-code-of-practice-0-to-25

House of Commons Education Committee (2019). Special educational needs and disabilities. Available at: ℘ https://publications.parliament.uk/pa/cm201919/cmselect/cmeduc/20/20.pdf

Writing a SEN Report and providing medical advice

See Fig. 13.1.

Details of child or young person		
Full name	Date of birth	NHS number
Ryan ABCD	7899	123 456
	Setting, school or college attended	
	Primary School	

2. Details of service involvement
Ryan has not previously been known to the Community Paediatric Service. The following report has been written following a clinic consultation on the 28th January and from reviewing documentation provided as listed in Section 8a.

3. Contextual information

Ryan has the following diagnoses and difficulties:

Austism Spectrum Disorder (ASD)

Sensory Porcessing difficulties

High levels of anxiety

Developmental coordination disorder (DCD, previously known as dyspraxia)

Ryan was diagnosed with ASD by the CDC in 2017 because of significant difficulties with social interaction, language, communication and flexibility.

Ryan has a high level of sensory needs and sensory sensitivities.

These needs have been assessed by an Occupational Therapist in 2017 and more recently by the Communication and Interaction Service and recommendations made to support him with these at home and at school.

Ryan can become highly anxious and distressed by small triggers.

He was previously coping in his educational setting. Often masking his anxiety, but he is no longer able to do. This means he can become highly distressed at school and this prevents him from learning and accessing the curriculum.

Difficulties with Ryan's fine motors skills and coordination skills have been highlighted since he started school. It was felt likely following his Occupational Therapy Assessment, that he has Developmental Coordination Disorder.

Situations, interpreting people's meaning and will often find social injustice when there isn't any and this can impact on his ability to interact with his peers.

He does have a friend at school and an older brother who he gets on with, but he can find it easier to communicate with his peers online, when he is just responding to a voice.

Cognition and Learning

Ryan is able to access learning if he is calm, however, if he is over whelmed by a situation or anxious, he cannot. This is significantly impacting on his ability to learn currently.

Social emotional and mental health

Ryan is highly anxious and has low self-esteem. He can misread people' intentions and will often see everyone as sister. He finds it difficult to switch of and it can sometimes be hard to work out what has triggered his anxiety.

Ryan's mother finds that making a kind gesture towards him can help distract him and alleviate his anxiety.

Ryan has particularly high level of anxiety in public situations.

He can suddenly freeze and go into a state of terror. When this happens his mother will reassure and comfort him. If his fear escalates he will cover his ears, he can then make a noise, get louder or shout and at worst will run away.

Separation from his parents is also another trigger for Ryan's anxiety and he prefers only his parents to look after him. His mother described that he constantly struggles with feeling safe.

Mobility posture and equipment needs

There were concerns about Ryan's movements, a tendency to fall over and poor sense of danger after he started school.

He can run, jump and climb well, but he has a tendency to fall over. He can ride a bike and use a hover board well. Ryan's mother described that has flat feet and poor core stability.

Ryan finds hand writing very difficult. He often types in school.

Ryan can struggle with coordination and knowing how much force to use for a task, as he doesn't know his own strength.

Ryan has previously been reviewed by an occupational therapist who felt he may have developmental coordination disorder.

Independence and self-care

Ryan can dress himself and put on his own shoes and socks. However, his sensory needs can impair his ability to carry this out as he is very sensitive to how clothes feel and hates wearing shoes. He can finish meals independently.

Ryan can go to the toilet to pass urine independently. However, opening his bowels can cause him emotional distress.

Other relevant issues (sleep/pain/sensory)

Sensory

Many of Ryan's sensory sensitivities have already been described.

Ryan's sensory difficulties have worsened over the last few years.

He can have meltdowns over clothes and shoes and now has one set of clothes that he will wear every day.

Ryan likes to have the TV on loudly, but other loud noises can be difficult for him and make him feel overwhelmed, for example, the noise at school. A number of sensory strategies and aids to support him have been suggested to help him cope at school, for example movement breaks, wobble cushions, weighted blankets, ear defenders and dark glasses.

Sleep

Ryan's mother sleeps with him and he uses a weighted blanket to help with sleep.

---

6. Health outcomes

Ryan to live a healthy lifestyle, including eating healthy foods and exercising. Ryan's weight should be monitored. He should have encouragement to be more active and exercise, and eat more healthily in order to lose weight

Ryan to receive support to improve his coordination and fine motor skills.

Ryan to feel less anxious so that he is able to not only access the curriculum and learn. But also interact with others and be able to do more of things he enjoys.

7(a) Education provision to meet needs and support outcomes

Ryan will need:

A learning environment that provides staff with relevant and specialist knowledge of ASD and associated anxiety.

Access to specialist behavioural support and advice for the teaching staff

A learning environment, tools and staff with relevant and specialist knowledge to support Ryan's sensory needs. These could include adaptations to the physical environment, for example, to lighting and acoustics or having a designated 'safe space.'

A learning environment that also support his coordination and fine motor needs.

7b. Health provision to meet needs and support outcomes	By whom
We would recommend Ryan attends a local optician to have his eyes tested annually	Parents to arrange
We would be grateful if Ryan's GP or the school nursing team could monitor Ryan's weight.	Community Services
The activities as recommended by to Occupational Therapist may be useful to support handwriting, fine motor and organisation skills and sensory needs:	Health Commissioned Services
I have referred Ryan to the CAMHS team for further support of his anxiety	Health commissioned Services
I have referred Ryan to the Integrated Therapies Team for further support with his motor and sensory needs	Health Commissioned Services

8a. List the repots/meeting that have contributed to this report (where applicable)	
Following documents were also available for this advice: ASD assessment Report, Communication and Interaction Team Report Educational Psychology Report Occupational Therapy Report	Dated: Dated: Dated: Dated:
8b. Service from which other advice should be south	
Educational Psychology Assessment	

Name of person completing the advice	Designation/Service/Agency Registrar in Community Paediatrics working with Dr Consultant Community Paediatrican
Address – Community Paediatrics,	Phone number Email
Signature	Date advice completed
	Date advice shared with family

Fig. 13.1 Health advice for a statutory EHC assessment.

School health promotion

- Schools play an important role in supporting the health and well-being of C&YP.
- In the decades between 1960 and 1990, a range of health services for children were offered in schools. These ranged from screening programmes (school entry, 10-year checks, and school leaving medicals), immunizations, and dental and audiology services to the management of medical problems.
- In the last two decades, there has been a shift in management of a range of common childhood conditions to primary care, community paediatrics, or hospital-based outpatient services.
- The concept of the 'school doctor' is now largely limited to a community paediatrician who supports the medical needs of children in special schools in partnership with health and education professionals.

Aims of a school health service

- Early identification and management of health problems that may interfere with the child's learning in school.
- Assessment of children with learning difficulties to exclude health problems as a contributing factor.
- Health promotion—prevention and early intervention services.
- Safeguarding children (see ➜ pp. 610–11).
- Support for parents and carers.

Health promotion in schools

Focusing on early intervention and prevention is both socially and economically more effective in the long term.

A needs assessment for a school (or a group of schools) will provide a clear picture of the school community, to enable identified needs to be met.

The key health priorities recommended in the Healthy Child Programme from 5 to 19 years are:

1. Identification and targeted support for C&YP with particular vulnerabilities:
   - C&YP with complex or enhanced needs (illness, disability, complex or long-term health needs including mental health problems).
   - C&YP whose family background puts them at higher risk (parents with learning difficulties, serious mental health, drug or alcohol problems).
   - C&YP not accessing existing services (refugee and asylum seekers, travellers, living in temporary accommodation).
   - C&YP with particular behaviour/lifestyle risks (not in education, employment, or training; engaging in risk-taking behaviour).
2. Screening programmes:
   - For primary school-aged children:
     - School entry: vision check, hearing test, and height and weight measurement.
   - For secondary school-aged young people:
     - Universal vision test no longer recommended.
     - Chlamydia screening offered to those who may have been sexually active (those under the age of 16 years need to be Fraser competent to consent).

3. Immunization programmes:
   • BCG, hepatitis B, and seasonal influenza vaccinations for individuals at high risk. Human papillomavirus vaccination offered to girls aged between 12–13 years (school year 8). Tetanus, diphtheria, and inactivated polio vaccine (Td/IPV) booster given between ages 13 and 18 years.
4. Promoting emotional health, psychological well-being, and mental health:
   • Early identification of children with emotional distress.
   • Improving access to mental health support through universal services.
5. Promoting healthy weight:
   • Promoting play and physical activity.
   • Good food habits at school and encouraging more children to access the midday school meal.
   • Signposting children and families to local weight management services.
6. Teenage pregnancy and sexual health:
   • Targeted support for young people most at risk of early sex and teenage pregnancy.
   • Information and advice about preventing sexually transmitted infections.

The UK Department of Education has developed a Healthy Schools Toolkit, designed to help schools to 'plan, do, and review' health and well-being improvements for their C&YP and to identify and select activities and interventions effectively.

Educational psychology

Background

- Educational psychologists are trained in normal child development, the psychology of learning and teaching, and the psychological aspects of teaching children with SEN.
- Educational psychologists work within local authorities, in partnership with families and other professionals, to help C&YP achieve their full potential. Educational psychologists support schools and local authorities to improve all children's experiences of learning.

Roles and service provisions for educational psychology

- Educational psychologists become involved with C&YP who have the most significant and complex difficulties which affect their learning and development. They always work in conjunction with the staff in the school for the child.
- Educational psychologists tackle challenges such as learning difficulties, social and emotional problems, issues around disability, as well as more complex developmental disorders. Specifically, they can support C&YP with their:
  - Concentration difficulties.
  - Emotional and behavioural needs.
  - Learning needs.
  - Physical disabilities.
  - Sensory needs such as problems with eyesight or hearing.
  - Social skills difficulties.
- They work in a variety of ways including observations, interviews, and assessments and offer consultation, advice, and training on how schools might help children to learn and develop.
- They research innovative ways and develop strategies to improve learning environment, advice on teaching approaches, curriculum materials, and behavioural support.
- Educational psychology service provisions in the UK may differ from area to area. In many cases, a school, cluster of schools, or local area will be assigned an educational psychologist.

Functions of educational psychology service

- Before an educational psychology assessment is offered, parents are asked permission for this work to take place.
- An educational psychologist's assessment may involve:
  - Talking to the child's teachers, parents/carers, and the child.
  - Observing the child in the classroom.
  - Looking at the child's work.
  - Analysing existing assessment information.
  - Questionnaires or specific assessment materials.
  - Considering information wider than the child such as the impact of an event at home.
- Educational psychology assessment is a vital part of the statutory EHC needs assessment in UK. The educational psychologist can also help by working in a multiprofessional network when there are safeguarding

concerns about a child. The educational psychologist can contribute by attending meetings such as annual SEN reviews, meetings where a child's school placement is in jeopardy, or reviews by social care colleagues.

Educational psychologists can offer
- Individual work with C&YP when additional needs are identified:
  - Assessments: cognitive assessments, dynamic or play-based assessments.
  - Interventions and therapeutic work: CBT-based interventions, solution-focused brief therapy, emotional coaching, whole class intervention.
- Whole school support: school development projects, soft systems methodology, and provision management.
- Staff support: training and interventions, well-being and stress management, motivational interview.
- Support for parents and carers: parents' workshop.

The educational psychology provisions in England are underlined by the SEND Code of Practice (see ➔ 'Further resources').

How educational psychologists can get involved

- Educational psychology involvement might be requested for children <5 years by the nursery or by a professional who is working closely with the child such as a SLT or the preschool teaching service (Portage).
- Once in school, if teachers have significant concerns about progress or behaviour these will have already been discussed with the parent and additional SEN school support will have been provided. If concerns about the child/young person persist following a period of targeted SEN school support, then the SEN coordinator may ask for advice from an educational psychologist.
- The SEN team may request an assessment of a child/young person's SEN. This usually only occurs when the child has received intensive intervention through the SEN procedures set out in the Code of Practice. If a formal assessment takes place to contribute towards an EHC plan, the educational psychologist will be one of the people who advise about the child's needs. Parents have a right to be involved during the assessment of their child.
- If a parent is concerned their child is struggling at school, they have the right to ask their education authority to find out whether their child has additional support needs and to request a specific assessment (which can include an educational psychology assessment).

Further resources

British Psychological Society: ℜ https://www.bps.org.uk
Department for Education, Department of Health and Social Care (2015). Special educational needs and disability code of practice: 0 to 25 years. Statutory guidance for organisations which work with and support children and young people who have special educational needs or disabilities. Available at: ℜ https://www.gov.uk/government/publications/send-code-of-practice-0-to-25

Schooling in special circumstances

Elective home education

- Parents have a right to educate their children at home.
- Educating children at home works well when it is a positive, informed, and dedicated choice.
- Most parents who take up the weighty responsibility of home education do a great job, and many children benefit from being educated at home.
- In past few years, there has been a very significant increase in the number of children being educated at home, and there is considerable evidence that many of these children are not receiving a suitable education. There is increasing concern that some children educated at home may not be in a safe environment.
- Local authorities have a moral and social obligation to ensure that a child is safe and being suitably educated.

Reasons for elective home education

- Ideological or philosophical views which favour home education.
- Religious or cultural beliefs, and a wish to ensure that the child's education is aligned with these.
- Dissatisfaction with the school system.
- Bullying at school.
- Health reasons, particularly mental health of the child.
- As a short-term intervention for a particular reason.
- A child's unwillingness or inability to go to school, including school phobia.
- SEN, or a perceived lack of suitable provision in the school system for those needs.
- Disputes with a school over the education.
- As a stop-gap while awaiting a place at a school other than the one allocated.

Hospital school

- A hospital school is an educational provision operated in a hospital, generally a children's hospital, which provides learning support to all primary and secondary grade levels throughout their stay in the hospital.
- Hospital school support the education of pupils who have an illness/diagnosis such as cancer which requires prolonged or recurring periods of absence from school.
- Pupils receive a minimum entitlement of 5 hours of teaching a week.
- Teachers at the hospital school liaise with and keep in close contact with a pupil's home school.
- If upon discharge pupils are still too unwell to attend their own school for longer periods, some hospital schools may work with the medical staff to make a home teaching referral so children may be taught at home until well enough to return to their own school.
- In the UK, these provisions are funded by the local authority.

Excluded children

- The UK government has issued guidance on the process and support for C&YP who are excluded from educational settings.
- Section 51A of the Education Act 2002 empowers the head teacher of a school to exclude a pupil on disciplinary grounds.

- Disruptive behaviour can be an indication of unmet needs. In case of behavioural concerns about a pupil at school, staff should try to identify whether there are any causal factors and intervene early in order to reduce the need for a subsequent exclusion.
- Permanent exclusion should only be used as a last resort, in response to a serious breach or persistent breaches of the school's behaviour policy.
- The decision to exclude a pupil must be lawful, reasonable, and fair.
- Schools should take reasonable steps to set and mark work for pupils during the first five school days of exclusion. Alternative provision must be arranged from the sixth day.
- Schools should have a strategy for reintegrating a pupil who returns to school following exclusion and for managing their future behaviour.
- Local authorities in the UK are responsible for arranging suitable full-time education for permanently excluded pupils.
- Excluded children are at high risk of sexual and drug exploitation as well as gang activities.

Looked after children

- Looked after children (see ➔ pp. 619–48) start with the disadvantage of their pre-care experiences and, often, have SEN. Local authorities in England are required to discharge their statutory duty under 22(3A) of the Children Act 1989 to promote the educational achievement of looked after children.
- Looked after children are significantly more likely to have SEN than their peers. Of those with SEN, a significant proportion will have EHC plans.
- Looked after children are at higher risk of poor educational achievement for following reasons:
  - Dealing with a parent's alcohol or substance abuse.
  - Chaotic home circumstances.
  - Problems associated with trauma or abuse experienced in the early years.
  - Moving home a lot and having to change schools.
  - Being bullied or stigmatized.
  - Finding it hard to control behaviour.
  - Poor school attendance.
  - Feeling depressed or anxious.
  - Having difficulty finding a quiet place to do homework and accessing the internet.
- Social workers, virtual school heads, independent review officers, school admission officers, and SEND departments should work together to ensure that, except in an emergency, appropriate education provision for a child is arranged at the same time as a care placement.
- All looked after children should have a Personal Education Plan (PEP) which is part of the child's care plan or detention placement plan.
- The duty to promote the educational achievement of a looked after child extends to looked after young people aged 16 or 17 preparing to leave care.

Further resources

Department for Education, Department of Health and Social Care (2014). Special educational needs and disability code of practice: 0 to 25 years. Statutory guidance for organisations which work with and support children and young people who have special educational needs or disabilities. Available at: ℘ https://www.gov.uk/government/publications/send-code-of-practice-0-to-25

National curriculum

The structure of the national curriculum in England is shown in Table 13.1.

P scales

- These are used to measure the progress made by C&YP with learning disabilities aged 5–16 who are working below national curriculum level 1.
- The P scales have eight levels starting at P1 and progressing to P8.

Table 13.1 Structure of the national curriculum in England

	Key stage 1	Key stage 2	Key stage 3	Key stage 4
Age (years)	5–7	7–11	11–14	14–16
Year groups	1–2	3–6	7–9	10–11
Core subjects				
English	✓	✓	✓	✓
Mathematics	✓	✓	✓	✓
Science	✓	✓	✓	✓
Foundation subjects				
Art and design	✓	✓	✓	
Citizenship			✓	✓
Computing	✓	✓	✓	✓
Design and technology	✓	✓	✓	
Languages		✓	✓	
Geography	✓	✓	✓	
History	✓	✓	✓	
Music	✓	✓	✓	
Physical education	✓	✓	✓	✓

Further resources

Department for Education (2013). National curriculum in England: framework for key stages 1 to 4. Available at: M https://www.gov.uk/government/publications/national-curriculum-in-england-framework-for-key-stages-1-to-4
Department for Education and Standards and Testing Agency (2017). Performance – P Scales – attainment targets for pupils with special educational needs. Available at: https://www.gov.uk/government/publications/p-scales-attainment-targets-for-pupils-with-sen
GOV.UK. The national curriculum: https://www.gov.uk/national-curriculum

Access arrangements

- These are available for all examinations in line with the Disability Discrimination Act 1995.
- These are pre-examination adjustments which can be applied for, to give all candidates the opportunity to demonstrate in examinations their skills, knowledge, and understanding of the work they have done.
- Applications for particular access arrangements are made on the basis of evidence of need.
- Need can include a disability, SEN such as dyslexia, a temporary difficulty such as a broken arm, or psychological problems such as bereavement.
- Applications should be applied for as early as possible, with supporting evidence of eligibility provided by a professional whose qualifications are acceptable to the Joint Council for Qualifications.

Various arrangements can be requested to meet individual SEN, such as:
- Alternative accommodation for the exam.
- Braille question papers.
- Extra time up to a maximum of 25%.
- A reader.
- A scribe.
- Supervised rest breaks.
- A word processor etc.

Further resources

British Psychological Society: ℘ http://www.bps.org.uk

Department for Education, Department of Health and Social Care (2014). Special educational needs and disability code of practice: 0 to 25 years. Statutory guidance for organisations which work with and support children and young people who have special educational needs or disabilities. Available at: ℘ https://www.gov.uk/government/publications/send-code-of-practice-0-to-25

Education Resources: ℘ http://www.teachernet.gov.uk

Every Child Matters: ℘ http://www.everychildmatters.co.uk

Joint Council for Qualifications. Access Arrangements. ℘ https://www.jcq.org.uk/exams-office/access-arrangements-and-special-consideration/

National Autistic Society. Early Bird support programmes: email earlybird@nas.org.uk; ℘ https://www.autism.org.uk/what-we-do/support-in-the-community/family-support

Further education for young adults with special educational needs

- With the right support and high aspirations, the vast majority of young people who have SEN or disabilities can make a successful transition into adulthood, whether into employment, further or higher education, or training.
- The UK government introduced the Children and Families Act 2014 with a focus on greater cooperation between education, health, and social care and a greater focus on the outcomes so that young adults with SEN can lead contended and fulfilled lives.
- Further education colleges, sixth form colleges, 16–19 academies, and independent specialist colleges approved under Section 41 of the Children and Families Act 2014 have specific statutory duties including to:
  - Have regard to the 0–25 years SEND Code of Practice.
  - Cooperate with the local authority on arrangements for C&YP with SEN.
  - Admit a young person if the institution is named in an EHC plan.
  - Use their best endeavours to secure the special educational provision that the young person needs.
  - Ensure that appropriately qualified staff provide the support needed.
- Colleges should ensure they have access to external specialist services and expertise. These can include, e.g. educational psychologists, CAMHS, specialist teachers and support services, supported employment services, and therapists.
- Colleges have a duty through their funding agreements to ensure that students are provided with independent careers advice. This duty applies for all students up to and including the age of 18 and to 19–25-year-olds who have EHC plans.
- There are a number of specialist colleges around the UK catering for young people with disabling conditions including Star College (age 16–25) near Cheltenham, Trelaw school (age 9–16) and college (16+) in Hampshire, and The Queen Elizabeth Foundation Banstead in Surrey (specializing in brain injury, 16+).

Parental perspective

- Parents of severely disabled young people often had to fight for their education (including funding agreement from local authorities for specialist provisions), medical care, and social care engagement.
- The prospect of the young adult leaving home and moving on to college or independent living is often a highly charged and emotional situation. Parents are torn between pride in and hope for their children who are 'moving on', and the pain of letting go.
- It should be approached with great sensitivity, recognizing the needs of the young adult to establish independence, the high degree of emotional investment on the part of parents, and the high potential for very enmeshed relationships.

Further resources

Association of National Specialist Colleges (Natspec): ✎ https://natspec.org.uk/

Autism Education Trust: ✎ https://www.autismeducationtrust.org.uk/

Department for Education (2014). Further education: guide to the 0 to 25 SEND code of practice. Advice for further education colleges, sixth form colleges, 16 to 19 academies, and independent specialist colleges approved under section 41 of the Children and Families Act 2014. Available at: ✎ https://assets.publishing.service.gov.uk/government/uploads/system/uploads/attach-ment_data/file/348883/Further_education__guide_to_the_0_to_25_SEND_code_of_practice.pdf

Livability: ✎ http://www.livability.org.uk

Further reading

Chapter 14

Working with multiagency professionals

Health visitors

- HVs are registered nurses/midwives who have additional training in community public health nursing.
- They provide a professional public health service based on best evidence of what works for individuals, families, groups, and communities; enhancing health and reducing health inequalities through a proactive, universal service for all children aged 0–5 years and for vulnerable populations targeted according to need.
- With public health issues like obesity becoming more prevalent, there is an increasing need for preventive strategies and HVs can play an especially important role in implementing various public health policies.
- A HV's role is particularly valuable in socially deprived areas where their input is most likely to have an impact on the overall health of communities.

Health visitor role

- HVs work with parents who have new babies, offering support and informed advice from the antenatal period until the child starts school at 5 years. They may work in teams or have sole responsibility for a caseload derived from the local area or a general practice list; they are usually based in children's centres, surgeries, community, or health centres.
- In England, the service follows what is known as the 'four, five, six' model. This encompasses four levels of service, five mandated contacts, and six high-impact areas.
- The four levels of service are:
  - Community-based knowledge of local resources, including children's centres and self-help groups.
  - Universal—five key visits.
  - Universal plus—provide families with access to expert advice and support on issues such as postnatal depression, weaning, and sleepless children.
  - Universal partnership plus—support families with children with complex needs, such as long-term conditions, both themselves and linking them with local services.
- The five mandated elements include:
  - Antenatal health promotion visits.
  - New baby review.
  - 6–8-week assessment.
  - 1-year assessment.
  - 2–2½-year review.
- The six high-impact areas HVs focus on:
  - Parenthood and early weeks.
  - Maternal mental health.
  - Breastfeeding.
  - Healthy weight.
  - Minor illnesses and accidents.
  - Healthy 2-year-olds and getting ready for school.

- As part of their day-to-day duties, HVs could:
  - Give advice to new parents on feeding babies, hygiene, safety, and sleeping.
  - Support parents with their children's development needs.
  - Coordinate child immunization programmes.
  - Organize special clinics or drop-in centres.
  - Support postnatal depression and parental mental and physical health.
  - Advise on behaviour issues—sleeping, eating, potty training, tantrums, etc.
  - Support children with special needs.
  - Advise on how to reduce the risk of accident and injury.
  - Work closely with social services and other organizations to safeguard and protect children.

Family Nurse Partnership (FNP)

- Works with parents aged 24 and under, providing them with a specially trained family nurse who visits them regularly, from early pregnancy until their child is 2 years old.
- FNP is a licensed programme in which families benefit most when the programme starts early in pregnancy and where the number of visits and content delivered follows those set out in programme model.
- By focusing on their strengths, FNP enables young parents to:
  - Develop good relationships with and understand the needs of their child.
  - Make choices that will give their child the best possible start in life.
  - Believe in themselves and their ability to succeed.
  - Mirror the positive relationship they have with their family nurse with others.

School health nursing team

Context

- Research in the US demonstrated that school nursing services are a cost beneficial investment of public money.
- School nurses or specialist community public health nurses in the UK are qualified nurses or midwives with specialist graduate-level education in community health and the health needs of school-aged C&YP.
- School health nurses are in a unique position within the community and education settings to support MDTs, with relationships within primary and secondary care.
- Use their autonomy, clinical skills, and professional judgement to improve the health and well-being of C&YP and reduce health inequalities.
- Promote emotional well-being through the school-aged years working alongside children and young people to support those with emotional and mental health difficulties.
- Are playing increasingly important role in children's safeguarding processes.
- Young people value the involvement of nurses in 'Sex and Relationships Education' and 'Personal, Social, and Health Education' sessions and often prefer talking to a nurse rather than a teacher about sensitive issues.
- Improves attendance in severe long-term conditions such as asthma and diabetes.

Range of school nurse's activities

- Have a crucial role in leading, coordinating, and delivering the Healthy Child Programme (age 5–19).
- Educating and training school staff about long-term conditions.
- Creating individual healthcare plans for long-term conditions such as asthma, epilepsy, anaphylaxis, diabetes, etc.
- Health promotion including promoting health and well-being, supporting accident prevention, reducing risk-taking behaviours, and contributing to 'Personal, Social, and Health Education'.
- Running clinics, conducting drop-in sessions, making and responding to referrals, delivering immunization sessions, supporting students with sexual health needs, conducting health screening sessions including the National Child Measurement Programme, and supporting parents and working with families.
- Identifying individual and population health needs by undertaking recommended health assessment and reviews including:
  - Using reception/year 1 (age 4–5) school entry assessment (transition from 0–5 HCP, school entry questionnaire).
  - Providing year 6/7 (age 10–12) assessment at transition from primary to secondary school.
  - Supporting mid-teens reviews when young people are embarking on the next transition stage.
  - Health protection by coordinating programmes such as chlamydia screening.
  - Safeguarding by working together to protect vulnerable children and contributing to safeguarding processes.

School Nursing Service model

The Department of Health and Public Health England set out a model of school nurses offering support at four levels.

- At the community level—early identification of risk factors in the school population and act upon health concerns to offer advice and guidance.
- At the level of universal services—assessment of health and well-being need and early identification of risk factors and providing health checks to indicate developmental concerns and delays, ensure support for health promotion, and change management activity around identified health issues.
- At the level of universal plus—using evidence-based interventions or specific packages of care for identified health need, provide referrals to appropriate specialist services such as Child and Adolescent Mental Health Services (CAMHS).
- At the level of universal partnership plus—promote health in school and community settings, inform other professionals about health needs of the child, young person, and family and use local multiagency tools for assessments.

Portage/Early Years SEN team

- A Portage/Early Years SEN team is a home-visiting educational service for preschool children with SEND and their families.
- Statutory guidance for SEND (2015) recommends that 'Where a child continues to make less than expected progress, despite evidence-based support and interventions that are matched to the child's area of need, practitioners should consider involving appropriate specialists, for example, health visitors, speech and language therapists, Portage workers, Educational Psychologists or specialist teachers'.
- Professionals working in Early Years teams are specialist advisory teachers who are qualified, skilled, and experienced in working with children (birth to 5 years) with SEN.
- Aims of the Portage/Early Years SEN service:
  - Work with families to help them develop a quality of life and experience, for themselves and their young children, in which they can learn together, play together, participate, and be included in their community in their own right.
  - Play a part in minimizing the disabling barriers that confront young children and their families.
  - Support the national and local development of inclusive services for children.
- These services support preschool children with SEND by:
  - Offering flexible and sensitive support to meet the learning and developmental needs of children and families.
  - Working in partnership with families and other professionals working with children such as therapists, paediatricians, and HVs to promote good inclusive practice.
  - Advice on external additional resources and assistance with accessing these, including the requesting of and involvement in an education, health, and care needs assessment if appropriate.
- Professionals working in Early Years' service use a broad range of assessment materials including observational records and developmental profiles/checklists to support and monitor their progress.

Further resources

Department for Education and Department of Health and Social Care (2014, updated 2020). Special educational needs and disability code of practice: 0 to 25 years. [Statutory guidance for organizations which work with and support children and young people who have special educational needs or disabilities.] ◌ https://www.gov.uk/government/publications/send-code-of-practice-0-to-25

National Portage Association: ◌ http://www.portage.org.uk

Children's community nursing

- Community children's nursing represents a diverse and dynamic approach to providing care to children within their own homes and support to their families.
- Community children's nursing requires integration and joint working across health, social care, education, and many other agencies.
- The CCN's role encompasses education, training, emotional support, and expert clinical care.
- CCNs provide continuity of care from hospital to home, especially in long-term conditions, and a single point of access, especially during periods of crises.
- The services provided may include a range of different activities including:
  - Continuing care for children and families with complex healthcare needs.
  - Children who need high levels of technological care.
  - A single visit for a specific purpose such as completing the course of parental antibiotics course after discharge from hospital.
  - Providing education and training to carers, e.g. administration of buccal midazolam, care of tracheostomy and gastrostomy, etc.
  - Liaison role between primary and secondary care.
- CCNs are able to meet the needs of the following four groups of children:
  - Children with acute and short-term conditions.
  - Children with long-term conditions such as CP, epilepsy, and those requiring gastrostomy feeds, stoma, and home ventilation by avoiding unnecessary hospitalization and providing better quality of life.
  - Children with disabilities and complex conditions, including those requiring continuing care and neonates.
  - Children with life-limiting and life-threatening illness, including those requiring palliative and end of life care.

Children and families social care team

- In the UK, children's social care workers are generally situated within or alongside broader children's services.
- Local authorities have specific duties to safeguard and promote the welfare of all children in their area.
- All decisions should be driven by the well-being of the child—core principles of the children's social care system in England.
- The Children Acts of 1989 and 2004 set out specific duties for local authorities:
  - Section 17 of the Children Act 1989 puts a duty on the local authority to provide services to children in need in their area.
  - Section 47 of the same Act requires local authorities to undertake enquiries if they believe a child has suffered or is likely to suffer significant harm.
- Children and family social care services in UK may include:
  - Services for looked after children, including fostering and residential care.
  - Court liaison and advisory services.
  - Adoption.
  - Child protection.
  - Family support.
  - Services for children with disabilities.
  - Youth offending team.
  - Parent and child assessment team.
- Children's social workers can support children and their parents if the child:
  - Needs support with maintaining their health or development.
  - Has a disability.
  - Is in need of protection.
  - Is fostered, adopted, or lives in residential care.
- A social worker can:
  - Do an assessment of the child's and the family's needs.
  - Provide immediate help.
  - Give information about other support organizations that could help.
  - Involve other professionals when assessing the help the child or parents may need.
- Referral to children's social care can be made by:
  - Parents or carers.
  - Other professionals including school staff, GP, or HV.
  - Anyone if concerned that a child is being abused or neglected.
- In the US, the Administration for Children & Families, a division of the US Department of Health & Human Services, promotes the economic and social well-being of families, children, individuals and communities with funding, strategic partnership, guidance, training, and technical assistance.

- Similarly, in Australia, the Department of Social Services helps to support families and children through programmes and services as well as benefits and payments.

Further resources

Children and young people's services: https://www.nhs.uk/conditions/social-care-and-support-guide/caring-for-children-and-young-people/children-and-young-peoples-services/

Working with voluntary and statutory organizations

(Also see ➡ p. 22.)

- In order to provide holistic and comprehensive support to children with special needs and their families, it is important that various agencies involved work together to deliver effective interventions.
- Health, social care, and education services have a direct role in the delivery of many of these interventions and in other areas, a role in collaborative work with other agencies, in lobbying for policy change, and in raising the profile of child health promotion.
- These agencies may represent statutory bodies, public sector, or voluntary organizations.
- Voluntary organizations are not-for-profit organizations set up and run by voluntary unpaid management committees. They differ from the private sector which is run for profit and the statutory sector which is set up by statute.

Provision of coordinated and responsive multiagency support to children and families in need

This requires:

- Establishing agreed clear aims, roles, responsibilities, and timetables between partners (see ➡ pp. 12–3).
- Recognition and acceptance of importance of all the agencies involved working together to achieve a shared goal.
- Commitment to joint working with open and clear communication.
- Acknowledgement of different constraints under which various agencies work.
- Appropriate sharing of information along with respect for each other's confidentiality protocols.
- Mutual respect for each other's roles and contributions.
- A multiagency steering group and commitment at all levels of the organizations involved.
- Support and training of staff in new way of working.
- Interprofessional programmes of continuing education.

Further resources

National Council for Voluntary Organisations: ✍ http://www.ncvo-vol.org.uk

Index

Notes Tables, figures and boxes are indicated by an italic *t*, *f* and *b* following the page number.